2995

Williams Obstetrics

A Study Guide

Charles R.B. Beckmann, M.D., M.H.P.E.
Department of Obstetrics and Gynecology
University of Illinois at Chicago

Barbara M. Barzansky, Ph.D., M.H.P.E.
Center for Education Development
University of Illinois at Chicago

Frank W. Ling, M.D.
Department of Obstetrics and Gynecology
University of Tennessee College of Medicine

with a Foreword by
Jack A. Pritchard, M.D.,
Paul C. MacDonald, M.D.,
and Norman F. Gant, M.D.
Editors, *Williams Obstetrics, 17th Edition*

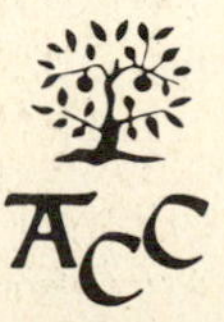

APPLETON-CENTURY-CROFTS/Norwalk, Connecticut

0-8385-9735-1

Notice: Our knowledge in the clinical sciences is constantly changing. As new information becomes available, changes in treatment and in the use of drugs become necessary. The author(s) and the publisher of this volume have taken care to make certain that the doses of drugs and schedules of treatment are correct and compatible with the standards generally accepted at the time of publication. The reader is advised to consult carefully the instruction and information material included in the package insert of each drug or therapeutic agent before administration. This advice is especially important when using new or infrequently used drugs.

85 86 87 88 89 / 10 9 8 7 6 5 4 3 2 1

Prentice-Hall International, Inc., London
Prentice-Hall of Australia, Pty. Ltd., Sydney
Prentice-Hall Canada, Inc.
Prentice-Hall of India Private Limited, New Delhi
Prentice-Hall of Japan, Inc., Tokyo
Prentice-Hall of Southeast Asia (Pte.) Ltd., Singapore
Whitehall Books Ltd., Wellington, New Zealand
Editora Prentice-Hall do Brasil Ltda., Rio de Janeiro
Prentice-Hall Hispanoamericana, S.A., Mexico

Library of Congress Cataloging in Publication Data
Beckmann, Charles R. B.
Williams Obstetrics, a study guide.
To be used with the textbook: Williams Obstetrics, 17th ed.
Includes index.
1. Obstetrics—Examinations, questions, etc.
I. Barzansky, Barbara M. II. Ling, Frank W. III. Williams,
J. Whitridge (John Whitridge), 1866–1931. Obstetrics.
IV. Title. [DNLM: 1. Obstetrics—examination questions.
WQ 100 W724w Suppl.]
RG532.B44 1985 618.2′0076 84-24490
ISBN 0-8385-9735-1

PRINTED IN THE UNITED STATES OF AMERICA

CONTENTS

FOREWORD

> The easiest and surest way of acquiring facts is to learn them in groups, in systems, and systematized knowledge is science. You can very often carry two facts fastened together more easily than one by itself, as a housemaid can carry two pails of water with a hoop more easily than one without it.
>
> Oliver Wendell Holmes
> *Scholastic and Bedside Teaching*

The above quotation remains as true today as when written more than one hundred years ago. With the influx of a seemingly endless supply of newer and newer information which may or may not withstand the light of truth or the test of time, the student of medicine is inundated today as never before with choices of the correct source of information. Most of us—medical students, house officers, and practitioners—remain true to our professions and actively seek new information which is grouped into "systems" and "systematized" into textbooks, if not into pure science.

The correct choice of an obstetrics textbook allows the beginning or continuing student to pursue new information which is added to established knowledge gained through the scientific method or, in many cases, through years of clinical experience. Thus, newer and ever newer information must be shifted, condensed, updated, and presented in understandable written and graphic form in textbooks; out-dated dogma, misinformation, or simply misapplication of information must be deleted and previous errors in understanding acknowledged and corrected. Most good textbooks have all of these characteristics. We believe that the Seventeenth Edition of *Williams Obstetrics* is such a textbook.

Thus, before learning begins, the correct sources of information must be grouped together and presented in concise and palatable form such as in the Seventeenth Edition of *Williams Obstetrics*. Then, as in the Holmes analogy, "this pail of water" can be more easily managed by combining it with a second "pail" which is not heavier or less manageable but may balance the first and make it easier to carry.

Such a balancing factor is this Study Guide, designed and written to be the companion to the Seventeenth Edition of *Williams Obstetrics*. The Study Guide is not intended to be an added weight but rather to balance and augment the process of learning, and we believe that this Study Guide accomplishes these objectives.

Jack A. Pritchard, M.D.
Paul C. MacDonald, M.D.
Norman F. Gant, M.D.

PREFACE

For decades *Williams Obstetrics* has been the standard against which medical students, residents, and practicing physicians have measured their knowledge of obstetrics. The task of acquiring this knowledge is increasingly formidable as the body and complexity of information concerning obstetrics increases.

Williams Obstetrics: A Study Guide is designed to help by providing study questions organized both by chapter and by concept-area or topic. The questions are written in simple formats (short answer, multiple choice, matching, true/false) so that the reader's efforts may be specifically directed toward learning and understanding the information in *Williams Obstetrics.* Each question is referenced to a page (or pages) in *Williams Obstetrics* and cross-referenced to related concepts.

We believe that the use of *Williams Obstetrics: A Study Guide* will ease and speed the reader's understanding and retention of the vital information provided in this classic textbook of obstetrics.

Charles R.B. Beckmann
Barbara M. Barzansky
Frank W. Ling

INSTRUCTIONS FOR USE

This book is designed to help you master the information contained in the Seventeenth Edition of *Williams Obstetrics.* Use of the Study Guide should help you efficiently organize and direct your learning, whatever the level of knowledge and experience that you possess.

ORGANIZATION OF THE STUDY GUIDE

As the Study Guide is a companion volume to *Williams Obstetrics,* no new information is presented beyond what is found in the recent edition of the text. The chapters in the Study Guide are numbered identically to the chapters in *Williams Obstetrics.* The Guide is divided into three basic sections:

- The first section contains a set of questions based on the content of each chapter in *Williams Obstetrics.* The questions are designed to emphasize and synthesize the major points covered in the chapter.
- The second section consists of the answers to the questions from each chapter. For each question, the page references to *Williams Obstetrics* where the information to answer the question may be found are included. In addition, the specific content areas (topics) relevant to the question are listed. The topics come from an analysis of both the subject matter of the question and the way that the subject matter is applied in practice (e.g., the topics listed for a question on cesarean delivery for a fetus in the breech position may include "breech presentation" as well as "cesarean delivery").
- The third section of the Study Guide is a "topics list" that serves as an index. For all the topics named in the second section, it enumerates the questions (by number) that include that topic.

QUESTION FORMATS

There are four basic types of questions utilized in the Study Guide: multiple choice, true–false, matching, and short answer. For the multiple choice items, one, more than one, or none of the options may be correct.

USE OF THE STUDY GUIDE

Based on the reader's level of expertise, there are several ways in which the Study Guide may be utilized. The beginning student in a clerkship in OB-Gyn should probably read the chapter in *Williams Obstetics* and then attempt to answer the questions in the Study Guide. For those questions that are incorrectly answered, the student should re-read the relevant pages and attempt to correct any misunderstandings before proceeding to the next chapter. The junior house officer might attempt to answer the questions in the Study Guide first, and then read the text to specifically correct any problem areas that are identified. For a senior house officer or a practitioner, it might be most appropriate to answer all the questions related to a topic of interest (e.g., fetal distress, prostaglandins, cesarean delivery). This approach will help the experienced individual synthesize the content in a given area that is presented throughout *Williams Obstetrics.*

QUESTIONS

1. OBSTETRICS IN BROAD PERSPECTIVE

1–1. Obstetrics is defined as the study of labor and delivery, both normal and abnormal.

a. True
b. False

1–2. The fertility rate is defined as the number of

a. Births per 1000 population
b. Births per 1000 women aged 15 to 44
c. Live births per 1000 women aged 15 to 44
d. Births per 100,000 women aged 15 to 44

1–3. The birth rate is defined as the number of

a. Births/1000 population
b. Births/10,000 population
c. Births/100,000 population
d. Live births/10,000 population
e. Live births/1000 women

Instructions for Items 1–4 to 1–6: Match the term with the appropriate definition.

a. Abortus
b. Stillbirth
c. Live birth

1–4. When the infant at birth or sometime after birth breathes spontaneously or shows another sign of life
1–5. A fetus removed or expelled from the uterus at 20 weeks or less of gestation
1–6. An infant who at birth shows no signs of life nor breathes spontaneously

1–7. Which of the following is a criterion for a live birth?

a. Presence of a heart beat
b. Presence of voluntary muscle movements
c. Spontaneous breathing
d. Weight at birth greater than 2500 g

1–8. The perinatal mortality rate is defined as

1–9. The stillbirth rate is synonymous with the

a. Neonatal mortality rate
b. Perinatal mortality rate
c. Fetal death rate
d. Reproductive mortality rate

Answers begin on page 197.

Instructions for Items 1–10 to 1–13: Match the term with the appropriate description.

a. Abortus
b. Preterm or premature infant
c. Term infant
d. Postterm infant
e. Low birth weight infant

1–10. An infant born any time after the 42nd week
1–11. An infant with a first recorded weight of less than 2500 g
1–12. An infant born before 38 completed weeks of gestation
1–13. An infant born no earlier than 38 completed weeks and no later than 42 completed weeks of gestation

1–14. A woman dies from complications of mitral stenosis during the course of her pregnancy. This would be defined as

a. A direct maternal death
b. An indirect maternal death
c. A nonmaternal death

1–15. The maternal death rate is defined as the number of maternal deaths per

a. 1000 pregnancies
b. 100,000 pregnancies
c. 1000 live births
d. 100,000 live births
e. 1000 births
f. 100,000 births

1–16. Reproductive mortality is defined as

1–17. Which of the following factors is directly related to the maternal mortality rate?

a. Age
b. Race
c. Parity
d. Socioeconomic status

1-18. Which of the following is a common cause of maternal mortality?

a. Hypertension
b. Diabetes
c. Infection
d. Hemorrhage

1-19. The most useful statistical index of the quality of obstetric care is the

a. Birth rate
b. Stillbirth rate
c. Neonatal mortality rate
d. Perinatal mortality rate
e. Maternal mortality rate

1-20. Which of the following statements about neonatal deaths is correct?

a. Currently there are more fetal deaths than neonatal deaths.
b. Most neonatal deaths occur during the second to the sixth months of life.
c. Neonatal death is more common in low birth weight infants.
d. Central nervous system injury is a significant cause of neonatal death.

1-21. Birth certificates serve to

a. Provide evidence of age
b. Provide evidence of citizenship
c. Provide evidence of family relationships
d. Provide vital statistics for health care planning

2. THE ANATOMY OF THE REPRODUCTIVE TRACT OF WOMEN

2-1. Which one of the following does not mean the same as the others?

a. Vulva
b. External generative organs
c. Organs providing for ovulation, fertilization, and implantation
d. Pudenda

2-2. Which of the following is a part of the vulva?

a. Labia majora
b. Labia minora
c. Clitoris
d. Vestibule
e. Vagina

2-3. Which of the following statements about the labia majora is correct?

a. The labia majora are embryologically homologous with the male scrotum.
b. The uterosacral ligaments terminate at the upper borders of the labia majora.
c. In multiparous women, the labia majora are more prominent than in nulliparous women.
d. In nulliparous women, the labia majora lie in close apposition.
e. Posteriorly, the labia majora merge into the perineum.

2-4. Which types of tissue are prominent in the labia majora?

a. Fat
b. Sebaceous glands
c. Muscle
d. Connective tissue

2-5. Which of the following statements about the labia minora is correct?

a. In nulliparous women, the labia minora usually project beyond the labia majora.
b. The labia minora are covered by stratified squamous epithelium.
c. There are numerous hair follicles in the labia minora.
d. Superiorly, the labia minora form the frenulum of the clitoris and the prepuce.
e. Inferiorly, the labia minora form the fourchet.

2-6. Which of the following statements about the clitoris is correct?

a. It is homologous to the male scrotum.
b. It contains many smooth muscle fibers.
c. The free end of the clitoris points toward the vaginal opening.
d. The glans is very sensitive to touch.
e. The vessels of the clitoris are connected with the vestibular bulbs.

2-7. Which of the following organs is erectile?

a. Clitoris
b. Frenulum
c. Labia majora
d. Labia minora

2-8. Which of the following are boundries of the vestibule?

a. Labia majora
b. Clitoris
c. Fourchet
d. Labia minora

2–9. The Bartholin glands

a. Are also termed the major vestibular glands
b. Are situated beneath the vestibule on either side of the vaginal opening
c. Do not possess a duct
d. Are sometimes partially covered by the vestibular bulbs
e. Can harbor bacterial pathogens

2–10. Which of the following structures is *not* richly supplied with nerve fibers?

a. Labia minora
b. Labia majora
c. Hymen
d. Clitoris

2–11. Which of the following statements about the hymen is correct?

a. Among women, there is a marked similarity in the shape and consistency of the hymen.
b. The surfaces of the hymen are covered by stratified squamous epithelium.
c. The hymen is comprised mainly of muscle.
d. In virgins, the hymen covers the labia minora.

2–12. Presence of an unruptured hymen is a sure indication that the patient is virginal.

a. True
b. False

2–13. The cicatrized nodules of various sizes which are hymenal remnants after childbirth are called ____________.

Instructions for Items 2–14 to 2–18: Refer to Figure 1. Match the letter with the appropriate description.

2–14. Site of the greatest concentration of genital corpuscles
2–15. Rich supply of sebaceous glands and hair follicles
2–16. Remnants of the relatively avascular connective tissue covering of the vaginal opening
2–17. Distensible posterior extension of the labia majora and minora
2–18. Distensible anterior extension of the labia majora and minora

2–19. Which of the following is a function of the vagina?

a. Excretory duct for the uterus
b. Female organ of copulation
c. Excretory duct for the bladder
d. Birth canal

Fig. 1

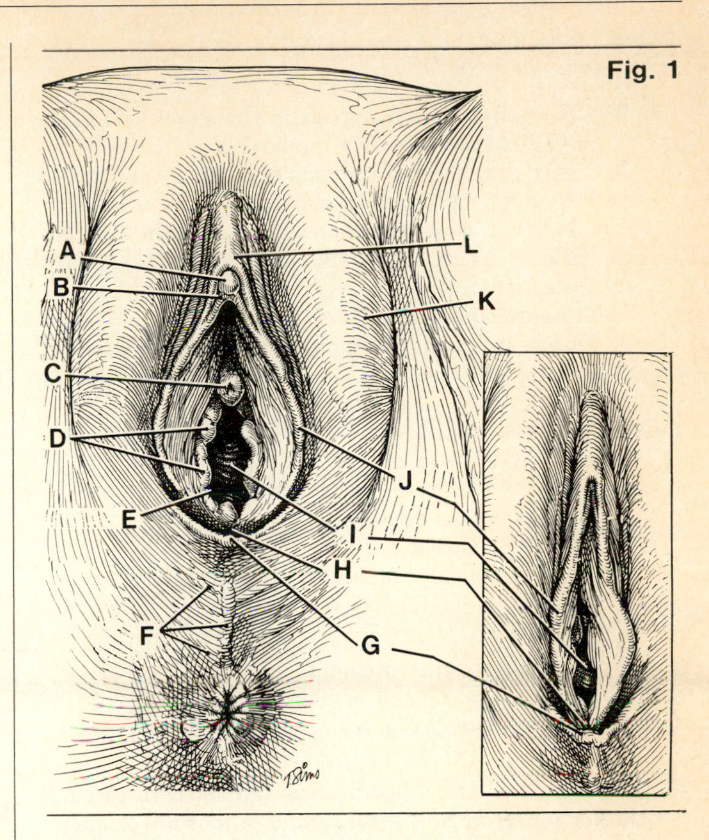

2–20. Which of the following statements about the vagina is correct?

a. It arises embryologically from the Müllerian ducts and the urogenital sinus.
b. It is in contact with both the rectum and bladder.
c. A transverse section of a nondistended vagina is H-shaped.
d. The vagina is distensible only during childbirth.
e. Vaginal length varies among women.

2–21. The upper one-quarter of the vagina is separated from the rectum by the rectouterine pouch, also called the ____________.

2–22. The anterior and posterior walls of the vagina are of equal length.

a. True
b. False

2–23. In which of the following situations are vaginal rugae *not* prominent.

a. In nulliparous women
b. In multiparous women
c. Before menarche
d. After menopause

2–24. Which of the following statements about the vagina is correct?

a. Glycogen begins to appear in the superficial layer of vaginal mucosa after menarche.
b. There are numerous glands present in the vagina.
c. Exfoliated vaginal epithelial cells can be utilized to identify various hormonal events of the ovarian cycle.
d. Uterine secretions contribute to vaginal moisture in nonpregnant women.
e. During pregnancy, vaginal secretions decrease.

Instructions for Items 2–25 to 2–27: Match the portion of the vagina with its arterial blood supply.

a. Inferior vesical arteries
b. Middle hemorrhoidal artery
c. Cervicovaginal branches of uterine arteries
d. Internal pudendal artery

2–25. Upper one-third of vagina
2–26. Middle one-third of vagina
2–27. Lower one-third of vagina

2–28. Which of the following vascular structures contained within the external genital organs are prone to rupture and hematoma formation during vaginal delivery?

a. Venous plexus of the labia majora
b. Vestibular bulbs
c. Venous plexus of the vagina
d. Venous plexus of the labia minora

2–29. Vessels from the venous plexus around the vagina eventually empty into the ________________ veins.

2–30. The lymphatics from the lower third of the vagina and the vulva drain into the

a. Inguinal nodes
b. Hypogastric nodes
c. Iliac nodes

2–31. The vagina contains a rich supply of special nerve endings (genital corpuscles).

a. True
b. False

Instructions for Items 2–32 to 2–33: Match the muscles with the appropriate support structures of the perineum.

a. Deep transverse perineal
b. Levator ani
c. Coccygeus
d. Constrictor of urethra

2–32. Pelvic diaphragm
2–33. Urogenital diaphragm

2–34. The perineal body is formed by which of the following muscles?

a. External anal sphincter
b. Bulbocavernosus muscles
c. Superficial transverse perineal muscles
d. Deep transverse perineal muscles

2–35. The entire surface of the uterus is covered by serosa or peritoneum.

a. True
b. False

Instructions for Items 2–36 to 2–39: Match the portion of the uterus with its correct description.

a. Cornua
b. Cervix
c. Fundus
d. Corpus

2–36. Upper triangular portion
2–37. Lower, fusiform (cylindrical) portion
2–38. Junction of superior and lateral margins
2–39. Convex segment between the insertion points of the fallopian tubes

2–40. In the nulliparous woman, the ratio of uterine body length to cervix length is approximately

a. 1:2
b. 1:1
c. 2:1

2–41. During pregnancy, which portion of the uterus forms the lower uterine segment?

a. External cervical os
b. Isthmus
c. Fundus
d. Cornua

2–42. Which of the following statements about the anatomy of the cervix is correct?

a. The external os approximates the level at which the peritoneum reflects on the bladder.
b. The posterior surface of the supravaginal segment is covered by peritoneum.
c. The cervix is attached laterally to the cardinal ligaments.
d. The portio vaginalis is synonymous with the internal os.

2–43. The appearance of the external cervical os can be sufficiently characteristic to allow an examiner to ascertain whether a woman has borne children by vaginal delivery.

a. True
b. False

2–44. Incompetent cervixes have a greater proportion of muscle fibers than normal cervixes.

a. True
b. False

2–45. Which of the following statements about the structure of the cervix is correct?

a. The cervix is composed mainly of smooth muscle cells.
b. A histologic section taken through the cervical canal resembles a section taken through the endometrium.
c. The endocervical mucosa consists of a single layer of ciliated columnar epithelial cells.
d. Occlusion of the ducts of cervical glands give rise to Nabothian cysts.

2–46. The peritoneum that forms the serosal layer of the uterus is not firmly adherent ______________.

2–47. Which of the following statements about the endometrium is correct?

a. In nonpregnant women, it varies in thickness from 0.5 to 5 mm.
b. The endometrium is attached to the underlying uterine submucosa.
c. The endometrial epithelium consists of a single layer of ciliated, columnar cells.
d. The endometrial glands secrete a thin, acidic fluid.

2–48. The blood supply of the uterus is derived from the

a. Uterine artery
b. Ovarian artery

2–49. Which of the following statements about the blood supply of the endometrium is correct?

a. The coiled arteries (arterioles) supply most of the midportion and the superficial third of the endometrium.
b. The basal arteries usually extend only into the basal layer of the endometrium.
c. The coiled arteries (arterioles) are responsive to hormone action.
d. The basal arteries are responsive to hormone action.

2–50. In pregnancy the myometrium increases mainly through hyperplasia.

a. True
b. False

2–51. Which of the following are portions of the broad ligament?

a. Mesosalpinx
b. Infundibulopelvic ligament
c. Cardinal ligament

Instructions for Items 2–52 to 2–55: Match the ligaments of the uterus with the appropriate statements.

a. Infundibulopelvic ligament
b. Cardinal ligament
c. Round ligament
d. Uterosacral ligament

2–52. Encloses the uterine vessels and the lower portion of the ureter
2–53. Encloses the ovarian vessels
2–54. Corresponds embryologically to the gubernaculum testis in the male
2–55. Forms the lateral boundaries of the pouch of Douglas

Instructions for Items 2–56 to 2–60: Refer to Figure 2. Match the letter with the appropriate structure.

Fig. 2

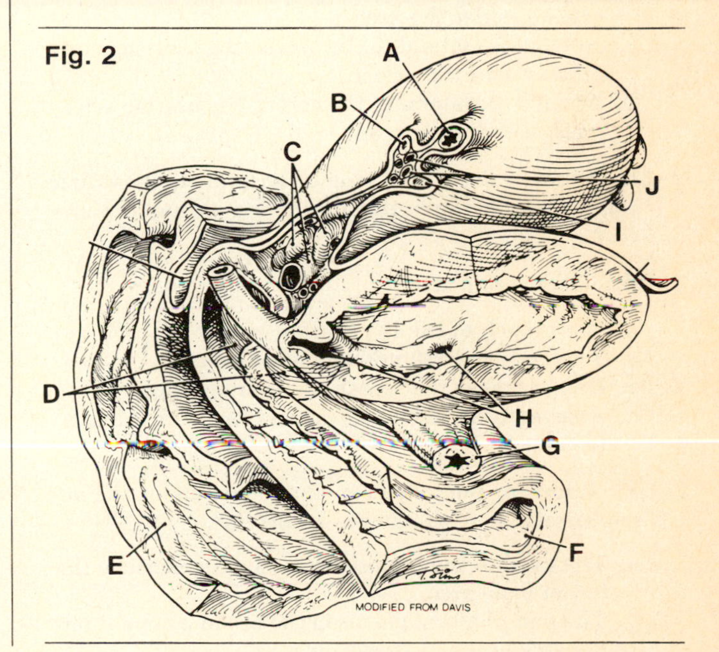

2-56. Cervix
2-57. Round ligament
2-58. Ovarian artery and veins
2-59. Urethra
2-60. Utero-ovarian ligament

2-61. In a nonpregnant woman, which of the following statements about the position of the uterus is correct?

a. The position of the body of the uterus varies with the degree of bladder or rectal distention.
b. The uterus is free to move in the anteroposterior plane.
c. Posture and gravity influence the position of the uterus.
d. The position of the uterus in a woman who is standing and a woman who is supine is the same.

2-62. The uterine artery is a branch of the ______________.

2-63. Which structures are supplied by branches of the uterine artery?

a. Vagina
b. Cervix
c. Body of uterus
d. Oviduct

2-64. Which of the following statements regarding the position of the ureter in relation to the uterine artery is correct?

a. About 2 cm lateral to the cervix, the uterine artery crosses under the ureter.
b. About 3 cm lateral to the cervix, the uterine artery crosses under the ureter.
c. About 2 cm lateral to the cervix, the uterine artery crosses over the ureter.
d. About 3 cm lateral to the cervix, the uterine artery crosses over the ureter.

2-65. What is the clinical significance of the anatomic relationship between the uterine vessels and the ureter?

2-66. The ovarian artery

a. Is a branch of the hypogastric artery
b. Traverses the infundibulopelvic ligament
c. Has branches that enter the ovarian hilum
d. Anastamoses with the ovarian branch of the uterine artery

2-67. Which of the following statements about the venous drainage of the uterus is correct?

a. The uterine vein empties into the hypogastric (internal iliac) vein.
b. The pampiniform plexus in the broad ligament terminates in the ovarian vein.
c. The right ovarian vein empties into the right renal vein.
d. The left ovarian vein empties into the left renal vein.

Instructions for Items 2-68 to 2-69: Match the segment of the uterus with its lymphatic drainage.

a. Hypogastric nodes
b. Periaortic nodes

2-68. Cervix
2-69. Body of uterus

2-70. Which of the following statements regarding the innervation of the genital organs is correct?

a. The nerve supply of the uterus is derived principally from the sympathetic nervous system.
b. Sensory fibers from the uterus are carried through the eleventh and twelfth thoracic nerve roots.
c. Sensory fibers from the cervix and upper portion of the birth canal pass through the second, third and fourth sacral nerves.
d. Sensory fibers from the lower portion of the birth canal pass through the pudendal nerve.

2-71. Which is the correct sequence of oviduct segments through which a sperm travels?

a. Infundibulum, ampulla, isthmus, interstitium
b. Interstitium, isthmus, ampulla, infundibulum
c. Isthmus, interstitium, infundibulum, ampulla
d. Ampulla, interstitium, infundibulum, isthmus

2-72. Which of the following statements about the structure of the oviducts is correct?

a. The musculature of the tube is usually arranged in two layers.
b. The tubal musculature undergoes rhythmic contractions that vary with the ovarian cycle.
c. The tubal muscular contractions are strongest during pregnancy.
d. The tubal mucosa undergoes cyclic histologic changes.
e. Histologic cross-sections taken at various points along the oviduct appear similar.

2-73. Tubal cilia produce a current in the direction of the uterine cavity.

a. True
b. False

2-74. Innervation of the oviduct is principally from the ______________ system.

a. Sympathetic
b. Parasympathetic

2-75. ______________ in the wall of the oviduct may contribute to the development of ectopic pregnancy.

2–76. Which of the following statements about the embryologic development of the uterus and oviducts is correct?

a. The uterus and oviducts arise from the Müllerian ducts.
b. The Müllerian ducts initially appear in the coelomic epithelium at the level of the fourth thoracic segment.
c. The two Müllerian ducts approach each other in the midline in the 6th week and begin to fuse a week later.
d. The uterine lumen is completed in the 7th week.
e. The vaginal canal is not patent in its entire length until the 6th month.

2–77. Which of the following statements about the anatomy of the ovary is correct?

a. A normal ovary in the childbearing years may be up to 5 cm long.
b. The ovary normally lies in the ovarian fossa of Waldeyer.
c. The ovary is attached to the broad ligament by the mesosalpinx.
d. The ovary is attached to the uterus by the suspensory ligament of the ovary.
e. The ovarian vessels are contained within the infundibulopelvic ligament.

Instructions for Items 2–78 to 2–83: Match the histologic finding with the appropriate portion of the ovary.

a. Cortex
b. Medulla

2–78. Ova
2–79. Connective tissue
2–80. Tunica albuginea
2–81. Germinal epithelium of Waldeyer
2–82. Arteries and veins
2–83. Smooth muscle fibers

2–84. The ovary is only supplied by sympathetic nerves.

a. True
b. False

2–85. When and where does the earliest sign of a developing gonad appear in the embryo?

2–86. The female primordial germ cells originate in the

a. Mesenchyme of the developing ovary
b. Yolk sac
c. Genital ridge
d. Germinal epithelium

2–87. Which of the following statements about the embryology of the testis is correct?

a. The testis is recognizable in the 7th week by the presence of well-defined sex cords.
b. Sex cords develop into seminiferous tubules and tubuli reti.
c. The mesonephric ducts become the vas deferens.
d. The rete establishes connection with the mesonephric tubules that develop into the epididymis.

2–88. In the developing ovary

a. The proliferation of germinal epithelium continues longer than in the testis
b. The medulla and cortex are not defined until the 5th month
c. The medulla makes up the bulk of the organ
d. There are distinct sex cords present from about the 3rd month
e. Synapsis is first visible in developing oogonia between the 3rd and 4th months

2–89. By 8 months, the ovary is attached to the body wall along the line of hilum by the ________.

2–90. In the young girl (before puberty), the primordial follicles nearest the central portion of the ovary are at the most advanced stages of development.

a. True
b. False

Instructions for Items 2–91 to 2–93: Match the embryologic remnant with its origin.

a. Wolffian (mesonephric duct)
b. Mesonephric tubules

2–91. Gartner duct
2–92. Paroophoron
2–93. Parovarium

3. THE HUMAN OVARY AND OVULATION

3–1. Cyclic, predictable spontaneous menses is strong evidence for ________________, which in turn implies normal sex hormone production.

3–2. Which of the following migration pathways of germ cells in the fetus is correct?

a. Epithelium of yolk sac, hindgut, gonadal ridge
b. Epithelium of yolk sac, gonadal ridge, hindgut
c. Gonadal ridge, epithelium of yolk sac, hindgut
d. Hindgut, epithelium of yolk sac, gonadal ridge

3–3. The number of germ cells in the ovary increases by

a. Mitosis
b. Meiosis

3–4. Ooogonia are formed in the ovaries until puberty.

a. True
b. False

Instructions for Items 3–5 to 3–8: Match the number of germ cells in the ovary with the appropriate age.

a. 400,000
b. 600,000
c. 2,000,000
d. 6,800,000

3–5. 2 months' gestation
3–6. 5 months' gestation
3–7. Birth
3–8. 10 years of age

Instructions for Items 3–9 to 3–14: Refer to Figure 3. Match the letter with the appropriate part of the maturing graafian follicle.

3–9. Granulosa cell layer
3–10. Theca interna
3–11. Theca externa
3–12. Cumulus oophorus
3–13. Ovum
3–14. Zona pellucida

Instructions for Items 3–15 to 3–17: Match the cell type with the part of the graafian follicle that it forms.

a. Ovarian stromal cell
b. Follicular cell

Fig. 3

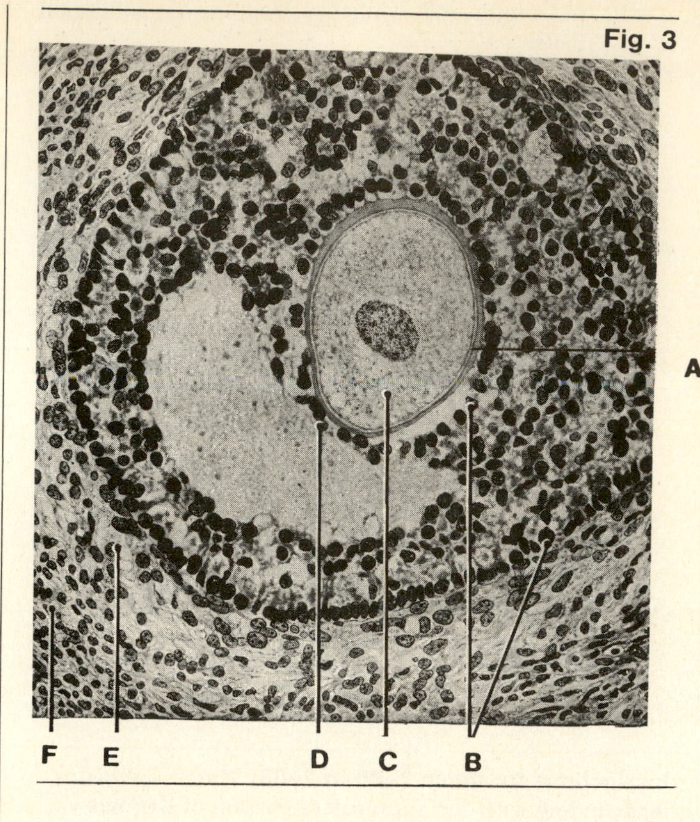

3–15. Theca externa
3–16. Cumulus oophorus
3–17. Membrana granulosa/granulosa cell layer

3–18. Primary oocytes are arrested in which stage of the first meiotic division?

a. Leptotene
b. Zygotene
c. Pachytene
d. Diplotene
e. Metaphase

3–19. Oocyte meiosis can be reinitiated by

a. In vitro culture
b. Gonadotropin stimulation
c. Low oxygen levels
d. Steroids

3–20. Which of the following is an action of FSH?

a. It increases aromatization of C_{19}-steroids in granulosa cells.
b. It primes cells to become competent to LH action.
c. It stimulates the production of LH receptors.
d. It stimulates the production of prolactin receptors.

3–21. In extraglandular sites, androstenedione is converted to

a. Estrone
b. Estriol
c. Estradiol
d. Testosterone

3–22. An increase in the production of androstenedione may result in which of the following clinical manifestations?

a. Virilization
b. Feminization
c. Masculinization
d. Infantilization

3–23. In women, ______________ is the almost exclusive source of cholesterol for progesterone biosynthesis.

a. De novo synthesis
b. High density lipoprotein (HDL)
c. Low density lipoprotein (LDL)

3–24. At ovulation, the ovum is extruded along with the

a. Zona pellucida
b. Corona radiata
c. Follicular fluid
d. Theca interna

3–25. The time of ovulation is better determined from the date of onset of the next menstrual period than from the previous menses.

a. True
b. False

3–26. A woman's normal menstrual cycle is 22 days in length. If her menstrual bleeding began on March 30, when did she last ovulate?

a. March 22
b. March 19
c. March 16
d. March 13

3–27. The temperature elevation seen just before or during ovulation is primarily caused by

a. Intraperitoneal irritation from the released ovum
b. A thermogenic effect of FSH
c. A thermogenic effect of progesterone
d. A thermogenic effect of estrogen
e. A sympathetic neural response to ovum release

3–28. Which of the following constitutes proof that ovulation has already occurred?

a. Biphasic basal body temperature chart
b. Maximal Spinnbarkeit
c. Ferning of dried mucus
d. Presence of a secretory endometrium
e. Elevated levels of plasma progesterone

3–29. The most predictable endocrine event that precedes ovulation is a rise in

a. Estradiol
b. FSH
c. LH
d. Progesterone

3–30. Which cells of the corpus luteum are physiologically active?

a. K cells
b. Theca interna cells
c. Granulosa cells
d. Fibroblasts in the central coagulum

3–31. Which of the following statements about corpus luteum regression is correct?

a. Complete regression occurs prior to menstruation.
b. Capillary proliferation continues throughout the menstrual cycle.
c. There is a loss of lipid-staining material throughout the corpus luteum.
d. Degenerative changes are postponed if pregnancy occurs.

3–32. A functional corpus luteum is required throughout pregnancy.

a. True
b. False

3–33. Surgical ablation of the corpus luteum of early pregnancy

a. Predisposes the patient to spontaneous abortion
b. Requires that the patient be treated with exogenous progestin
c. Removes the sole endogenous source of progesterone
d. Interferes with implantation of the embryo

3–34. If pregnancy does not occur, the corpus luteum is replaced by a connective tissue structure called the ______________.

3–35. During the process of follicular atresia, the

a. Ovum undergoes cytolysis
b. Membrana granulosa degenerates
c. Theca lutein cells proliferate
d. Granulosa lutein cells proliferate

3–36. Which of the following hormones is produced by the ovary?

a. Estrogens
b. Androgens
c. Progesterone
d. Relaxin

3–37. Which of the following is a common estrogen in humans?

a. Estradiol-17β
b. Androstenedione
c. Estriol
d. Estrone

3–38. The principal metabolites of estrone and estradiol-17β are called ______________.

3–39. Extraglandular estrogen is derived by the conversion of androstenedione to

a. Estrone
b. Estradiol-17β
c. Estriol
d. Catechol estrogen

3–40. Extraglandular estrogen production normally is the primary source of estrogen in

a. Prepubertal children
b. Reproductive age women
c. Postmenopausal women
d. Men

3–41. The plasma prehormone, androstenedione, originates by direct secretion from the

a. Ovary
b. Endometrium
c. Adrenal cortex
d. Peripheral fat deposits

3–42. In the ovary, estrogen may be synthesized de novo from acetate or cholesterol.

a. True
b. False

3–43. Which of the following biosynthetic pathways is utilized in the ovary for the production of estradiol-17β?

a. Androstenedione ⟶ estrone ⟶ estradiol-17β
b. Androstenedione ⟶ testosterone ⟶ estradiol-17β
c. 17-hydroxypregnenolone ⟶ dehydroepiandrosterone ⟶ estradiol-17β

Instructions for Items 3–44 to 3–48: Refer to Figure 4. Match the compound with the appropriate structure.

3–44. Cholesterol
3–45. Estradiol
3–46. Androstenedione
3–47. Progesterone
3–48. Testosterone

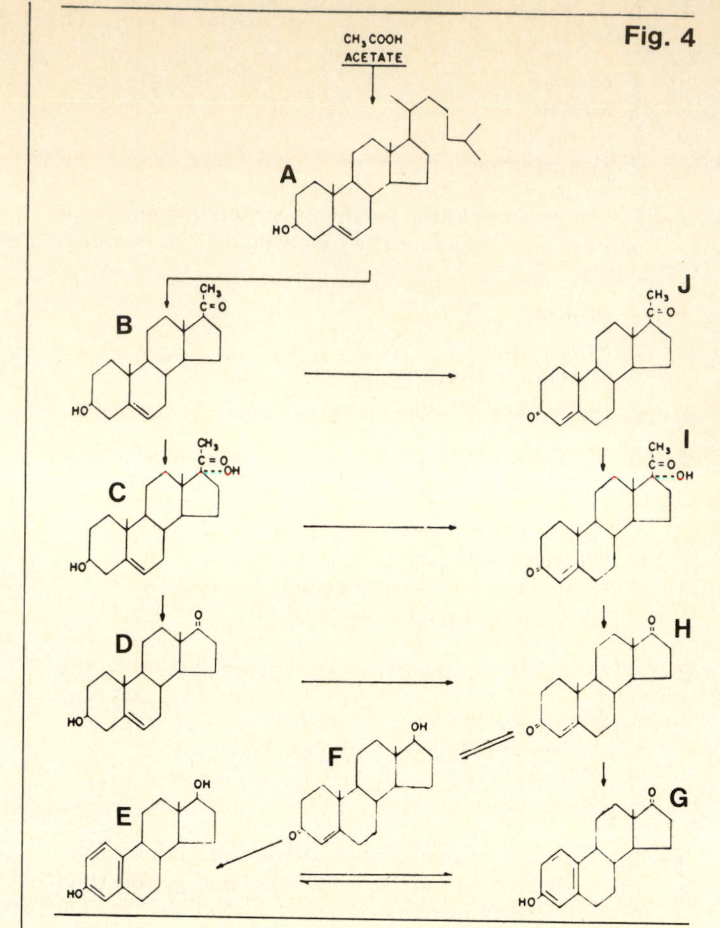

3–49. The principal estrogen secreted by the ovary is

a. Estrone
b. Estradiol-17β
c. Estriol
d. Estrone glucuronide

3–50. The estrogens that circulate in blood are principally ______________ (1), whereas the metabolites found in urine are principally ______________ (2).

a. Sulfuric acid conjugates
b. Glucuronic acid conjugates

3–51. Urinary estrogen concentrations represent what percent of total daily estrogen production?

a. <5 percent
b. 15 percent
c. 50 percent
d. 75 percent

3–52. Estradiol-17β has a selective affinity for which of the following structures?

a. Cervix
b. Vagina
c. Endometrium
d. Myometrium
e. Fallopian tubes

3–53. Estrogen

a. Causes the Müllerian ducts and the genital tubercle to differentiate along female lines
b. Stimulates the growth of spiral arterioles in the uterus
c. Stimulates the cervical epithelium to secrete mucus
d. Causes thickening of the vaginal epithelium
e. Stimulates the secretion of FSH by the pituitary
f. Stimulates the growth of the ovarian follicle

3–54. Progesterone is the principal hormone secreted by the corpus luteum.

a. True
b. False

3–55. The major urinary metabolite of progesterone is ________________.

3–56. In the blood of ovulatory women, the maximum concentration of progesterone and its metabolites is found

a. At the time of ovulation
b. 3 days after ovulation
c. 1 week after ovulation
d. 2 weeks after ovulation

Instructions for Items 3–57 to 3–61: Match the hormone with its action.

a. Estrogen
b. Progesterone

3–57. Promotes linear bone growth
3–58. Inhibits the contractility of uterine smooth muscle
3–59. Increases the respiratory rate
3–60. Triggers the release of LH, which brings about ovulation
3–61. Prepares the endometrium for blastocyst implantation

3–62. During pregnancy, endogenous progesterone can be supplied by

a. The placenta
b. The corpus luteum
c. Peripheral sources

3–63. Despite adequate ATP and actomyosin, progesterone can inhibit myometrial contractility by decreasing ________________.

3–64. Which of the following is characteristic of the fallopian tube mucosa during the luteal phase?

a. Changes occur that are indicative of secretory activity.
b. There is an increased content of glycogen.
c. There is an increase in muscular contractions.

3–65. Progesterone causes the production or secretion of cervical mucus that is scanty, viscid, impermeable to spermatozoa and full of leukocytes.

a. True
b. False

Instructions for Items 3–66 to 3–68: Match the hormone with its effects on the breasts.

a. Estrogen
b. Progesterone

3–66. Responsible for acinar and lobular development
3–67. Acts on ductal epithelium
3–68. Inhibits the action of prolactin in α-lactalbumin synthesis

Instructions for Items 3–69 to 3–72: Match the hormone with its principal site of synthesis.

a. Ovary
b. Adrenal gland
c. Extraglandular sites

3–69. Androstenedione
3–70. Dehydroisoandrosterone
3–71. Dehydroisoandrosterone sulfate
3–72. Testosterone

3–73. Androstenedione serves as a precursor for

a. Estrogen
b. Testosterone
c. Dehydroisoandrosterone

3–74. Sources of relaxin include the

a. Placenta
b. Decidua
c. Corpus luteum

3–75. Which of the following statements about relaxin is correct?

a. Receptors for relaxin are found in the myometrium.
b. Relaxin induces myometrial quiescence.
c. Relaxin is potentiated by prolactin.
d. Relaxin effects are resistant to oxytocin.
e. Relaxin effects can be overridden by $PGF_2\alpha$.

3–76. Changes in which gland are primarily responsible for the onset of puberty?

a. Hypothalamus
b. Pituitary
c. Ovary
d. Adrenal

3–77. FSH

a. Causes growth of the ovarian follicle
b. Causes an increase in ovarian weight
c. Is essential for the production of estrogen in the ovary

3–78. After the menopause, the secretion of estrogens is ______ (1) and the secretion of FSH is ______ (2).

a. Increased
b. Decreased

3–79. The plasma level of LH peaks

a. Approximately 12 hours prior to ovulation
b. At the time of ovulation
c. Approximately 12 hours after ovulation

3–80. The preovulatory LH surge is dependent upon a

a. Rise in circulating FSH
b. Rise in circulating progesterone
c. Rise in circulating estrogen
d. Fall in circulating estrogen
e. Fall in circulating progesterone

3–81. Prolactin

a. Is a luteotropic hormone
b. Secretion is episodic
c. Secretion is stimulated by TRH (thyrotropin-releasing hormone)
d. Secretion is associated with a decrease of gonadotropin secretion

3–82. The clinical picture of amenorrhea and galactorrhea is associated with which of the following?

a. Tranquilizers
b. Reserpine
c. Inhibition of dopamine synthesis
d. Elevated levels of prolactin

3–83. The substance in the ovarian follicle that specifically regulates the secretion of FSH is called ______.

Instructions for Items 3–84 to 3–87: Match the hormone with its effect on folliculostatin production.

a. Increases
b. Decreases

3–84. Progesterone
3–85. Androstenedione
3–86. Testosterone
3–87. Estradiol-17β

3–88. A cybernin is defined as ______.

4. THE ENDOMETRIUM AND MENSTRUATION: UNIQUE PROPERTIES

4–1. Which of the following statements about estradiol-17β is correct?

a. It is the most potent natural estrogen.
b. It enters the endometrial cell by simple diffusion.
c. It is involved in the synthesis of receptor molecules for progesterone.
d. It is involved in the synthesis of receptor molecules for estradiol-17β.

4–2. Progesterone negates the effects of estrogen by

a. Bringing about a decrease in the production of estradiol-17β receptors
b. Causing a decrease in intracellular estradiol-17β concentration
c. Increasing the sulfurylation of estrogen
d. Competitively occupying estrogen receptors

4–3. The absence of progesterone receptors in a breast tumor indicates that the tumor is more likely to be responsive to endocrine ablation procedures.

a. True
b. False

4–4. Menstruation is ultimately due to

a. Estrogen withdrawal
b. Estrogen stimulation
c. Progesterone withdrawal
d. Progesterone stimulation

4–5. Ovarian cycle events occur ______________ the corresponding menstrual cycle events.

a. Before
b. Coincident with
c. After

Instructions for Items 4–6 to 4–8: Match the phase of the ovulatory ovarian cycle with the characteristics of the endometrium.

a. Early follicular
b. Late follicular
c. Luteal

4–6. Significant gland mitoses, no visible secretion in gland lumena, little stromal edema, considerable stromal mitoses
4–7. Increasing numbers of gland mitoses, no visible secretion in gland lumena, some stromal edema, low level of stromal mitoses
4–8. Sharply decreasing number of gland mitoses, considerable secretion in gland lumena, significant stromal edema, decreasing stromal mitoses

4–9. The follicular phase of the menstrual cycle is commonly synonymous with the

a. Preovulatory phase of the ovarian cycle
b. Postovulatory phase of the ovarian cycle
c. Proliferative phase of the endometrial cycle
d. Secretory phase of the endometrial cycle

4–10. Which of the following statements about the proliferative phase of the endometrial cycle is correct?

a. It is associated with the follicular phase of the ovarian cycle.
b. It coincides with the time of graafian follicle growth and maturation in the ovary.
c. Estrogen is the predominant hormone acting during the phase.

Instructions for Items 4–11 to 4–14: Match the phase of the menstrual/endometrial cycle with the appropriate histologic description.

a. Secretory phase
b. Proliferative phase
c. Premenstrual phase

4–11. Development of coiled or spiral arterioles
4–12. Basal, compact, and spongy zones of endometrium become well defined
4–13. "Dating" of endometrium not possible
4–14. Infiltration of the stroma by polymorphonuclear leukocytes occurring

Instructions for Items 4–15 to 4–19: Match the stage of the endometrial cycle with its histologic characteristics.

a. Early proliferative
b. Late proliferative
c. Early secretory
d. Late secretory
e. Premenstrual

4–15. Extremely vascular, rich in glycogen, stromal cells undergoing hypertrophic changes, spiral arterioles become highly tortuous
4–16. Glands narrow and tubular, glandular epithelium low columnar, deep stromal cells densely packed
4–17. Three zones (basal, spongy, and compact) become well defined, stromal edema prominent
4–18. Infiltration of stroma by polymorphonuclear or mononuclear leukocytes
4–19. Glandular epithelium becomes taller and pseudostratified, glands of deeper zone become crowded and tortuous

4–20. The menstrual phase of the normal menstrual cycle is

a. Preceded by corpus luteum regression
b. Preceded by falling levels of progesterone and estrogen
c. Preceded first by spiral arteriole vasoconstriction and slowed circulation and then by vasodilation and increased blood flow
d. Characterized by predominantly venous bleeding

4–21. The decidua (the specialized endometrium of pregnancy)

a. May be the source of amnionic fluid prolactin
b. Serves as an allograft model
c. Has high levels of phospholipase A_2 activity
d. Contains a low concentration of arachidonic acid

4–22. Which of the following statements about the synthesis and action of prostaglandins is correct?

a. They cannot be synthesized from the esterified form of arachidonic acid.
b. Their synthesis is dependent on the action of phospholipase A_2.
c. They can precipitate the initiation of menstruation in nonpregnant women.
d. They can cause symptoms of dysmenorrhea when administered in large doses.

4–23. Which of the following are potentially normal events during the menstrual cycle?

a. The follicular phase may vary in length from 1 to 3 weeks.
b. There may be bleeding during anovulatory cycles.
c. Bleeding ("placental sign") may result from the implantation of the fertilized ovum.

4–24. A 26-year-old woman who has been using oral contraceptives for 3 years has been menstruating regularly. This woman is most probably ovulating normally.

a. True
b. False
c. Cannot be determined from the data available

4–25. Which of the following statements concerning cervical mucus secretion is correct?

a. Secretion is maximal at the time of ovulation.
b. Spinnbarkeit is minimal at the time of ovulation.
c. Cervical mucus secretion is the result of estrogenic stimulation.
d. Maximal secretion of cervical mucus coincides with the maximal secretion of the endometrial glands.

4–26. In which of the following situations is a well-developed "fern pattern" likely to be seen when cervical mucus is spread on a glass slide?

a. During pregnancy
b. When the sodium chloride concentration is less than 1 percent
c. During the late secretory portion of the menstrual cycle
d. When estrogen, but not progesterone, is being produced

Instructions for Items 4–27 to 4–28: Match the hormone with its effect on the sodium chloride concentration of cervical mucus.

a. Estrogen
b. Progesterone

4–27. Results in raised sodium chloride concentration
4–28. Results in lowered sodium chloride concentration

Instructions for Items 4–29 to 4–32: Match the stage of the menstrual cycle with the cellular characteristics of the vagina.

a. Follicular phase
b. Luteal phase

4–29. Leukopenia
4–30. Increased number of basophilic cells
4–31. Enlarged, flattened superficial cells
4–32. Increased number of leukocytes

4–33. Which of the following statements regarding menarche is correct?

a. Menarche always occurs between the ages of 11 and 14.
b. Menarche is a sign of puberty.
c. Menarche occurs at an earlier age now than 30 years ago.
d. Menarche is indicative of sexual maturity.

Instructions for Items 4–34 to 4–37: Match the term with its definition.

a. Menarche
b. Puberty
c. Menopause
d. Climacteric

4–34. Cessation of menses
4–35. Transition between childhood and maturity
4–36. Onset of first menstruation
4–37. "Change of life"

4–38. Which of the following statements about the normal menstrual cycle is correct?

a. There is marked variation among women in the length of the menstrual cycle.
c. There is often considerable variation in the length of a given woman's menstrual cycles.
c. There is considerable variation among women in the duration of menstrual flow.
d. There is usually considerable variation in the duration of a given woman's menstrual flow.

4–39. A marked irregularity in the length of a patient's menstrual cycles usually means that she is sterile.

a. True
b. False

4–40. The normal menstrual cycle is usually characterized by

a. A highly coagulable menstrual discharge
b. A usual flow duration of 4 to 6 days
c. An average weight gain of 1 to 2 pounds
d. A yearly iron loss of 150 to 400 mg

4–41. A premenstrual weight gain of 3 to 5 pounds is a common physiologic phenomenon.

a. True
b. False

5. GAMETOGENESIS AND THE DEVELOPMENT OF THE OVUM

5–1. The unique process by which either mature ova or spermatids are produced through reduction and division is called ______________.

5–2. The number of autosomes in mature gametes is

a. 48
b. 46
c. 23
d. 22
e. 2
f. 1

5–3. What is the number of chromosomes in a primitive germ cell (oogonium or spermatogonium)?

a. 48
b. 46
c. 24
d. 22
e. 2
f. 1

5–4. The basic difference between mitosis and meiosis is the prolonged prophase in mitosis, where pairing of homologous chromosomes occurs.

a. True
b. False

Instructions for Items 5–5 to 5–8: Match the stage of meiosis with the appropriate events.

a. Leptotene
b. Zygotene
c. Pachytene
d. Diplotene

5–5. Homologous chromosomes aligned in synapsis
5–6. Chromatids in tetrads, joined at the centromere
5–7. 46 chromosomes appear as single slender threads
5–8. Homologous strands separate

5–9. The acellular glycoprotein layer deposited by follicular cells around the primary oocyte is called the ______________.

5–10. Which of the following events occurs during the maturation phase of oogenesis?

a. The germ cells divide mitotically.
b. The cells enter prophase of the first meiotic division.
c. A ring of granulosa cells surrounds the oogonium.
d. Definitive oocytes are formed within the primary follicles.

5–11. Which of the following is the correct sequence of events in the development of the human ovum?

a. Migration, division, maturation
b. Migration, maturation, division
c. Division, maturation, migration
d. Maturation, division, migration
e. Maturation, migration, division

5–12. As a result of the second meiotic division, each daughter cell contains __________ chromosomes?

a. 46
b. 44
c. 23
d. 22

5–13. In oogenesis, the haploid number of chromosomes first appears in the

a. Primitive germ cell
b. Primary oocyte
c. Secondary oocyte
d. Oogonium

5–14. If x is the amount of DNA in a mature oocyte, the amount of DNA present at the end of the first meiotic division is

a. x
b. $2x$
c. $3x$
d. $4x$

5–15. Oocyte maturation inhibitor, a substance in follicular fluid that inhibits oocyte maturation, is believed to be

a. Cyclic AMP
b. A cybernin
c. LH
d. FSH

5–16. Which of the following is formed as a result of the first meiotic division?

a. Primary oocyte
b. Secondary oocyte
c. First polar body
d. Second polar body

5–17. When does the human ovum undergo the second maturation division?

5–18. The ovum is capable of being fertilized up to __________ hours after ovulation?

a. 8
b. 18
c. 24
d. 48
e. 72

5–19. What are the locations of the primordial germ cells in developing embryos?

a. Cortex of testis, cortex of ovary
b. Medulla of testis, cortex of ovary
c. Cortex of testis, medulla of ovary
d. Medulla of testis, medulla of ovary

5–20. The solid sex cords in the developing testis form lumina and transform into seminiferous tubules

a. At about 7 months' gestation
b. At about 8 months' gestation
c. At the time of birth
d. After birth

Instructions for Items 5–21 to 5–24: Match the process with the appropriate description.

a. Oogenesis
b. Spermatogenesis

5–21. First meiotic division has a long prophase where exchange of genetic material between homologous chromosomes occurs
5–22. The two meiotic divisions result in four equally sized products
5–23. There is a sevenfold increase in size of the developing gamete
5–24. Primordial germ cells enter the developing gonad during the 5th week

Instructions for Items 5–25 to 5–29: Match the chromosomal complement with the appropriate developmental stage.

a. 46, XY
b. 23, X
c. 23, Y

5–25. Spermatogonium
5–26. Primary spermatocyte
5–27. Secondary spermatocyte
5–28. Spermatid
5–29. Spermatozoon

5–30. Approximately what percent of sperm in the ejaculate reaches the site of ovum fertilization?

a. 100 percent
b. 10 percent
c. 1 percent
d. 0.1 percent
e. 0.01 percent

5–31. The time from insemination to arrival of sperm at the site of fertilization is compatible with migration by flagellar action.

a. True
b. False

5–32. Which of the following statements about fertilization is correct?

a. At the time of fertilization, the oocyte is usually in the ampulla of the fallopian tube.
b. The oocyte must complete the second meiotic division prior to fertilization.
c. The zona pellucida must disappear for fertilization to occur.
d. Only one sperm can enter the ovum at the time of fertilization.

5–33. The incidence of Down syndrome in the general population is ____(1)____, but in women at age 40 it is ____(2)____.

5–34. The risk of chromosomal aberrations in the offspring of men over 40 is __________ than average.

a. Greater
b. No different
c. Less

Instructions for Items 5–35 to 5–38: Match the type of cell division with the appropriate event.

a. Mitosis
b. Meiosis

5–35. Division of oogonia to form primary oocytes
5–36. Division of primary oocytes to form mature oocytes
5–37. Division of zygote
5–38. Exchange of material between homologous chromosomes

Instructions for Items 5–39 to 5–40: Match the stage of development with the appropriate events.

a. Blastocyst
b. Embryo
c. Fetus

5–39. The major organ systems are formed
5–40. Implantation occurs

5–41. Place the following developmental stages into the correct chronologic sequence.

a. Fetus
b. Morula
c. Blastomere
d. Embryo
e. Zygote
f. Blastocyst

5–42. Which of the following statements about implantation is correct?

a. The fertilized ovum undergoes cleavage for 3 days in the fallopian tube.
b. After entering the uterine cavity, the blastocyst remains free (i.e., does not implant) for 1 or 2 days.
c. The zona pellucida disappears before implantation occurs.
d. The pole of the blastocyst with the inner cell mass implants first.

5–43. Which of the following statements about the inner cell mass is correct?

a. It forms the embryo.
b. It develops into the cytotrophoblast.
c. It induces a decidual reaction in surrounding maternal tissues.
d. It gives rise to extraembryonic mesoderm.

5–44. Development of syncytiotrophoblast is required for

a. Formation of new cytotrophoblast cells
b. Successful invasion of the endometrium
c. Elicitation of a decidual response
d. Formation of the amnion

5–45. The body stalk, which connects the chorion and embryo, develops into the ________________.

Instructions for Items 5–46 to 5–53: Refer to Figure 5. Match the letter with the appropriate structure.

Fig. 5

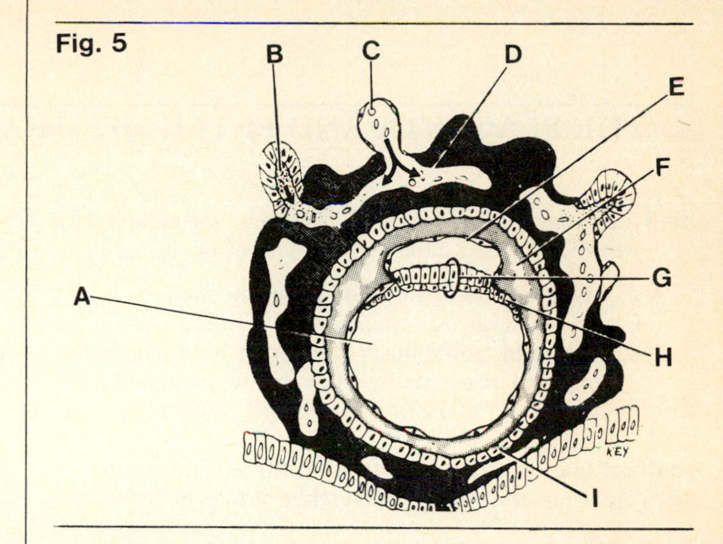

5–46. Embryonic disc
5–47. Amnionic cavity
5–48. Maternal blood in lacunar network
5–49. Extraembryonic endoderm
5–50. Cytotrophoblast
5–51. Lacunar network
5–52. Primitive yolk sac
5–53. Extraembryonic coelom developing in extraembryonic mesoderm

Instructions for Items 5–54 to 5–60: Match the germ layer with the structures derived from it.

a. Ectoderm
b. Mesoderm
c. Endoderm

5–54. Epidermis
5–55. Lining of the GI tract
5–56. Nervous system
5–57. Vascular system
5–58. Skeletal muscle
5–59. Liver
5–60. Dermis

5–61. Which of the following statements about the notochord is correct?

a. It arises as a forward extension of the primitive streak.
b. It constitutes the primordial supporting structure of vertebrates.
c. It disappears early in embryonic life.
d. Remnants of notochord persist in the adult as the nucleus pulposus of the intervertebral discs.

5–62. Differentiation of the embryo proceeds from the cephalic end to the caudal end.

a. True
b. False

5–63. Somites

a. Are derived from lateral mesoderm
b. Give rise to skeletal and connective tissues
c. Begin at the level of the developing neck

6. THE PLACENTA AND FETAL MEMBRANES

6–1. Primary placental villi become secondary villi when ______ (1) and tertiary villi after ______ (2).

a. Solid trophoblastic columns are formed
b. Angiogenesis occurs in situ
c. The solid trophoblast is invaded by a mesenchymal cord, presumably from the cytotrophoblast

Instructions for Items 6–2 to 6–4: Match the event with the time after fertilization when it occurs.

a. 7 days
b. 10 days
c. 12 days
d. 14 days
e. 17 days

6–2. Placental circulation established
6–3. Maternal arterial blood enters intervillous spaces
6–4. Villi distinguishable in the placenta

6–5. Which of the following statements about chorionic villi is correct?

a. Chorionic villi are not recognizable until about 4 weeks after fertilization.
b. Incomplete or absent angiogenesis may present as hydatidiform mole.
c. Villi in contact with the decidua basalis proliferate to form the chorion frondosum.
d. An extension of the syncytiotrophoblast anchors the villi to the decidua at the basal plate.

Instructions for Items 6–6 to 6–7: Match the component with its correct location.

a. Cytotrophoblast cells
b. Decidua of basal plate
c. Trophectoderm
d. Chorionic plate

6–6. Floor of intervillous space
6–7. Roof of intervillous space

6–8. At 19 days postfertilization, which of the following does *not* describe human embryonic development?

a. The embryo is at the primitive streak stage.
b. The decidua basalis is present.
c. The decidua capsularis is present.
d. The embryo is trilaminar.
e. A choriovitelline placenta has formed.

Instructions for Items 6–9 to 6–10: Match the descriptions of components of the chorion at 3 weeks after fertilization.

a. Cuboidal cells
b. Clear cytoplasm
c. Light, vesicular nuclei
d. Dark nuclei
e. Granular cytoplasm

6–9. Cytotrophoblast
6–10. Syncytiotrophoblast

6–11. The chorionic villi in contact with the decidua basalis proliferate to form the ______ (1) whereas the villi in contact with the decidua capsularis degenerate, which results in the ______ (2).

a. Chorion laeve
b. Chorion frondosum

6–12. Which of the following statements about the chorion is correct?

a. Villi are distributed over the entire periphery of the chorionic membrane throughout pregnancy.
b. The chorion laeve comprises only a small portion of the chorion.
c. Prostaglandin synthesis at parturition is associated with the amniochorion.
d. The amniochorion in the human is formed from the amnion and the chorion frondosum.
e. The amniochorion is not formed until near the end of the third trimester.

6–13. The amniochorion functions in solute and fluid transport.

a. True
b. False

6–14. A placental cotyledon is formed from ______________.

6–15. The number of placental cotyledons increases steadily until the last month of pregnancy.

a. True
b. False

6–16. Which of the following changes is seen in the placenta as pregnancy advances?

a. Volume of cytotrophoblast cells decreases
b. Syncytium thickens
c. Syncytium forms knots
d. Stroma becomes denser
e. Number of Hofbauer cells increases

6–17. Which of the following statements about the decidua is correct?

a. The decidua is the endometrium of pregnancy.
b. The decidual reaction occurs in response to estrogen.
c. The decidual reaction occurs in response to human placental lactogen.
d. The decidual reaction is completed prior to nidation.
e. Decidual cells arise from stromal cells of the endometrium.

6–18. Which of the following occurs in the decidua as pregnancy progresses?

a. The decidua thickens to a depth of 2 cm or more.
b. The decidua basalis overlies the developing embryo and separates it from the rest of the uterine cavity.
c. The decidua capsularis is formed directly beneath the site of implantation.
d. The uterine cavity is obliterated after the fusion of the decidua capsularis and parietalis (vera).

Instructions for Items 6–19 to 6–23: Refer to Figure 6. Match the letter with the appropriate description.

6–19. Decidua vera
6–20. Decidua capsularis
6–21. Decidua basalis
6–22. Chorion frondosum
6–23. Chorion laeve

Fig. 6

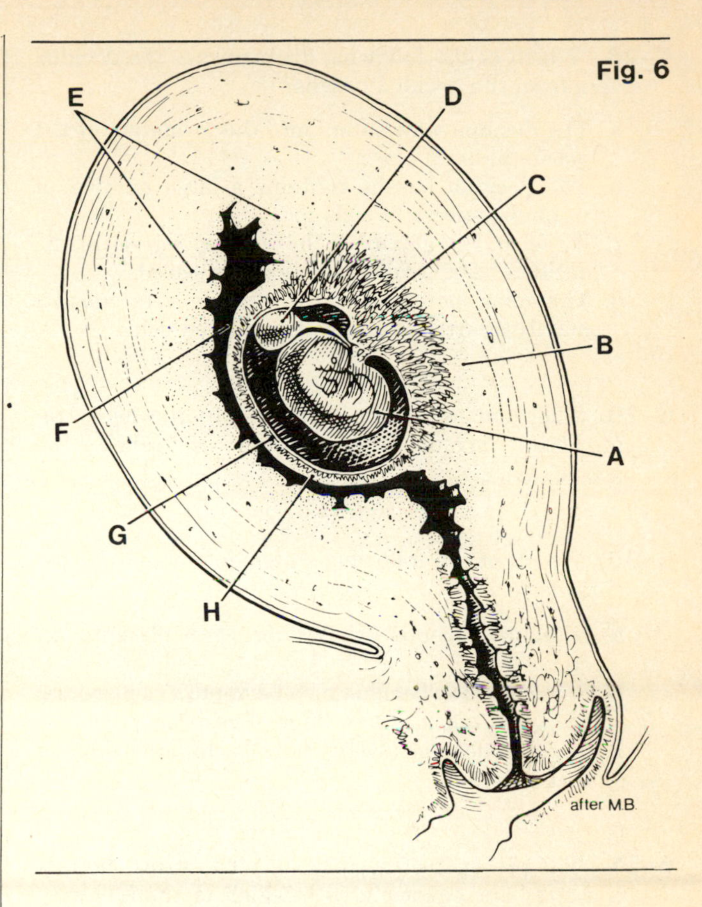

6–24. The correct sequence of layers, starting from the surface, in the decidua vera and the decidua basalis is

a. Compacta, spongiosa, basalis
b. Compacta, basalis, spongiosa
c. Spongiosa, compacta, basalis
d. Spongiosa, basalis, compacta
e. Basalis, compacta, spongiosa
f. Basalis, spongiosa, compacta

6–25. After delivery, which of the following portions of the decidua remains to give rise to the new endometrium?

a. Zona compacta
b. Zona spongiosa
c. Zona functionalis
d. Zona basalis

Instructions for Items 6–26 to 6–27: Match the decidual zone with the appropriate histologic description.

a. Zona compacta
b. Zona spongiosa
c. Zona basalis

6–26. Large distended glands, minimal stroma
6–27. Large closely-packed polygonal cells, numerous small round cells

6–28. Which of the following distinguishes the decidua vera from the decidua basalis?

a. The decidua vera enters into the formation of the placental basal plate.
b. The decidua basalis contains a large number of trophoblastic giant cells.
c. By term, the glands of the zona spongiosa in the decidua basalis have largely disappeared.
d. The zona spongiosa of the decidua vera consists mainly of arteries and widely dilated veins.

6–29. The zone of fibrinoid degeneration where trophoblasts invade the decidua is called the ________________.

6–30. Which of the following statements about the decidua is correct?

a. Nitabuch layer is usually absent in placenta accreta.
b. Some necrotic decidua may be found in a placental specimen taken at any stage of gestation.
c. Necrotic decidua always indicate threatened or actual abortion.

6–31. The presence of necrotic decidua during the first trimester is compatible with which of the following possibilities?

a. Threatened abortion
b. Incomplete abortion
c. Septic abortion
d. Completed abortion
e. Normal pregnancy

6–32. Which of the following statements about prolactin and the decidua is correct?

a. Prolactin occurs in high concentration in amnionic fluid.
b. Amnionic fluid prolactin concentration is decreased when a pregnant woman is treated with bromocriptine.
c. Dopamine increases decidual prolactin secretion.
d. Thyrotropin-releasing hormone decreases decidual prolactin secretion.
e. Arachidonic acid decreases decidual prolactin secretion.
f. Pituitary and decidual prolactin are immunologically and biologically distinguishable.

6–33. Which of the following statements about the biochemistry of the decidua is correct?

a. Relaxin is produced in the decidua.
b. 1,25-dihydroxyvitamin D_3 is produced in the decidua.
c. Throughout pregnancy, there are elevated levels of polyamines in maternal fluids.
d. The enzyme ornithine carboxylase has been identified in the decidua of women.
e. Diamine oxidase levels rise significantly in midpregnancy.

6–34. Which of the following statements about the trophoblast is correct?

a. Mitotic figures are completely absent from cells in the cytotrophoblast.
b. The syncytium is derived from cytotrophoblast and is a mitotic end stage.
c. Langhans cells are connected with each other and with the syncytium by desmosomes.
d. As the syncytium matures, the fine structural changes are reflective of loss of functional capability.

6–35. The number of layers in the histologic placental "barrier" may be directly equated with the functional efficiency of the placenta.

a. True
b. False

6–36. Studies indicate that the site of placental steroid production is the ________________.

6–37. Which of the following describes the typical human placenta at term?

a. Discoid shape
b. 20 cm diameter
c. 10 cm thickness
d. 500 g weight
e. Succenturiate lobe

Instructions for Items 6–38 to 6–41: Refer to Figure 7. Match the letter with the appropriate part of the placenta and uterus.

6–38. Myometrium
6–39. Chorionic plate with fetal blood vessels
6–40. Placental villi
6–41. Decidua basalis

6–42. Which fetal vessel carries blood with the highest oxygen content?

a. Umbilical artery
b. Aorta
c. Umbilical vein
d. Pulmonary artery
e. Pulmonary vein

Fig. 7

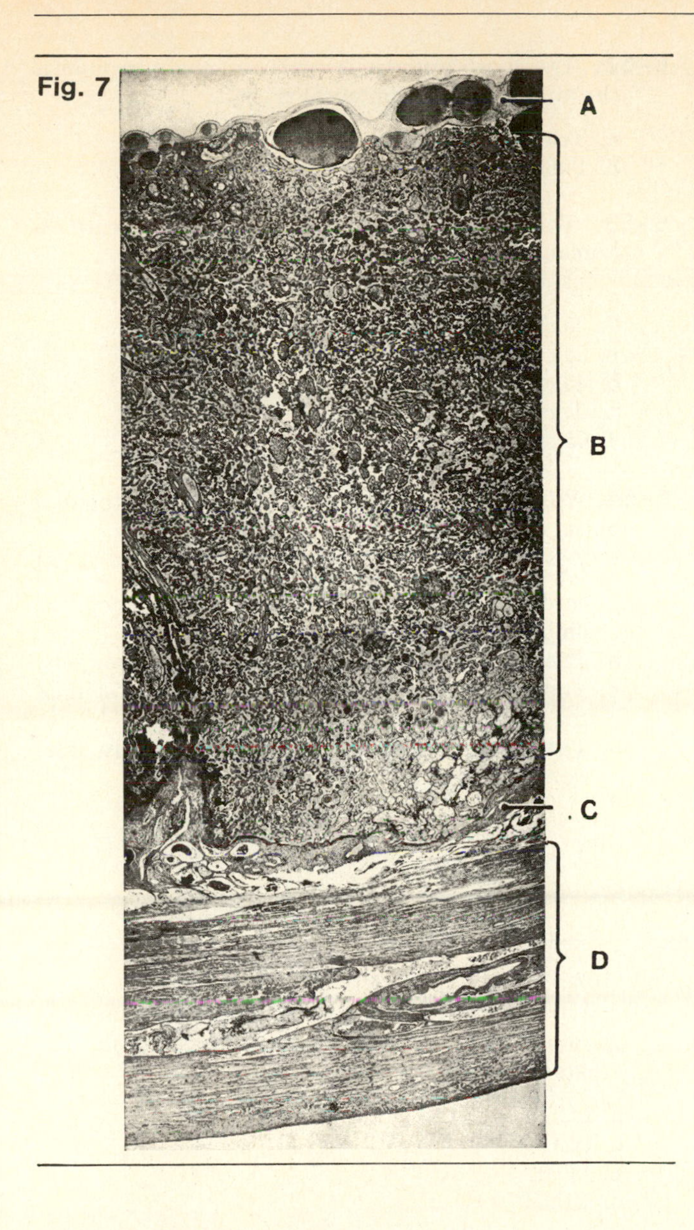

6–43. Which of the following statements about placental circulation is correct?

a. Maternal blood enters the intervillous space via spiral arteries (arterioles).
b. Maternal blood traverses the placenta in preformed channels.
c. Maternal blood traverses the placenta as a result of the negative pressure of the maternal venous system relative to that of the maternal arterial system.
d. The arterial entrances and the venous exits are scattered at random over the entire base of the placenta.
e. The spiral arteries (arterioles) are generally perpendicular and the placental veins parallel to the uterine wall.
f. Countercurrent flow plays an important part in the mechanism of placental circulation.

6–44. Which of the following statements about the effect of uterine contractions on placental circulation is correct?

a. The arrangement of spiral arterioles and placental veins facilitates maternal blood loss from the placenta during contractions.
b. Drainage through veins is decreased during contractions.
c. The amount of blood entering the intervillous space is decreased during contractions.
d. Distention of the placenta with blood during contractions results in an increase in the dimensions of the placenta.

6–45. The regulation of blood flow in the intervillous space is dependent on which of the following factors?

a. Arterial blood pressure
b. Countercurrent flow
c. Intrauterine pressure
d. Uterine contraction pattern

6–46. Which of the following progressive changes in uteroplacental circulation occurs during gestation?

a. There is an intraarterial accumulation of trophoblasts.
b. There is a decrease in the number of arterial openings into the intervillous space.
c. There is an extension of trophoblasts proximally from the terminal portions of uteroplacental arteries.
d. The normal muscular and elastic tissue of the wall of spiral vessels is replaced by fibrous tissue and fibrinoid.
e. A prominent venous plexus develops between the decidua basalis and the myometrium.

6–47. The ability of the placenta and fetus to "defy the laws" of transplantation immunology has been adequately explained by which of the following?

a. The placenta's ability to absolutely separate the maternal and fetal circulations.
b. The antigenic immaturity of the fetus.
c. The presence of a diminished maternal immune response.

6–48. Which of the following statements about placental immunology is correct?

a. The fetus demonstrates antigenic competency.
b. The trophoblast demonstrates antigenic incompetency.
c. The presence of the disease erythroblastosis fetalis defies the fact that the placenta maintains an absolute integrity of the fetal and maternal circulations.
d. The uterus is an immunologically privileged site.
e. The trophoblast provides a physical "immunologic barrier."

6–49. Which of the following statements about the amnion is correct?

a. Near the end of the first trimester, the amnion physically unites with the chorion to produce a single membrane, the amniochorion.
b. The amnion is highly innervated.
c. The number of blood vessels in the amnion increases as gestation proceeds.
d. Amnionic caruncles represent sites of incomplete attachment of the amnion to the chorion.
e. The amnion contains glycerophospholipids rich in arachidonic acid and the enzyme phospholipase A_2.

6–50. Which vessels are normally found in the umbilical cord at term?

a. Right umbilical artery
b. Left umbilical artery
c. Right umbilical vein
d. Left umbilical vein

6–51. When the intraabdominal portion of the duct of the umbilical vesicle remains patent it is called ______________.

6–52. The most common vascular anomaly in man is the absence of one umbilical artery.

a. True
b. False

6–53. The average length of the umbilical cord in humans is

a. 15 cm
b. 25 cm
c. 35 cm
d. 45 cm
e. 55 cm
f. 65 cm

6–54. Which of the following statements about the umbilical cord is correct?

a. False knots (nodulations on the surface of the cord) are the result of folding and tortuosity of the umbilical vessels.
b. The matrix of the cord consists of Wharton jelly.
c. The umbilical artery has a smaller diameter than the umbilical vein.
d. The umbilical vein empties directly into the inferior vena cava.

7. THE PLACENTAL HORMONES

7–1. Which of the following statements about the history of human chorionic gonadotropin (hCG) is correct?

a. Human chorionic gonadotropin was first identified in humans.
b. The "Ascheim-Zondek" ("A-Z") and "Friedman" tests involve the induction of ovulation in induced ovulators by hCG in the urine of pregnant women.
c. In 1938, Gey and others demonstrated the production of chorionic gonadotropin by cultured trophoblastic cells.

7–2. Which of the following statements about the biochemistry of hCG is correct?

a. It is a glycoprotein with a high carbohydrate content.
b. It is composed of two similar subunits, designated alpha and beta.
c. The two subunits are covalently linked.
d. The molecular weight of hCG is approximately 37,000 to 38,000.
e. The syntheses of the alpha and beta chains of hCG are regulated by separate mRNAs.
f. Biologic activity of hCG requires the bonding of the alpha and beta subunits, neither of which is active alone.

7–3. Which of the following glycoprotein hormones has an alpha subunit significantly different from the others?

a. hCG
b. hLH
c. hFSH
d. hTSH

7–4. The beta subunit of hCG is most similar to the beta subunit of

a. hLH
b. hTSH
c. hFSH

7–5. The beta subunit of glycoprotein hormones confers their characteristic biologic activity.

a. True
b. False

7-6. Which of the following statements about the synthesis of hCG is correct?

a. Human chorionic gonadotropin is produced principally by cells in the cytotrophoblast.
b. The greatest concentration of hCG in the plasma of pregnant women is found at 8 to 10 weeks' gestation.
c. The alpha and beta subunits of hCG are synthesized as larger presubunits.
d. The synthesis of the alpha subunit is the rate-limiting step in the synthesis of hCG.

7-7. Which of the following statements about the secretion of hCG is correct?

a. The amounts of alpha and beta subunits in the placenta and plasma of pregnant women are essentially equal.
b. The alpha and beta subunits are secreted separately and also as the hCG hormone.
c. The rate of secretion of hCG may be subject to trophic regulation.

7-8. The most apparent function of hCG is ________.

7-9. Which of the following statements about the activity of hCG is correct?

a. The half-life of hCG is approximately 24 to 37 hours.
b. The half-life of hCG is long compared with that of LH.
c. The high concentration of hCG at 8 to 10 weeks' gestation may ultimately result in a reduction in the rate of corpus luteum progesterone secretion.
d. In the human ovary primed by FSH, hCG can be used as an LH surrogate to induce ovulation.
e. The life span of a corpus luteum induced by LH and one induced by hCG are approximately equal.
f. A role for hCG in the provision of immunologic privilege to the trophoblast has been suggested.

7-10. Which of the following is relevant in the use of bioassays and immunoassays for hCG in pregnancy testing?

a. Cross-reactivity of the alpha subunits of glycoprotein hormones causes a lack of specificity in immunoassays for hCG.
b. The present specificity of immunologic pregnancy tests is primarily a result of the development of antibodies to the beta subunit of hCG.
c. Antibodies to the beta subunit of hCG cross-react significantly with the beta subunit of LH.

7-11. Which of the following statements about hCG levels in urine is correct?

a. Urinary excretion of hCG is maximal between the 60th and 70th day of gestation.
b. A nadir in urinary excretion is reached between the 100th and 130th days.
c. The level of urinary excretion rises about the 200th day and maintains a high level throughout the rest of pregnancy.
d. Women at the same phase of gestation excrete similar amounts of hCG.

7-12. Which of the following statements about hCG levels is correct?

a. The concentrations of the alpha and beta subunits of hCG rise steadily until about 30 weeks' gestation and remain at a plateau for the remainder of pregnancy.
b. Significantly higher levels of hCG are found in multiple gestations.
c. Levels of hCG are lower in an Rh-sensitized pregnancy.
d. Levels of hCG are higher in women with hydatidiform mole.

7-13. The renal clearance of hCG as the native molecule accounts for ________ percent of the total metabolic clearance rate (MCR), the remainder being metabolized by pathways other than renal excretion.

a. 10
b. 30
c. 50
d. 70
e. 90

7-14. Human chorionic gonadotropin can act on the fetal testes as an LH surrogate to promote male sexual differentiation and testosterone synthesis and secretion.

a. True
b. False

7-15. Which of the following statements about the synthesis of human placental lactogen (hPL) is correct?

a. It is concentrated in the syncytiotrophoblast.
b. It consists of a single polypeptide chain with a molecular weight of about 22,000.
c. It is immunochemically similar to human growth hormone.
d. The synthesis of hPL is stimulated by cAMP and insulin.
e. The secretion of hPL is stimulated by PGE_2 and $PGF_{2\alpha}$.
f. The production rate of hPL near term is the greatest of any known hormone.

7–16. Human placental lactogen

a. Can be detected in the serum of pregnant women about 4 weeks after fertilization
b. Has a plasma level in maternal blood that is proportional to placental mass
c. Has a plasma concentration that is lower than the concentration in amnionic fluid
d. Is found in high levels in the fetal circulation
e. Is found in low levels in maternal urine
f. Is concentrated in fetal tissues, where its main metabolic effects are manifest

7–17. The highest level of hPL is found in the

a. Cord blood
b. Maternal urine
c. Maternal blood
d. Fetal urine
e. Amnionic fluid

7–18. Possible actions of hPL include

a. Increasing the levels of circulating free fatty acids
b. Inhibiting both the uptake of glucose and gluconeogenesis in the mother
c. Decreasing the maternal levels of insulin
d. Ensuring a mobilizable source of amino acids for transport to the fetus

7–19. Human placental lactogen has been demonstrated to be a requirement for a normal pregnancy outcome.

a. True
b. False

7–20. The plasma levels of ACTH in pregnant women before labor are significantly higher than in nonpregnant women.

a. True
b. False

7–21. There is evidence that the placenta is a source of which of the following hormones?

a. ACTH
b. LHRH
c. TRH
d. CRF

7–22. Which of the following statements about pregnancy "specific" proteins is correct?

a. These proteins were identified by use of antibodies developed in animals against the serum of pregnant women.
b. Approximately five of these proteins have been discovered.
c. The functions of these proteins have not as yet been well defined.

7–23. The mechanisms of estrogen synthesis in the normal pregnant woman are essentially the same as those in the normal premenopausal nonpregnant woman.

a. True
b. False

7–24. Which of the following statements about the production of estrogen in pregnancy is correct?

a. Pregnancy is a normo-estrogenic state relative to the nonpregnant state.
b. The placenta is the site of origin of estrogens during pregnancy.
c. The prehormones used to synthesize estrogens are produced by cytotrophoblast cells.
d. Maternal urinary estriol originates by conversion of fetal products.
e. Estriol is formed primarily by the conversion of estrone and estradiol-17β.

7–25. Bilateral oophorectomy performed in the second trimester will result in spontaneous loss of the pregnancy due to the lack of circulating estrogens produced by the ovary.

a. True
b. False

7–26. Which of the following statements is the *principal* reason for the increase in urinary estriol during pregnancy?

a. Alteration in the fractional conversion of estrone and estradiol-17β to estriol in the mother.
b. Alteration in the fractional conversion of estrone and estradiol-17β to estriol in the fetus.
c. Placental formation of estriol from 16α-hydroxydehydroisoandrosterone sulfate.
d. De novo synthesis of estriol from acetate and cholesterol.

7–27. In the placenta, the synthesis of estrogen from acetate or cholesterol is not possible because ____________.

Instructions for Items 7–28 to 7–31: Match the hormone with its predominant site of origin.

a. Estradiol-17β
b. Estrone
c. Estriol
d. Dehydroisoandrosterone sulfate

7–28. Placenta
7–29. Extraglandular origin, nonpregnant
7–30. Ovary, nonpregnant
7–31. Fetal adrenal cortex

7–32. Which of the following is a potential precursor of estrogens produced by the placenta?

a. Dehydroisoandrosterone sulfate
b. Dehydroisoandrosterone
c. Testosterone
d. Androstenedione

7–33. The *principal* circulating precursor of placental estrone and estradiol-17β is

a. Dehydroisoandrosterone sulfate
b. Dehydroisoandrosterone
c. Testosterone
d. Androstenedione

7–34. Which of the following statements about dehydroisoandrosterone sulfate (DS) and its metabolism is correct?

a. In pregnancy, DS is derived primarily from the fetal adrenal cortex.
b. The rich supply of placental sulfatase allows the use of DS in estrogen production.
c. The concentration of DS in the plasma of pregnant women increases as pregnancy progresses.
d. The increased clearance of DS in pregnancy is attributable to its conversion to estradiol-17β and its metabolism via increased 16α-hydroxylation in the maternal compartment.
e. The placental clearance of maternal DS is decreased in women who will develop pregnancy-induced hypertension.

7–35. The estriol in the urine of pregnant women can be accounted for by the metabolism of estrone and estradiol-17β.

a. True
b. False

7–36. Which of the following occurs when a woman is pregnant with an anencephalic fetus?

a. The rate of formation of placental estriol is lower than in a normal pregnancy.
b. Production of estrogens can almost totally be accounted for by placental utilization of maternal dehydroisoandrosterone sulfate.
c. Administration of ACTH results in decreased urinary estriol levels.
d. Administration of a potent glucocorticosteriod results in decreased placental production of estrogens.

7–37. In a pregnant woman with Addison's disease, there is an equivalent decrease in all types of estrogens excreted in the urine.

a. True
b. False

7–38. In a woman with an androgen-secreting ovarian tumor, a female fetus is only rarely virilized because ________________.

7–39. Which of the following statements about the fetal adrenal gland is correct?

a. A large portion of the gland is occupied by the fetal zone.
b. The weight of the gland at term approximates the weight of an adult adrenal gland.
c. There is a rapid involution of fetal adrenal cortex after birth.
d. Fetal adrenal growth and steroid secretion is controlled by a single trophic stimulus similar to that which is present in the adult.

Instructions for Items 7–40 to 7–42: Match the structure with the appropriate function.

a. Fetal adrenal cortex
b. Maternal adrenal cortex

7–40. Site of origin of placental estrogen precursors
7–41. Important in fetal lung maturation
7–42. Important in the initiation of labor

7–43. Administration of glucocorticoids to the mother can result in decreased levels of

a. Fetal pituitary ACTH
b. Fetal cortisol
c. Progesterone

7–44. The primary pathway for production of fetal cortisol is ________________.

7–45. Which of the following statements about the biosynthetic activities of the fetal adrenal gland is correct?

a. LDL-cholesterol is a primary source of precursors for fetal adrenal steroidogenesis.
b. Cortisol biosynthesis from cholesterol and pregnenolone is enhanced.
c. The output of steroids from the fetal adrenal gland greatly exceeds that in the adult.
d. The majority of cholesterol utilized for fetal steroidogenesis is transferred from the mother.
e. The fetal adrenal gland secretes large amounts of dehydroisoandrosterone sulfate.

7–46. Which of the following substances probably has an important trophic influence upon the fetal adrenal gland?

a. Chorionic ACTH
b. Progesterone
c. LDL-cholesterol
d. Fetal pituitary prolactin
e. Urinary estriol

7-47. When hyperprolactinemic patients with elevated levels of dehydroisoandrosterone sulfate (DS) are treated with bromocriptine, the plasma DS level

a. Increases
b. Decreases
c. Remains unchanged
d. Fluctuates widely

7-48. After birth there is a(n) ______ (1) in the concentration of prolactin in plasma and a(n) ______ (2) in the size and rate of secretion of the adrenal glands.

a. Increase
b. Decrease

7-49. Which of the following statements about the use of estriol levels as a test of fetal well-being is correct?

a. Fetal death is accompanied by a reduction in the levels of urinary estrogens.
b. Plasma estriol levels correlate well with urinary estriol levels.
c. The use of plasma estriol levels has the advantage of ease and reliability of sample collection.
d. Estriol levels have been proven to be a reliable indicator of placental functions.

7-50. A single measurement of urinary estriol which falls outside the normal range is a reliable indicator of fetal jeopardy or death.

a. True
b. False

7-51. The usefulness of maternal estriol levels as a test of fetal well-being must be interpreted in light of which of the following?

a. There is a narrow range of normal values in serum and urine.
b. Single measurements outside the "normal" range are very reliable.
c. Estriol production can be independent of placental function.
d. Estriol levels may be lowered due to drug ingestion.
e. Lower estriol levels may be due to lack of placental sulfatase activity.
f. Elevated estriol levels may be seen in multiple gestations.

Instructions for Items 7-52 to 7-56: Match the cause of altered estriol levels with the appropriate result.

a. Decreased estriol levels
b. Increased estriol levels

7-52. Maternal ingestion of aspirin
7-53. Acute pyelonephritis
7-54. Fetal anencephaly
7-55. Rh sensitized mother with an erythroblastic fetus
7-56. Maternal ingestion of glucocorticosteroids

7-57. Lack of placental sulfatase activity is associated with pregnancies resulting in male infants who develop the skin disorder ______.

7-58. Which of the following statements about estetrol is correct?

a. Estetrol is 15α-hydroxyestriol.
b. Estetrol is derived principally from estriol via the utilization of fetal precursors.
c. Estetrol is produced almost exclusively by the fetus.
d. The measurement of estetrol has not, so far, proved advantageous over that of estriol in the evaluation of fetal well-being.

7-59. Maternal urinary estriol levels provide clinically indispensable insight into the fetal condition in high-risk pregnancies.

a. True
b. False

7-60. Which of the following statements about progesterone synthesis in pregnancy is correct?

a. It occurs in cytotrophoblast cells.
b. The principal precursor is maternal plasma cholesterol.
c. The fetus produces little or no precursor to progesterone.
d. The rate of progesterone secretion is dependent on uteroplacental blood flow.
e. Immediately after fetal death there is a significant decrease in plasma levels of progesterone.

Instructions for Items 7-61 to 7-65: Match the hormone with its rate of synthesis in the normal pregnant woman.

a. Estradiol-17β
b. Estriol
c. Progesterone
d. Deoxycorticosterone
e. Human placental lactogen

7-61. 3 to 12 mg/day
7-62. 15 to 20 mg/day
7-63. 50 to 100 mg/day
7-64. 250 to 600 mg/day
7-65. 1 g/day

7-66. The vast majority of which of the following placental steroids enters the maternal circulation?

a. Estradiol-17β
b. Estriol
c. Estrone
d. Progesterone

8. THE MORPHOLOGIC AND FUNCTIONAL DEVELOPMENT OF THE FETUS

8–1. Gestational age is calculated from the

a. Time of ovulation
b. Time of fertilization
c. First day of the last menstrual period
d. Last day of the last menstrual period

8–2. Which of the following terms are synonymous?

a. Gestational age
b. Ovulation age
c. Fertilization age
d. Menstrual age

8–3. In a woman with a 28-day menstrual cycle, implantation usually occurs ________ weeks after the 1st day of the last menstrual period (LMP)?

a. 1
b. 2
c. 3
d. 4

8–4. Place the following developmental events in correct chronologic sequence.

a. Ovulation
b. Implantation
c. Blastocyst formation
d. Fertilization
e. Primitive villi formation

8–5. After which of the following events is the fertilized ovum referred to as an embryo?

a. Entrance into the uterus
b. Formation of a blastocyst
c. Implantation
d. Development of chorionic villi

8–6. Which of the following statements about the beginning of the 5th week after the onset of the LMP is correct?

a. Most pregnant women will have a positive pregnancy test at this time.
b. The embryonic disc is well defined.
c. The body stalk has differentiated.
d. Chorionic villi have formed.
e. The intervillous space contains maternal blood.

8–7. Most body structures have been formed by the end of the embryonic period.

a. True
b. False

Instructions for Items 8–8 to 8–12: Match the time after ovulation with the developmental events that have occurred.

a. Week 4
b. Week 6
c. Week 8
d. Week 10
e. Week 14
f. Week 18

8–8. Fingers and toes present
8–9. Heart and pericardium very prominent
8–10. Fetal sex can be determined by examination of external genital organs
8–11. Centers of ossification have appeared in most bones
8–12. Some scalp hair visible

8–13. The average crown-rump length of the fetus at term is approximately ________ (1) cm and the average fetal term weight is approximately ________ (2) g.

8–14. Which of the following statements about fetal measurement is correct?

a. Sitting height is synonymous with crown-rump length.
b. Standing height is a more accurate measurement than sitting height.
c. Length is a more accurate criterion of fetal age than weight.
d. Length and weight increase linearly throughout gestation.

8–15. Which of the following statements about fetal weight is correct?

a. Male birth weights tend to be higher than female birth weights.
b. Socioeconomic factors affect fetal growth rate.
c. Size of parents is unrelated to birth weight.
d. Parity of the mother affects birth weight.

8–16. Which of the following statements about the fetal head is correct?

a. A large proportion of the head at term is represented by the face.
b. The irregular spaces where sutures meet are protected by a cartilage roof.
c. The bones of the fetal skull are rigidly united.
d. All bones of the skull are paired.
e. As a rule, the infants of multiparas have larger heads than those of nulliparas.

8–17. Which of the following sutures is midline?

a. Lambdoidal
b. Sagittal
c. Frontal
d. Coronal
e. Temporal

8–18. With a vertex presentation, all sutures are palpable during labor except the

a. Frontal
b. Sagittal
c. Coronal
d. Lambdoid
e. Temporal

Instructions for Items 8–19 to 8–22: Match the fontanel with the appropriate description.

a. Anterior (greater)
b. Posterior (lesser)
c. Temporal (Casserian)

8–19. Situated at the intersection of the sagittal and lambdoid sutures
8–20. Situated at the junction of the lambdoid and temporal sutures
8–21. Situated at the junction of the sagittal and coronal sutures
8–22. May be readily felt during labor

Instructions for Items 8–23 to 8–25: Match the diameter of the infant's head with the appropriate description.

a. Occipitofrontal
b. Biparietal
c. Bitemporal
d. Occipitomental
e. Suboccipitobregmatic

8–23. The greatest transverse diameter of the head
8–24. Measured from the chin to the most prominent portion of the occiput
8–25. Measured from the root of the nose to the most prominent portion of the occipital bone

8–26. The greatest circumference of the head corresponds to the plane of the $\underset{1}{\underline{\qquad}}$ diameter and the smallest circumference corresponds to the plane of the $\underset{2}{\underline{\qquad}}$ diameter.

8–27. All fetal heads at the same gestational age are equally able to adapt to the maternal pelvis by molding.

a. True
b. False

8–28. Fetal age can be accurately determined from the external appearance of the brain.

a. True
b. False

8–29. Which of the following statements about placental transfer is correct?

a. The placenta supplies materials for fetal growth and removes the products of fetal catabolism.
b. There is continuous direct communication between fetal blood in chorionic villi vessels and maternal blood in the intervillous space.
c. The escape of fetal erythrocytes into the maternal circulation is the mechanism by which Rh sensitization occurs.
d. A large number of maternal erythrocytes can be found in the fetal circulation.

8–30. Which of the following variables influences the effectiveness of the human placenta as an organ of transfer?

a. The plasma concentration of a substance
b. The rate of maternal blood flow in the intervillous space
c. The area available for exchange across the villous epithelium
d. The characteristics of the tissue barrier between the intervillous space and the fetal capillaries
e. The placental capacity for active transfer
f. The amount of placental metabolism of the transferred substance
g. The area available for exchange across the fetal capillaries in the placenta
h. The concentration of the substance in fetal blood
i. The rate of fetal blood flow through villous capillaries

8–31. Which of the following statements about blood flow in the intervillous space is correct?

a. The intervillous space combines functions of the lung, gastrointestinal tract, and kidney.
b. Most of the 1600 cc/min of uteroplacental blood flow goes through the intervillous space.
c. Blood flow through the intervillous space is decreased during contractions in proportion to the contraction intensity.
d. Blood pressure within the intervillous space is less than uterine arterial pressure but greater than uterine venous pressure.
e. Maternal posture affects pressure in the intervillous space.
f. During normal labor, the rise in fetal blood pressure parallels the pressure in the intervillous space.

8–32. Substances passing from maternal blood in the intervillous space to fetal blood must cross the

a. Maternal capillary wall
b. Trophoblast
c. Stroma
d. Fetal capillary wall

8–33. Which of the following changes affecting placental permeability occurs as pregnancy progresses?

a. The syncytiotrophoblast disappears
b. The number of cytotrophoblast cells decreases
c. The walls of villous capillaries become thinner
d. The relative number of fetal vessels increases in relation to the villous connective tissue

8–34. Which of the following statements about diffusion through the placenta is correct?

a. Substances with molecular weights under 1500 daltons readily diffuse through placental tissue.
b. Diffusion is the only mechanism of transport for low molecular weight substances.
c. Oxygen and water are transferred by diffusion.
d. Anesthetic gases apparently cross the placenta by simple diffusion.

8–35. No substance of very high molecular weight (>150,000 daltons) can traverse the placenta.

a. True
b. False

8–36. Which of the following statements about oxygen transfer to the fetus is correct?

a. The oxygen saturation of maternal blood in the intervillous space resembles that in maternal capillaries.
b. The oxygen saturation of maternal blood in the intervillous space is less than that of maternal arterial blood.
c. The average oxygen saturation of intervillous space blood is approximately 90 percent.
d. The partial pressure of intervillous space blood is 65 to 75 mm Hg.

8–37. Mechanisms which compensate for the relatively low Po_2 of umbilical vein blood include

a. Increased fetal cardiac output
b. Higher fetal hemoglobin concentration
c. Increased oxygen-carrying capacity of fetal hemoglobin
d. A larger fetal heart in proportion to the body than in the adult

8–38. Which of the following statements about the transfer of carbon dioxide is correct?

a. Carbon dioxide traverses the chorionic villus more rapidly than does oxygen.
b. Fetal blood has more affinity for carbon dioxide than does maternal blood.
c. Maternal hyperventilation favors carbon dioxide transfer from the fetus to the mother.
d. Carbon dioxide traverses the placenta by selective transport.

8–39. Which of the following support the concept of selective transfer by the placenta?

a. Different rates of transfer for the two histidine isomers
b. Different ascorbic acid concentrations in mother and fetus
c. Unidirectional iron transfer
d. Metastatic malignant melanomas of maternal origin in the fetus
e. Intrauterine infections

8–40. Which of the following statements about fetal circulation is correct?

a. The umbilical vein ascends along the anterior abdominal wall.
b. The ductus venosus is a branch of the portal sinus.
c. The oxygen content of blood in the inferior vena cava is greater than that in the superior vena cava.
d. Most of the blood from the superior vena cava passes through the foramen ovale.
e. Blood ejected from the left ventricle perfuses the brain and heart.

8–41. Blood ejected from the right ventricle into the pulmonary trunk is shunted to the descending aorta through the ______________.

8–42. Place the following fetal vessels in order from lowest to highest oxygen concentration.

a. Blood in inferior vena cava
b. Blood in umbilical vein
c. Blood in superior vena cava
d. Blood in umbilical artery

8–43. Which of the following characterizes fetal circulation?

a. Pulmonary vascular resistance high
b. Pulmonary blood flow high
c. Ductus arteriosus resistance high
d. Umbilicoplacental resistance low

8–44. Which of the following factors plays a role in regulating blood flow through the ductus arteriosus?

a. Difference in pressure between the pulmonary vein and aorta
b. Difference in pressure between the pulmonary artery and aorta
c. Oxygen tension of blood passing through the ductus arteriosus
d. pH of blood passing through the ductus arteriosus
e. Effect of prostaglandins on the ductus arteriosus

8–45. Inhibitors of prostaglandin synthetase may be used postnatally to induce closure of a patent ductus arteriosus.

a. True
b. False

8–46. Which of the following takes place as a result of lung expansion at birth?

a. Pressure in the right ventricle decreases.
b. Pressure in the pulmonary artery decreases.
c. Foramen ovale immediately closes.
d. There is a temporary reflux blood flow from the right ventricle to the right atrium.

Instructions for Items 8–47 to 8–49: Match the fetal vessel with its remnant in the adult.

a. Umbilical vein
b. Ductus venosus
c. Umbilical artery
d. Ductus arteriosus

8–47. Umbilical ligament
8–48. Ligamentum teres
8–49. Ligamentum venosum

8–50. Which of the following statements about fetal blood is correct?

a. Sites of hematopoiesis include the yolk sac, liver, and bone marrow.
b. All fetal erythrocytes are nucleated.
c. The hematocrit at term is slightly less than that of the adult male.
d. The reticulocyte count decreases as pregnancy progresses.
e. The life span of fetal erythrocytes is shorter than erythrocytes in the adult.

Instructions for Items 8–51 to 8–55: Match the type of hemoglobin with its composition.

a. Hemoglobin A_2
b. Hemoglobin A
c. Gower-2
d. Hemoglobin F
e. Gower-1

8–51. $\epsilon,\epsilon,\epsilon,\epsilon$
8–52. $\alpha,\alpha,\epsilon,\epsilon$
8–53. $\alpha,\alpha,\gamma,\gamma$
8–54. $\alpha,\alpha,\beta,\beta$
8–55. $\alpha,\alpha,\delta,\delta$

8–56. Hemoglobin A, the main adult hemoglobin, is present in the fetus after what week of pregnancy?

a. 5
b. 11
c. 16
d. 21

8–57. Fetal hypoxia can be intensified as a result of maternal hyperthermia because ________.

8–58. Which of the following statements about the fetal hematopoietic process is correct?

a. At term, the fetal hemoglobin concentration is higher than the maternal concentration.
b. The higher viscosity of fetal erythrocytes is offset by their increased deformability.
c. The fetoplacental blood volume at term is approximately 125 cc/kg.
d. The increased oxygen affinity of the fetal erythrocyte compared to the maternal erythrocyte is a result of decreased 2,3-diphosphogylcerate binding.
e. The concentration of hemoglobin F falls steadily during pregnancy to about 10 percent of the total at term.
f. The fetus is able to respond to anemia with increased production of erythropoietin.

8–59. Which fetal organ appears to be an important source of erythropoietin?

a. Liver
b. Kidney
c. Adrenal gland
d. Pituitary gland

Instructions for Items 8–60 to 8–64: Match the level of blood coagulation factors at the time of birth compared with a few weeks after birth.

a. Increased
b. Decreased
c. Unchanged

8–60. Factor II
8–61. Factor VII
8–62. Factor IX
8–63. Factor XIII
8–64. Fibrinogen

8–65. Platelet counts in cord blood are in the normal range for a nonpregnant adult.

a. True
b. False

8–66. Thrombin time (time for conversion of plasma fibrinogen to fibrin clot when thrombin is added) in the neonate is ________ as compared to older children and adults.

a. Prolonged
b. The same
c. Shortened

8–67. The measurement of Factor ________ coagulation activity in cord blood is of value for making a diagnosis of hemophilia.

8–68. Which immunoglobulins are found in lower concentrations in cord sera than in maternal sera?

a. IgA
b. IgG
c. IgM

8–69. IgM levels are increased in the fetus when ______.

8–70. Fetal urine is ______ relative to fetal plasma.

a. Hypertonic
b. Isotonic
c. Hypotonic

8–71. Which of the following statements about the fetal urinary system is correct?

a. Failure of the pronephros or mesonephros to develop properly may result in anomolous development of the urinary system.
b. The kidneys are functionally mature by 28 weeks of gestation.
c. The fetus at term produces about 650 ml of urine per day.
d. A diuretic administered to the mother has no effect on fetal urine formation.
e. Fetal glomerular filtration rates are reduced in growth-retarded infants.
f. Fetal glomerular filtration rates are reduced in cases of polyhydramnios.

8–72. Normal fetal kidney function is essential for survival in utero.

a. true
b. False

8–73. Which of the following statements about the development of the fetal respiratory system is correct?

a. The forces that promote deflation or collapse of the air-containing lung result from surface tension at the alveolar air-tissue interface.
b. The surface active components of the alveoli are attributable primarily to the properties of surfactant.
c. The principal surface active component of surfactant is the lecithin, dipalmityl phosphatidylcholine.
d. Respiratory distress syndrome is caused by a deficiency in surfactant production.
e. Surfactant is formed primarily in type II pneumocytes.

8–74. Phosphatidylcholines (lecithin) comprise what percent of surfactant glycerophospholipids?

a. 20
b. 40
c. 60
d. 80

8–75. Infants born before the appearance of ______ in surfactant are at increased risk for the development of respiratory distress syndrome, even when their lecithin levels are normal for mature lungs.

8–76. An increasing ratio of ______ (1) relative to that of ______ (2) is an index of fetal lung maturation.

8–77. Phosphatidic acid forms the backbone for which of the following?

a. Phosphatidylglycerol
b. Phosphatidylcholine
c. Phosphatidylinositol
d. Dipalmityl phosphatidylcholine

8–78. There is considerable evidence that the enzyme ______ occupies a central regulatory role in the biosynthesis of the glycerophospholipids of surfactant.

8–79. As the fetal lung matures, the concentration of phosphatidylinositol in surfactant ______ (1) and the concentration of phosphatidylglycerol ______ (2).

a. Decreases
b. Remains the same
c. Increases

8–80. Infants of diabetic mothers can be at greater risk for development of respiratory distress syndrome because their surfactant is rich in ______ (1) and deficient in ______ (2).

8–81. Which of the following statements about the control of surfactant production is correct?

a. Glucocorticosteroids, administered in large doses to women at any stage of pregnancy, will cause an increased production of surfactant.
b. Glucocorticosteroids, administered in large doses to mothers during the 29th to 33rd week of gestation result in a reduced incidence of respiratory distress syndrome.
c. Respiratory distress syndrome is always present in infants whose capacity to secrete cortisol is limited.
d. Increased surfactant synthesis in the third trimester may be causally linked to prolactin production.
e. Infants of mothers treated with bromocriptine while pregnant will suffer iatrogenic respiratory distress syndrome.
f. Infants whose mothers are heroin addicts demonstrate an increased incidence of respiratory distress syndrome.

8–82. Fetal chest wall movements have been detected at ________ weeks of gestation?

a. 8
b. 11
c. 14
d. 17
e. 20

8–83. Which of the following statements about fetal respiration is correct?

a. Fetal respiratory movements sufficiently intense to cause movement of amnionic fluid into and out of the lungs occur by the 4th month in utero.
b. The normal human fetus demonstrates irregular breathing movements in utero, typically with a frequency from 30 to 70 per minute.
c. Asphyxia in utero results in the initiation of gasping fetal respiratory efforts.
d. Crying in utero is a common phenomenon.
e. Fetal hiccuping in utero has been identified.

8–84. Which of the following statements about the fetal digestive system is correct?

a. By the 11th week of gestation, the small intestine undergoes peristalsis.
b. Fetal swallowing is developed in the 4th month.
c. Late in pregnancy, the volume of amnionic fluid is affected by fetal swallowing.
d. The amnionic fluid swallowed supplies most of the caloric requirements of the fetus.

8–85. Which of the following statements about meconium is correct?

a. Meconium consists of undigested debris from amnionic fluid and the products of secretion, excretion, and desquamation from the gastrointestinal tract.
b. The color of meconium is partially due to biliverdin.
c. Fetal hypoxia is associated with the release of meconium into the amnionic fluid.

8–86. Which of the following statements about bilirubin is correct?

a. The more immature the fetus, the more deficient the system to conjugate bilirubin.
b. Relatively more bilirubin is produced in the fetus than in the mother.
c. The fetal liver has a considerable ability to conjugate bilirubin.
d. Transfer of unconjugated bilirubin across the placenta is unidirectional from the fetus to the mother.
e. Conjugated bilirubin is not exchanged to any significant degree between the fetus and the mother.

8–87. Which of the following statements about fetal insulin is correct?

a. Plasma insulin is detectable by 8 weeks of gestation.
b. Insulin containing granules can be identified in the fetal pancreas by 9 weeks of gestation.
c. The fetal pancreas responds to hyperglycemia by increasing plasma insulin levels.
d. Serum insulin levels are high in infants of diabetic mothers.
e. Fetal insulin helps meet the requirements of a diabetic mother.

8–88. The lack of fetal pancreatic α-cell response to hypoglycemia is a consequence of inadequate hormone production.

a. True
b. False

8–89. Which of the following have been identified in the fetal pituitary gland by 10 weeks of gestation?

a. Growth hormone
b. ACTH
c. Prolactin
d. LH
e. FSH

8–90. Fetal growth hormone has been shown to be required for normal fetal growth and development.

a. True
b. False

8–91. Which of the following statements about fetal thyroid function is correct?

a. Until midpregnancy, secretion of thyroid-stimulating hormone and thyroid hormones is low.
b. Maternal thyrotropin readily crosses the placenta.
c. Long-acting thyroid stimulators (LATS) cross from mother to fetus when the maternal concentration is high.
d. The fetal thyroid concentrates iodine more avidly than the maternal thyroid.
e. Maternal thyroid secretion can compensate for inadequate fetal synthesis.
f. Thyrotropin secretion increases markedly after birth.

8–92. Fetal parathyroid glands elaborate parathormone by what time in gestation?

a. End of the first trimester
b. End of the second trimester
c. Middle of the third trimester
d. End of the third trimester

8–93. The lack of urine-concentrating ability in the newborn is felt to be due to the lack of fetal production of ________.

8–94. The fetal testis is capable of synthesizing testosterone by ____________ weeks of gestation?

a. 5
b. 10
c. 20
d. 28
e. 36

Instructions for Items 8–95 to 8–99: Match the events with the time in gestation when they occur.

a. 2 months
b. 3 months
c. 4 months
d. 5 months
e. 6 months
f. 7 months

8–95. Complete finger closure is achieved
8–96. Ability to suck is present
8–97. Eye sensitive to light
8–98. Mouth opens in response to stimuli
8–99. Fetus responsive to variations in taste

8–100. Which of the following statements about the fetal immune system is correct?

a. The fetus is immunologically incompetent until after birth.
b. Synthesis of components of complement has been demonstrated in the first trimester.
c. In the absence of antigenic stimulus to the fetus, fetal immunoglobulins consist of IgG synthesized by the mother.
d. In response to antigenic stimulus, IgM is the dominant immunoglobulin produced by the fetus.
e. Hemolytic disease of the newborn results from transfer of maternal IgA to the fetus.

8–101. Which of the following statements about fetal nutrition and metabolism is correct?

a. Due to the relatively large amount of yolk in the human ovum, the fetus is independent of the mother for nutrition until the 2nd month of gestation.
b. Stored maternal glycogen is the main source of glucose for maternal and fetal needs during pregnancy.
c. Glucose transfer across the placenta appears to be carrier mediated.
d. The uptake of amino acids by the placenta is solely a result of diffusion.
e. Placental lactogen acts to block the maternal peripheral uptake and utilization of free fatty acids.
f. Glycerol and neutral fats cross the placenta by active transport.

8–102. The plasma levels of glucose in pregnant women are relatively constant.

a. True
b. False

8–103. Which of the following conditions is significantly associated with small for gestational age or growth-retarded infants?

a. Maternal diabetes
b. Severe maternal vascular disease
c. Inadequate maternal nutrition
d. Decreased uteroplacental blood flow
e. Rh isoimmunization
f. Impaired placental transport mechanisms

8–104. Which of the following is a function of amnionic fluid?

a. Medium for fetal movement
b. Cushions fetus against injury
c. Assists in maintaining constant temperature
d. Dilates cervical canal during labor

8–105. Prolonged pregnancies result in hydramnios.

a. True
b. False

8–106. Which of the following changes occur in amnionic fluid as pregnancy progresses?

a. Phospholipids accumulate
b. Osmolarity increases
c. Particulate matter increases
d. Urea, creatinine, and uric acid concentrations increase

8–107. The fetal organ systems that affect amnionic fluid composition and volume are the ____________.

Instructions for Items 8–108 to 8–110: Match the amount of amnionic fluid with the condition with which it is associated.

a. Oligohydramnios
b. Hydramnios

8–108. Fetal esophageal atresia
8–109. Fetal renal agenesis
8–110. Early and prolonged rupture of the membranes

8–111. Fetal pulmonary hypoplasia may result from

a. Oligohydramnios
b. Hydramnios

8–112. Both the primary and secondary sex ratios in humans are unity.

a. True
b. False

8–113. A fetus with an XY chromosome complement and with no testis will develop as a

a. Male
b. Female

8–114. Which of the following statements about fetal sex differentiation is correct?

a. Genetic sex is determined at the time of fertilization.
b. The Y chromosome directs testicular differentiation.
c. Müllerian duct regression factor is synthesized by the fetal testis.
d. Müllerian duct regression factor acts locally.
e. Virilization of the external genitalia is brought about by 5α-dihydrotestosterone.

8–115. Ambiguous genitalia are caused by an abnormal in utero concentration of ________.

Instructions for items 8–116 to 8–122: Match the category of abnormal sexual differentiation with the appropriate description.

a. Female pseudohermaphroditism (Category 1)
b. Male pseudohermaphroditism (Category 2)
c. Dysgenetic gonads and true hermaphroditism (Category 3)

8–116. Müllerian duct regression factor is not produced
8–117. Müllerian duct regression factor is produced
8–118. Karyotype is 46,XX
8–119. Uterus, fallopian tubes, and upper vagina present
8–120. Testis may be present
8–121. Ovaries are present
8–122. No gonads are present

8–123. In female pseudohermaphroditism androgenic excess most commonly occurs due to oversecretion by what gland?

8–124. The female fetus is usually protected from virilization by maternal androgen excess because of the ________.

8–125. With appropriate therapy, all patients with female pseudohermaphroditism can be normal, fertile women.

a. True
b. False

8–126. Diminished masculinization may be caused by

a. Inadequate production of testosterone
b. Diminished responsiveness to normal quantities of androgen
c. Increased production of estrogen
d. Increased responsiveness to normal levels of estrogen

8–127. Which of the following are characteristic of testicular feminization?

a. Female phenotype
b. No Wolffian duct structures
c. Rise of testosterone levels at the time of puberty
d. Virilization occurs after puberty
e. Increased estrogen secretion by the testis

8–128. Reifenstein's syndrome is ________.

8–129. Turner syndrome is an example of what category of sexual differentiation abnormalities?

a. Female pseudohermaphroditism
b. Male pseudohermaphroditism
c. Dysgenetic gonads and true hermaphroditism

8–130. At birth, if a uterus is present in an infant with genital ambiguity, a possible diagnosis is

a. True hermaphroditism
b. Female pseudohermaphroditism
c. Male pseudohermaphroditism
d. Gonadal dysgenesis

8–131. If the urethra opens onto the perineum, the infant should be designated

a. Male
b. Female

9. MATERNAL ADAPTATION TO PREGNANCY

9–1. Myometrial enlargement during pregnancy is primarily the result of smooth muscle

a. Hyperplasia
b. Hypertrophy

9–2. Which of the following statements about the uterus in pregnancy is correct?

a. There is an accumulation of fibrous tissue, particularly in the external muscle layer.
b. The amount of elastic tissue is increased.
c. There is a relative decrease in the size and number of lymphatics in the uterus.
d. Hypertrophy of the nerve supply of the uterus occurs.
e. There is an increase in the size and number of blood vessels in the uterus.

9–3. Hypertrophy of the uterus in the first 2 months of pregnancy results mainly from mechanical pressure caused by the products of conception.

a. True
b. False

9–4. Polyamine levels in the urine of normal pregnant women are maximal at ________ weeks of gestation.

a. 6 to 8
b. 13 to 14
c. 18 to 20
d. 28 to 30

9–5. Uterine enlargement in pregnancy is most marked in the

a. Cervix
b. Lower uterine segment
c. Fundus
d. Uterine cornua

9–6. The portion of the uterus surrounding the placental site enlarges more rapidly than does the myometrium distal to the site of implantation.

a. True
b. False

9–7. In what ways does the uterus and its anatomic relationships change as pregnancy progresses?

a. With the pregnant woman standing, the abdominal wall supports the uterus.
b. With the pregnant woman supine, the uterus rests on the vertebral column and adjacent great vessels.
c. The uterus usually undergoes levorotation due to pressure from the inferior vena cava.
d. As the uterus enlarges, it displaces the intestines laterally and superiorly.

9–8. Which of the following statements about uterine contractions is correct?

a. Uterine contractions begin in the first trimester.
b. Uterine contractions may first be felt by an examiner during the third trimester.
c. Braxton Hicks contractions increase in frequency during the last 2 weeks of pregnancy.
d. Late in pregnancy, Braxton Hicks contractions can cause discomfort.
e. Late in pregnancy, Braxton Hicks contractions may assume some rhythmicity.

9–9. Uteroplacental blood flow near term is approximately ________ cc/min.

a. 100
b. 300
c. 500
d. 700
e. 900

9–10. Uterine contractions cause a decrease in uterine blood flow roughly proportional to the intensity of the contraction.

a. True
b. False

9–11. Which of the following statements about uteroplacental blood flow in animal models is correct?

a. The majority of uterine blood flow is directed to the endometrium and placenta.
b. There is vasodilation in addition to an increased number of vessels.
c. Estrogen stimulation can increase placental blood flow.
d. Epinephrine and norepinephrine can induce an increase in placental perfusion.
e. Similar to humans, pregnant sheep are relatively refractory to the pressor effects of angiotensin II.

9–12. Increased vascularity and edema of the cervix bring about what two early signs of pregnancy?

9–13. Which of the following statements about the cervical mucosa in pregnancy is correct?

a. Cervical glands undergo both hypertrophy and hyperplasia.
b. Proliferation of glands and endocervical epithelium commonly extends to the portio vaginalis.
c. Eversions of the cervix are usually an inflammatory response.
d. Ferning of cervical mucus usually heralds a poor pregnancy outcome.
e. The mucus plug which obstructs the cervical canal usually first appears during the second trimester.

9–14. Which of the following statements about ovarian function during pregnancy is correct?

a. Maturation of new follicles continues during pregnancy.
b. The corpus luteum of pregnancy functions maximally for about 7 weeks after the last menstrual period.
c. Usually only a single corpus luteum of pregnancy is found in the ovaries of pregnant women.
d. Ovulation continues throughout pregnancy.

9–15. Relaxin

a. Is a protein hormone secreted by the corpus luteum during pregnancy
b. Is synthesized in the largest amounts by the decidua
c. Is secreted throughout pregnancy
d. Is essential for the maintenance of human pregnancy

9–16. The luteoma of pregnancy

a. Is a true neoplasm
b. Generally regresses after delivery
c. May give rise to maternal virilization
d. May give rise to fetal virilization

9–17. A decidual reaction on or within the ovary or uterine serosa is common in pregnancy.

a. True
b. False

9–18. Which of the following changes occurs in the oviduct during pregnancy?

a. The musculature undergoes marked hypertrophy.
b. The epithelium proliferates significantly.
c. Decidual cells may develop in the stroma of the endosalpinx.
d. A continuous decidual membrane is formed.

9–19. Which of the following changes in the vagina occurs during pregnancy?

a. There is an increased vascularity.
b. The vaginal mucosa thins.
c. There is smooth muscle hypertrophy.
d. The length of the vaginal wall increases.

9–20. The characteristic violet color of the vagina during pregnancy is referred to as ______________.

9–21. Which of the following statements about vaginal secretions in pregnancy is correct?

a. The pH ranges from 3.5 to 6.0.
b. The pH predisposes to bacterial infection of the vagina.
c. Lactic acid is produced from glycogen by the action of *Lactobacillus acidophilus.*
d. There is an increase in both cervical and vaginal secretions.

9–22. Striae gravidarum

a. Occur in all pregnant women
b. Appear as reddish slightly depressed streaks
c. From previous pregnancies appear as glistening, silvery lines
d. Rarely occur in nulliparous women

9–23. The separation of the rectus muscles in the midline during pregnancy is termed ______________.

Instructions for Items 9–24 to 9–26: Match the skin change in pregnancy with the appropriate description.

a. Linea nigra
b. Chloasma

9–24. Abdominal skin markedly pigmented at the midline
9–25. Irregular brownish patches of varying size on face and neck
9–26. May be stimulated by the use of oral contraceptives

Instructions for Items 9–27 to 9–30: Match the cutaneous vascular change in pregnancy with the appropriate description.

a. Vascular spiders
b. Palmar erythema

9–27. More frequent in white women than in black women
9–28. Probably due to the hyperestrogenemia of pregnancy
9–29. Usually disappears shortly after the termination of pregnancy
9–30. Also designated as nevus or telangiectasis

9–31. Which of the following is a common sign or symptom related to the breasts that occurs at some time during pregnancy?

a. Tenderness
b. Tingling
c. Nipples larger, darker, more erectile
d. Colostrum expressed
e. Striations

9–32. The hypertrophic sebaceous glands scattered through the areolae of the breasts during pregnancy are termed the ______________.

9–33. The average weight gain in pregnancy is probably about ____________ pounds.

9–34. Which of the following statements about water metabolism in pregnancy is correct?

a. Increased retention of water is normal in pregnancy.
b. Demonstrable pitting edema of the ankles at the end of the day is abnormal and pathologic.
c. It is not unusual for a woman to retain 6.5 liters of extra fluid in a normal pregnancy.
d. Weight loss during the first 10 days after delivery in normal primiparas averages 5 pounds.

9–35. The fetus and placenta account for about 90 percent of the total protein increase normally induced by pregnancy.

a. True
b. False

9–36. Both fasting plasma glucose and plasma free fatty acids are decreased in pregnancy.

a. True
b. False

9–37. Which of the following statements about carbohydrate metabolism in pregnancy is correct?

a. Pregnancy is potentially diabetogenic.
b. Human placental lactogen promotes lipolysis and opposes the action of insulin.
c. Progesterone and estrogen produce an increased plasma insulin response to glucose.
d. Accelerated degradation of insulin by placental insulinase contributes appreciably to the diabetogenic state.
e. Both pancreatic β-cell and α-cell sensitivity to a glucose challenge is significantly increased during pregnancy.

9–38. The hypoglycemic effect of tolbutamide in normal pregnant women is ____________ its effect in nonpregnant women.

a. Greater than
b. Equal to
c. Less than

9–39. Which plasma lipids increase appreciably during pregnancy relative to the nonpregnant state?

a. Free fatty acids
b. Serum phospholipids
c. Esterified cholesterol
d. Total cholesterol

9–40. Which of the following statements about fat metabolism in pregnancy is correct?

a. Starvation causes more intense ketonemia in pregnant women than in nonpregnant women.
b. Storage of fat occurs primarily near term.
c. Fat is deposited more peripherally than centrally.
d. Progesterone may act to reset a hypothalamic "lipostat."
e. Breast feeding significantly alters the rate at which plasma lipids decrease postpartum.

9–41. Which of the following factors affects the acid-base equilibrium of the pregnant woman?

a. There is normally a maternal respiratory alkalosis due to hyperventilation.
b. There is a moderate reduction in plasma bicarbonate.
c. The affinity of maternal hemoglobin for oxygen is increased (Bohr effect).
d. An increase in 2, 3-diphosphoglycerate in maternal erythrocytes facilitates oxygen release to the fetus.

Instructions for Items 9–42 to 9–46: Indicate how serum levels of the following are altered during pregnancy as compared with the nonpregnant state.

a. Increased
b. Decreased
c. Unchanged

9–42. Copper
9–43. Sodium
9–44. Magnesium
9–45. Phosphorus
9–46. Potassium

9–47. Which of the following statements about maternal blood volume in pregnancy is correct?

a. A fetus is essential for the development of hypervolemia.
b. Blood volume increases an average of 50 percent above nonpregnant levels.
c. Maternal blood volume increases linearly throughout pregnancy.
d. The increase in blood volume results from an increase in both plasma and erythrocytes.

9–48. The increase in the volume of circulating erythrocytes in pregnancy occurs ____________ the increase in plasma volume.

a. Before
b. At the same time as
c. After

9–49. The increase in the volume of circulating erythrocytes is approximately ____________ percent.

9–50. Which of the following statements about erythrocytes in pregnancy is correct?

a. The increase in the volume of circulating erythrocytes is due to prolongation of erythrocyte life span.
b. The cell volume is increased.
c. Erythroid hyperplasia is present in the bone marrow.
d. The reticulocyte count is elevated in pregnancy.
e. Erythropoietin levels are decreased in pregnancy.

9–51. A hemoglobin concentration of 10.5 g/dl late in pregnancy should be considered

a. Normal
b. Abnormal and due to iron deficiency
c. Abnormal and due to physiologic hypervolemia

9–52. The total iron requirement during a normal singleton pregnancy is approximately

a. 0.1 g
b. 1 g
c. 10 g
d. 100 g

9–53. Approximately half the iron required in a normal pregnancy is used in the production of maternal erythrocytes.

a. True
b. False

9–54. Which of the following statements about iron requirements in pregnancy is correct?

a. In a normal pregnancy, exogenous iron is not usually required.
b. Iron absorption from the intestine is increased in pregnancy.
c. Hemoglobin production in the fetus is impaired if the mother is iron deficient.
d. In the absence of added exogenous iron, the maternal hemoglobin concentration falls during the second half of pregnancy.

9–55. The average blood loss during and after vaginal delivery of a single fetus is approximately

a. 200 ml
b. 400 ml
c. 600 ml
d. 800 ml
e. 1000 ml

9–56. The average blood loss associated with cesarean section is __________ the blood loss associated with vaginal delivery of twins.

a. Less than
b. The same as
c. Greater than

9–57. Which of the following statements about changes in maternal blood volume near the time of delivery is correct?

a. Some hemoconcentration occurs during labor.
b. Blood volume is reduced during and soon after labor.
c. Excess circulating hemoglobin yields iron for storage through accelerated erythrocyte destruction.
d. Blood volume returns to the nonpregnant level by 5 days postpartum.

9–58. During labor and the early puerperium, the blood leukocyte count is ______________ the leukocyte count during pregnancy.

a. Less than
b. The same as
c. Greater than

9–59. Starting early in pregnancy, alkaline phosphatase activity in leukocytes is increased.

a. True
b. False

Instructions for Items 9–60 to 9–67: Match the blood coagulation factor with its activity in pregnancy relative to the nonpregnant state.

a. Increased
b. Decreased
c. Unchanged

9–60. Factor I (plasma fibrinogen)
9–61. Factor II (prothrombin)
9–62. Factor VII (proconvertin)
9–63. Factor VIII (antihemophiliac globulin)
9–64. Factor IX (Christmas factor)
9–65. Factor X (Stuart factor)
9–66. Factor XI (plasma thromboplastin antecedent)
9–67. Factor XIII (fibrin-stabilizing factor)

Instructions for Items 9–68 to 9–71: Match the procedure with its rate in pregnancy as compared to the nonpregnant state.

a. Increased
b. Decreased
c. Unchanged

9–68. Sedimentation rate
9–69. Quick one-stage prothrombin time
9–70. Partial thromboplastin time
9–71. Clotting time of whole blood in a plain glass tube

9–72. Which of the following statements about coagulation in pregnancy is correct?

a. There is a decrease in platelets per unit volume.
b. High molecular weight soluble fibrin-fibrinogen complexes circulate in normal pregnancy.
c. Antithrombin III levels are higher in pregnancy.
d. There is a decreased capacity for neutralizing heparin.
e. All of the pregnancy-induced changes in levels of coagulation factors can be duplicated in nonpregnant women by administration of estrogen-progestin oral contraceptives.

9–73. Which of the following statements about fibrinolytic activity in pregnancy is correct?

a. During normal pregnancy, the level of maternal plasminogen (profibrinolysin) in plasma is increased.
b. An increase in profibrinolysin can be induced by estrogen treatment.
c. The measured time for clotted plasma to dissolve is decreased compared to the normal nonpregnant state.
d. Plasma fibrinolytic activity increases after delivery.
e. Fibrin degradation products usually rise after delivery.

9–74. During pregnancy, the heart is

a. Displaced to the right
b. Displaced upward
c. Slightly rotated in its long axis
d. Displaced due to the progressive elevation of the diaphragm

9–75. During pregnancy, it is easier to identify moderate degrees of cardiomegaly by physical examination or by simple roentgenographic studies than it is to identify this condition in the nonpregnant state.

a. True
b. False

Instructions for Items 9–76 to 9–80: Match the effect of pregnancy on the following.

a. Increased
b. Decreased
c. Unchanged

9–76. Cardiac volume
9–77. Ventricular wall mass
9–78. Stroke volume
9–79. Inotropic state of the myocardium
9–80. Heart rate

9–81. Which of the following changes in cardiac sounds may be present in a normal pregnancy?

a. Split first heart sound
b. Split second heart sound
c. Loud third heart sound
d. Systolic murmur
e. Loud, persistent diastolic murmur
f. Continuous murmurs

9–82. Which of the following changes can normally be found in an electrocardiogram taken during pregnancy?

a. Prolonged P-R interval
b. Shortened QRS complex
c. Flattened T waves
d. Slight left axis deviation

9–83. Which of the following statements about cardiac output in pregnancy is correct?

a. Cardiac output increases in the first trimester and remains elevated throughout pregnancy.
b. In late pregnancy, cardiac output is greater if a woman is supine than if she is in the lateral recumbent position.
c. In response to physicial activity, cardiac output is greater late in pregnancy than in the nonpregnant woman.
d. Cardiac output progressively increases in the first and second stages of labor.

9–84. Blood pressure in the brachial artery is highest when the gravida is in the ____________ position.

a. Lateral recumbent
b. Supine
c. Sitting

9–85. During pregnancy, arterial blood pressure decreases to a nadir during the second trimester or early third trimester and rises thereafter.

a. True
b. False

9–86. Which of the following statements about venous pressure in pregnancy is correct?

a. The antecubital venous pressure increases progressively during pregnancy.
b. The femoral venous pressure measured in the supine position remains unchanged.
c. Except in the lateral recumbent position, blood flow in the legs is retarded.
d. The enlarged uterus may occlude the pelvic veins and inferior vena cava.

9-87. Retarded blood flow and increased venous pressure contribute to which of the following conditions?

a. Preeclampsia
b. Dependent edema
c. Varicose veins
d. Hemorrhoids
e. Striae

9-88. Potential effects of a pregnant woman lying in the supine position near term include

a. Decreased venous return
b. Decreased cardiac output
c. Aortic compression
d. Arterial hypotension

9-89. In the pregnant woman, brachial artery pressure provides a reliable estimate of uterine artery pressure.

a. True
b. False

9-90. Compared to a woman in the supine position, a woman in the lateral recumbent position has

a. A lower blood pressure in the brachial artery
b. A higher cardiac output
c. An increased blood flow in the veins of the legs
d. An increased venous pressure in the legs

9-91. In pregnancy, the blood flow to the skin is

a. Increased
b. Decreased

9-92. Which of the following anatomic changes occurs during pregnancy?

a. The transverse diameter of the thoracic cage increases.
b. The thoracic circumference increases.
c. The level of the diaphragm rises.
d. The diaphragm is "splinted."

Instructions for Items 9-93 to 9-99: How does pregnancy affect the following pulmonary functions?

a. Increased
b. Decreased
c. Unchanged

9-93. Maternal arteriovenous oxygen difference
9-94. Maximum breathing capacity
9-95. Functional residual capacity
9-96. Lung compliance
9-97. Airway conductance
9-98. Tidal volume
9-99. Total pulmonary resistance

9-100. The increased respiratory effort in pregnancy is mostly induced by ______________.

9-101. Which of the following statements about the urinary system in pregnancy is correct?

a. The kidney increases in size.
b. The increases in glomerular filtration rate and renal plasma flow persist to term.
c. Water and sodium excretion are affected by posture late in pregnancy.
d. Amino acids and water-soluble vitamins are excreted in the urine of pregnant women in much higher amounts than in the urine of nonpregnant women.

9-102. The most useful measure of renal function during pregnancy is

a. Plasma urea concentration
b. Plasma creatinine concentration
c. Creatinine clearance
d. Urine concentration tests
e. Dye excretion tests

9-103. During pregnancy, urine concentration tests may give misleading results because ______________.

9-104. Which of the following statements about glucosuria in pregnancy is correct?

a. It is caused by increased glomerular filtration.
b. It is caused by decreased renal tubular absorption.
c. The possibility of diabetes mellitus can be ignored in a patient with minimal glucosuria.

9-105. Proteinuria is a fairly common, normal occurrence during pregnancy.

a. True
b. False

9-106. Which of the following statements about the urinary collecting system is correct?

a. The ureters are compressed at the pelvic brim by the uterus after is has risen out of the pelvis.
b. Ureteral dilation is usually greater on the right.
c. Progesterone may play a role in the development of a hydroureter.
d. The ureters are elongated during pregnancy.
e. After delivery, the urinary tract does not usually return to prepregnancy dimensions.

9-107. Which of the following statements about the bladder in pregnancy is correct?

a. Most anatomic changes occur in the first half of pregnancy.
b. The trigone becomes deeper and wider.
c. Late in pregnancy, the bladder becomes edematous and probably more prone to infection.
d. Urethral pressure and length are increased in all pregnancies.

9–108. Which of the following changes occurs in the gastrointestinal tract during pregnancy?

a. Tone is decreased.
b. Motility is decreased.
c. Gastric-emptying time is increased.
d. Intraesophageal pressures are higher than in nonpregnant women.

9–109. During pregnancy, the appendix is progressively displaced ________.

9–110. In human pregnancy, the liver both increases in size and changes in histologic appearance.

a. True
b. False

Instructions for Items 9–111 to 9–114: How does pregnancy affect the following?

a. Increased
b. Decreased
c. Unchanged

9–111. Total serum alkaline phosphatase activity
9–112. Plasma albumin concentration
9–113. Plasma cholinesterase activity
9–114. Serum leucine aminopeptidase activity

9–115. For which conditions does pregnancy serve as a predisposing factor?

a. Hemorrhoids
b. Tooth decay
c. Heartburn (pyrosis)
d. Swelling of gums
e. Gallstones

9–116. In normal pregnancy, the pituitary enlarges enough to significantly reduce the visual fields.

a. True
b. False

9–117. Which of the following statements about the pituitary gland in pregnancy is correct?

a. Pituitary microadenomas may enlarge significantly during pregnancy.
b. The maternal pituitary gland is essential for the maintenance of pregnancy.
c. The level of growth hormone is decreased in pregnancy and remains low after delivery for quite some time.
d. The prolactin level at term may be ten times the nonpregnant level.
e. Plasma prolactin decreases immediately postpartum except in the lactating woman.

9–118. Prolactin levels in both fetal plasma and amnionic fluid peak at 20 weeks' gestation.

a. True
b. False

9–119. Which of the following statements about β-endorphins in pregnancy is correct?

a. β-endorphin is a fragment of β-lipotrophin.
b. Maternal plasma levels of β-endorphin, β-lipotrophin, and γ-lipotrophin steadily increase in pregnancy.
c. The level of β-endorphin is lower in women who receive no analgesics than in women who have epidural anesthesia.
d. β-endorphin levels may be pathologically raised by fetal acidosis.

9–120. Which of the following statements about the thyroid in pregnancy is correct?

a. The thyroid enlarges through hyperplasia in pregnancy.
b. Goiter is a normal occurrence in pregnancy.
c. Abortion is frequently the result of a lack of increase of thyroxine early in pregnancy.
d. Increased thyroid activity in women with hydatidiform mole is due to the action of chronic gonadotropin.

9–121. Complete the following table by filling in whether the value is *increased* or *not increased.*

Test	Normal Pregnancy	Estrogen Administration	Hyperthyroidism
Basal metabolic rate	(a)	(b)	(c)
Total thyroxine	(d)	(e)	(f)
Thyroxine-binding globulin	(g)	(h)	(i)
Free thyroxine	(j)	(k)	(l)
Free triiodothyronine	(m)	(n)	(o)

9–122. Thyroxine, thyroxine-binding capacity, and triiodothyronine resin uptake values in cord serum are ________ (1) those in maternal serum, and ________ (2) levels in nonpregnant adults.

a. Less than
b. The same as
c. Greater than

9–123. Which of the following are clearly elevated in pregnancy?

a. Parathyroid hormone
b. Plasma-ionized calcium
c. Calcitonin
d. Plasma 1,25-dihydroxyvitamin D

9–124. Which of the following statements related to the adrenal gland in pregnancy is correct?

a. Adrenal secretion of cortisol is doubled in pregnancy.
b. The levels of ACTH are high initially, then gradually decrease as pregnancy progresses.
c. Renin and angiotensin are normally elevated, especially in the latter half of pregnancy.
d. Deoxycorticosterone markedly increases in maternal plasma during the third trimester.

9–125. Which of the following statements about the musculoskeletal system in pregnancy is correct?

a. There is a progressive maternal lordosis.
b. Traction on the ulnar and median nerves increases.
c. There is increased mobility of the sacroiliac and sacrococcygeal joints.
d. There is decreased mobility of the pubic joints.

9–126. Musculoskeletal disorders of pregnancy are due solely to hormonal changes in the mother.

a. True
b. False

9–127. True precocious puberty is becoming much more frequent as the average age of menarche is decreasing.

a. True
b. False

9–128. Maternal and fetal complications in women over 40 years of age are ________ in patients less than 40.

a. More frequent than
b. As frequent as
c. Less frequent than

10. DIAGNOSIS OF PREGNANCY

10–1. Which of the following is a positive sign of pregnancy?

a. Softening of the lower uterine segment
b. Uterine enlargement
c. Fetal heart tone identification
d. Perception of fetal movement by the examiner
e. Ultrasonographic/radiographic identification of fetus

10–2. The normal fetal heart rate ranges from ________.

10–3. Fetal heart activity can be identified by 8 weeks' gestation using which of the following?

a. Auscultation with a stethoscope
b. Instruments employing the Doppler principle
c. Real time sonography
d. Echocardiography

10–4. Which of the following may interfere significantly with correct identification of fetal heart action?

a. Maternal tachycardia
b. Fetal tachycardia
c. Maternal bradycardia
d. Fetal bradycardia
e. Funic souffle
f. Uterine souffle

Instructions for Items 10–5 to 10–12: Match the sounds heard on auscultation of the abdomen with the appropriate descriptions.

a. Funic (umbilical souffle)
b. Uterine souffle
c. Intrauterine fetal movement
d. Intestinal peristalsis or gas/fluid movement

10–5. Soft blowing sound synchronous with maternal pulse
10–6. Sharp whistling sound synchronous with fetal pulse
10–7. Gurgling sound
10–8. Irregular, sharp sound not synchronous with maternal or fetal pulse
10–9. Caused by rush of blood through umbilical arteries
10–10. Produced by blood rushing through dilated uterine vessels
10–11. Heard in 15 percent of pregnancies
10–12. May be heard in women with leiomyoma uteri

10–13. Which of the following statements about fetal movement is correct?

a. Fetal movement can be felt by an examiner throughout the second trimester.
b. Fetal movement may vary in intensity.
c. Fetal movement may be visible through the maternal abdominal wall.
d. Fetal movement may be simulated by muscular contractions of the maternal abdominal wall.
e. Fetal movement may be simulated by maternal intestinal peristalsis.

10–14. Which of the following statements about the ultrasonographic evaluation of pregnancy is correct?

a. By 4 to 5 weeks from the LMP, a normal intrauterine pregnancy may often be detected.
b. By 6 weeks from the LMP, a small white gestational ring may be seen, but its absence this early in pregnancy does not raise doubts about the pregnancy.
c. By 8 weeks from the LMP, the embryo (fetal pole) may usually be identified.
d. By 11 weeks from the LMP, fetal heart motion can usually be identified by real time ultrasonography.
e. By the 11th week, the fetal head and thorax can be identified.

10–15. Which of the following is characteristic of gestations in which there is a blighted ovum?

a. Spontaneous abortion will utimately occur.
b. Ultrasonography shows an unusually small gestational sac.
c. Ultrasonography shows a loss of definition of the gestational sac.
d. Ultrasonography shows strong echoes emanating from the fetus after 8 weeks' gestation.

10–16. Which of the following may be determined using ultrasonography at some time during pregnancy?

a. Gestational age of fetus
b. Number of fetuses
c. Presenting part
d. Some fetal anomalies
e. Presence of hydramnios
f. Rate of fetal growth

10–17. To date, no adverse effects on the human fetus have been identified from exposure to energies comparable to those used for clinical ultrasonographic examinations.

a. True
b. False

10–18. Positive identification of pregnancy, based on visualization of the fetal skeleton by x-ray, cannot be made until about ________________ weeks of gestation.

10–19. Which of the following is *not* a probable sign of pregnancy?

a. Nausea and vomiting
b. Changes in size/shape of uterus
c. Changes in cervix
d. Ballottement
e. Abdominal enlargement
f. Braxton Hicks contractions
g. Outlining of fetus
h. Results of endocrine tests

Instructions for Items 10–20 to 10–23: Match the description of the abdomen with the types of pregnancy with which it is most often associated.

a. Nulliparous
b. Multiparous

10–20. Uterus usually palpable abdominally by 12 weeks of gestation
10–21. Abdominal enlargement pronounced due to loss of muscle tone
10–22. Presence of a pendulous abdomen
10–23. Significant changes in abdominal shape due to body position.

10–24. Which of the following statements about changes in the uterus and cervix during pregnancy is correct?

a. During the first few weeks of pregnancy, the increase in size is limited to the anteroposterior diameter.
b. At about 4 weeks after the LMP, Hegar's sign becomes manifest.
c. Hegar's sign is not diagnostic of pregnancy.
d. The cervix normally remains firm and closed until labor ensues.
e. In certain inflammatory conditions, the cervix may soften during pregnancy.
f. Oral contraceptive use may cause softening and congestion of the cervix.

10–25. Which of the following is not characteristic of Braxton Hicks contractions?

a. Palpable
b. Painless
c. Irregular
d. Enhanced by massage
e. Confined to the third trimester

10–26. Near midpregnancy, sudden pressure exerted on the uterus may cause the fetus to sink in the amnionic fluid. The rebound, which may be felt by the examiner, is termed ________________________.

10–27. Outlining "a fetus" by palpation through the maternal abdominal wall is not a positive sign of pregnancy because ________________________.

10–28. Hormonal tests commonly used in the clinical laboratory absolutely identify the presence or absence of pregnancy.

a. True
b. False

10–29. Most chemical tests for the detection of pregnancy involve the identification of ________________ in blood or urine.

10–30. Which of the following statements about pregnancy tests is correct?

a. Radioreceptor assays, using bovine corpus luteum plasma membranes, are specific for hCG.
b. Antibodies against the entire hCG molecule do not recognize LH.
c. In immunoassay procedures, the principle of hemagglutination inhibition of erythrocytes may be employed.
d. In radioassays, the results are based on the competition between radiolabeled hCG and hCG in the sample to be tested.

10–31. In early pregnancy, the concentration of hCG in maternal plasma doubles about every ________ days.

a. 0.5
b. 1.5
c. 3
d. 5
e. 7

10–32. Human chorionic gonadotropin can be first detected by radioimmunoassay ________ the embryo can first be visualized by ultrasonography.

a. Earlier than
b. At the same time as
c. Later than

10–33. Which of the following statements about false results of pregnancy tests is correct?

a. At the time of menopause, the elevated levels of pituitary gonadotropins may be the cause of false-positive tests.
b. False-negative tests are more likely in the 5th month of pregnancy than in the 3rd month.
c. A tubal pregnancy may be associated with a false-negative result.
d. Freezing of urine may give rise to false-positive tests.

10–34. In home pregnancy tests, the false-negative rate is ________ the false-positive rate.

a. Lower than
b. The same as
c. Higher than

10–35. Which of the following statements about progesterone or synthetic progestin-induced withdrawal bleeding is correct?

a. It is able to specifically differentiate pregnancy from other etiologies of amenorrhea.
b. It requires an estrogen-primed endometrium.
c. It requires high levels of endogenous progesterone production.
d. It is a safe procedure with no potentially harmful fetal effects.

10–36. Which of the following statements about hCG levels in ectopic pregnancy is correct?

a. Sensitive assays for hCG show positive results in at least 80 percent of cases.
b. Normal levels of hCG are never found in ectopic pregnancy.
c. A doubling of plasma hCG concentration every 2 days is associated with an ectopic pregnancy in about 20 percent of cases.
d. Falling levels of hCG over time distinguish impending spontaneous abortion from ectopic pregnancy.

10–37. Due to the half-life of hCG, if postabortion monitoring for hCG is indicated, how long after the procedure should this be conducted?

a. 1 to 2 days
b. 3 to 4 days
c. 5 to 7 days
d. 2 to 3 weeks
e. 4 to 6 weeks

10–38. Which of the following constitutes presumptive evidence of pregnancy?

a. Cessation of menses
b. Discoloration of vaginal mucosa
c. Breast changes
d. Skin changes
e. Self-awareness of being pregnant
f. Nausea and vomiting
g. Perception of fetal movement
h. Constipation
i. Fatigue
j. Urinary disturbance
k. Poor libido

10–39. Which of the following statements about pregnancy, menstruation, and vaginal bleeding is correct?

a. In a woman with spontaneous, cyclic, predictable menstruation, a delay in the onset of menstruation greater than 3 days is strongly suggestive of pregnancy.
b. Gestation must be preceded by menstruation.
c. Macroscopic vaginal bleeding may occur in pregnancies with normal outcomes.
d. Bleeding during pregnancy is more common in primaparas than in multiparas.
e. Bleeding per vagina during pregnancy should be regarded as abnormal.

10–40. Breast changes similar to those seen in pregnancy may occasionally be found in which of the following situations?

a. Tranquilizer ingestion
b. Prolactin-secreting pituitary tumor
c. Pseudocyesis
d. Repeated breast stimulation

10–42. Increased skin pigmentation and the appearance of abdominal striae, common to pregnancy, may also be seen in users of oral steroidal contraceptives.

a. True
b. False

10–43. Which of the following statements about the symptoms of pregnancy is correct?

a. "Morning sickness" usually begins prior to the first missed period.
b. "Morning sickness" usually lasts 6 to 12 weeks.
c. Increased frequency of urination, unassociated with urinary tract infection, is more common at the beginning and end of pregnancy.
d. Easy fatigability is a characteristic of late pregnancy.
e. Sensations of fetal movement usually begin around 20 weeks after the LMP.

10–44. Which of the following conditions simulates the menstrual pattern of pregnancy?

a. Adenomyosis
b. Hematometra
c. Leiomyomata
d. Pelvic extrauterine mass

10–45. Which of the following statements about pseudocyesis (spurious pregnancy) is correct?

a. It is more common in women with an intense desire for children and in women nearing menopause.
b. Patients often experience morning sickness.
c. Abdominal distention may be present.
d. An enlarged, soft uterus may be present.
e. There may be a perception of fetal movement.
f. Irregular menses or amenorrhea may be present.

Instructions for Items 10–46 to 10–50: Match the physical finding with its most typical appearance in nulliparous and/or multiparous women.

a. Nulliparous
b. Multiparous

10–46. Pink abdominal striae present
10–47. Labia majora in close apposition
10–48. Abdominal wall lax or pendulous
10–49. Myrtiform caruncles present
10–50. Vagina narrow with well-developed rugae

10–51. Which of the following statements about fetal death is correct?

a. In the early months of pregnancy, hCG level is the most sensitive test for fetal death.
b. Fetal death may be suspected when the uterus fails to increase in size or begins to decrease in size.
c. The absence of fetal heart tones in auscultation with a stethoscope is positive proof of fetal demise.
d. Real time ultrasonographic examination can serve to accurately identify the presence of fetal heart action.

10–52. Which of the following is *not* a radiologic sign characteristic of fetal death?

a. Hyperextension of neck
b. Skull bone overlap
c. Exaggerated spinal curve
d. Gas in fetus
e. Transverse lie

11. THE NORMAL PELVIS

11–1. The mechanisms of labor are essentially processes of ______________ of the fetus to the bony passage through which it must pass.

11–2. The ______________ demarcates the false pelvis from the true pelvis.

Instructions for Items 11–3 to 11–6: Match the anatomic site with the appropriate boundary of the false pelvis.

a. Anterior
b. Inferior
c. Posterior
d. Lateral

11–3. Lumbar vertebrae
11–4. Linea terminalis
11–5. Abdominal wall
11–6. Iliac fossae

11–7. Complete the following table by listing the boundaries of the true pelvis.

Boundary	Anatomic Constituents
Anterior	______ (a)
Posterior	______ (b)
Lateral	______ (c)
Superior	______ (d)
Inferior	______ (e)

11–8. Which of the following statements about the true pelvis is correct?

a. The true pelvis is shaped like a truncated oblique cylinder.
b. The anterior and posterior walls of the true pelvis are almost always of equal height.
c. The walls of the true pelvis are partly ligamentous.
d. With a woman in the upright position, the upper portion of the pelvic canal is directed downward and forward and the lower portion directed downward and backward.
e. Normally, the side walls of the true pelvis converge slightly.
f. The angle of the pubic arch is usually 90 to 100 degrees.
g. The distance between the ischial spines is usually the smallest diameter of the pelvic cavity.

11–9. Which of the following statements about the sacrum is correct?

a. It forms the posterior wall of the pelvis.
b. The upper anterior margin of the sacrum (the first sacral vertebra) is called the promontory.
c. Normally, the sacrum is flat.
d. The sacrum has no relevance in clinical pelvimetry.

11–10. Which of the following statements about the pelvic inlet is correct?

a. Typically, the pelvic inlet is ovoid in shape.
b. The obstetric conjugate is the shortest distance from the sacral promontory to the symphysis pubis.
c. The obstetric conjugate is the same as the true conjugate.
d. The oblique diameters of the pelvic inlet average about 10 cm each.

11–11. The obstetric conjugate can be measured directly.

a. True
b. False

11–12. How is the length of the obstetric conjugate determined?

11–13. It is the measurement of the anteroposterior diameter of the plane of greatest pelvic dimensions that determines the ability of the fetus to pass through the birth canal.

a. True
b. False

11–14. Fill in the following chart describing the boundaries and diameters of some of the planes of the pelvis.

Boundaries	Pelvic Inlet	Pelvic Outlet
Anterior	______ (a)	______ (b)
Lateral	______ (c)	______ (d)
Posterior	______ (e)	______ (f)
Anterior-posterior diameter	______ (g)	______ (h)
Transverse diameter	______ (i)	______ (j)

Fig. 8

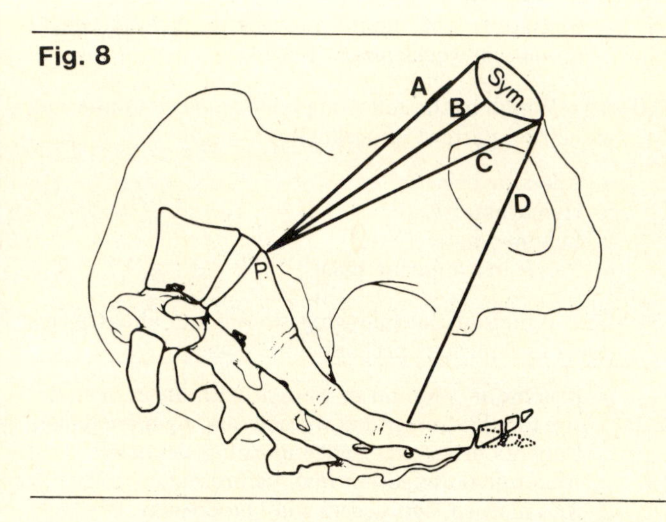

Instructions for Items 11–15 to 11–18: Refer to Figure 8. Match the letter with the correct anteroposterior diameter of the pelvis.

11–15. Anteroposterior diameter of midpelvis
11–16. Obstetric conjugate
11–17. True conjugate
11–18. Diagonal conjugate

11–19. Which term is not synonymous with the others?

a. Interspinous diameter
b. Plane of least pelvic dimensions
c. Transverse diameter of midplane
d. Plane of greatest pelvic dimensions

11–20. Placing which *two* of the following landmarks in a vertical plane reproduces the normal position of the pelvis in an erect woman?

a. Anterior superior spines of ilium
b. Ischial tuberosities
c. Sacral promontory
d. Ischial spines
e. Pubic tubercles

11–21. Which of the following is *not* involved in the anterior junction of the pelvic bones?

a. Inferior pubic ligament
b. Superior pubic ligament
c. Arcuate ligament
d. Symphysis pubis
e. Sacroiliac joint

11–22. Which of the following statements about the pelvic joints in pregnancy is correct?

a. The fibroelastic nature of the junction of the pelvic bones at the symphysis pubis allows a certain degree of motion.
b. The sacroiliac joints remain immobile during pregnancy.
c. An upward gliding displacement of the sacroiliac joint during pregnancy results in an increase in the diameter of the inlet of the pelvis.
d. Relaxation is due to the weight of the enlarged uterus.
e. Relaxation of the symphysis pubis begins during the third trimester.
f. The diameter of the pelvic outlet may be increased by pelvic mobility.

11–23. Placing a woman in an extreme position of hyperextension (Walcher position) increases the length of the obstetric conjugate.

a. True
b. False

11–24. Which of the following statements concerning the Caldwell-Moloy classification of pelvic shapes is correct?

a. The shape of the posterior and anterior segments of the pelvic inlet are important determinants.
b. Anterior and posterior segments are divided by a line through the greatest transverse diameter of the inlet.
c. The anterior segment determines the type of pelvis.

Instructions for Items 11–25 to 11–28: Match the Caldwell-Moloy classification of pelvic shape with appropriate description.

a. Gynecoid
b. Android
c. Anthropoid
d. Platypelloid

11–25. Round shape, transverse and anterior-posterior diameters of inlet about equal
11–26. Flattened oval shape, transverse diameter of inlet greater than anterior-posterior diameter
11–27. Heart shape, anterior-posterior diameter of inlet greater than transverse diameter
11–28. Oval shape, anterior-posterior diameter of inlet greater than transverse diameter

Instructions for Items 11–29 to 11–32: Match the pure Caldwell-Moloy type with its frequency in a population of white women.

a. Gynecoid
b. Android
c. Anthropoid
d. Platypelloid

11–29. 25 percent
11–30. 50 percent
11–31. 33 percent
11–32. Less than 3 percent

11–33. In nonwhite women, which are the *two* most frequent pelvic types?

a. Gynecoid
b. Android
c. Anthropoid
d. Platypelloid

11–34. Most pelves are pure Caldwell-Moloy types.

a. True
b. False

11–35. Which pure pelvic shape (Caldwell-Moloy classification) has the poorest prognosis for vaginal delivery?

a. Gynecoid
b. Android
c. Anthropoid
d. Platypelloid

11–36. Which of the following statements concerning clinical measurement of the anteroposterior diameter of the pelvic inlet is correct?

a. Palpation of the entire anterior sacral surface is easily accomplished.
b. Evaluation of mobility of the coccyx is considered a part of the routine evaluation.
c. To reach the sacral promontory, it is commonly necessary for the examiner to depress his/her elbow and to thereby exert enough pressure to forcibly indent the perineum.
d. The procedure described in answer (c) commonly causes discomfort to the patient.

11-37. If the diagonal conjugate is greater than 11.5 cm, it is usually justifiable to assume that the pelvic inlet is adequate for vaginal delivery.

a. True
b. False

11-38. Engagement is defined as ____________.

11-39. What type of examination can ascertain engagement?

a. Abdominal palpation
b. Rectal examination
c. Vaginal examination

11-40. Fixation of the fetal head is synonomous with engagement.

a. True
b. False

11-41. Which of the following statements relating to engagement is correct?

a. If the lowest part of the occiput is at or below the level of the ischial spine, the head is usually but not always engaged.
b. Absence of engagement at the onset of labor indicates pelvic contraction.
c. Engagement commonly occurs prior to the onset of labor.
d. Engagement is conclusive evidence of an adequate pelvic inlet for this fetus.

11-42. Which of the following terms are synonymous?

a. Transverse diameter of the outlet
b. Biischial diameter
c. Intertuberous diameter
d. Plane of least pelvic dimensions

11-43. The diameter between the ischial tuberosities should be at least ____________ cm to be considered normal.

a. 4
b. 6
c. 8
d. 10

11-44. Midpelvic capacity may be precisely determined by

a. The clinical measurement of ischial spine prominence
b. The clinical measurement of side wall convergence
c. The clinical measurement of sacral concavity
d. X-ray examination

11-45. Which of the following factors important for the outcome of labor is amenable to reasonably precise roentgenologic measurement?

a. Size and shape of bony pelvis
b. Size of fetal head
c. Presentation of fetus
d. Position of fetus
e. Moldability of fetal head

11-46. Which of the following pelvic diameters is *only* obtainable by x-ray pelvimetry?

a. Transverse diameter of the pelvic inlet
b. Obstetric conjugate
c. True conjugate
d. Transverse diameter of midpelvis
e. Interischial spinous diameter

11-47. X-ray pelvimetry may be indicated in which of the following circumstances?

a. Previous injury to bony pelvis
b. Breech presentations where vaginal delivery is considered
c. Failure to progress in labor (cephalopelvic disproportion)
d. All anticipated cesarean sections

11-48. Which parameters differentiate a man's pelvis from a woman's?

a. Weight
b. Angle of pubic arch
c. Shape of inlet
d. Size of inlet

11-49. Which of the following statements about the pelvis of a child is correct?

a. At birth, it is entirely cartilaginous.
b. Complete union in the acetabulum does not occur until puberty or later.
c. Ossification of innominate bones may occur after puberty.

11-50. Which of the following mechanical forces is important in bringing about the final shape of the pelvis?

a. Body weight
b. Upward and inward pressure from the head of the femur
c. Cohesive force of the symphysis pubis
d. Downward pressure of the sacrum

12. PRESENTATION, POSITION, ATTITUDE, AND LIE OF THE FETUS

12–1. The position which a fetus assumes in late pregnancy is called its ______________________.

12–2. Which of the following is a description of typical fetal posture in late pregnancy?

a. The back is convex.
b. The head is extended.
c. The thighs are flexed.
d. The legs are bent at the knee.
e. The arms are crossed over the thorax.

12–3. The characteristic fetal posture in late pregnancy results solely from a process of accommodation to the uterine cavity.

a. True
b. False

12–4. The lie of the fetus is defined as the __________.

12–5. Which of the following fetal lies is most unstable?

a. Longitudinal
b. Oblique
c. Transverse

12–6. What percentage of fetal lies are longitudinal?

a. 50 percent
b. 75 percent
c. 99 percent

12–7. In longitudinal lies, the presenting part can be the

a. Head
b. Breech
c. Shoulder

Instructions for Items 12–8 to 12–11: Refer to Figure 9. Match the letter with the appropriate type of cephalic presentation.

12–8. Vertex
12–9. Face
12–10. Sinciput
12–11. Brow

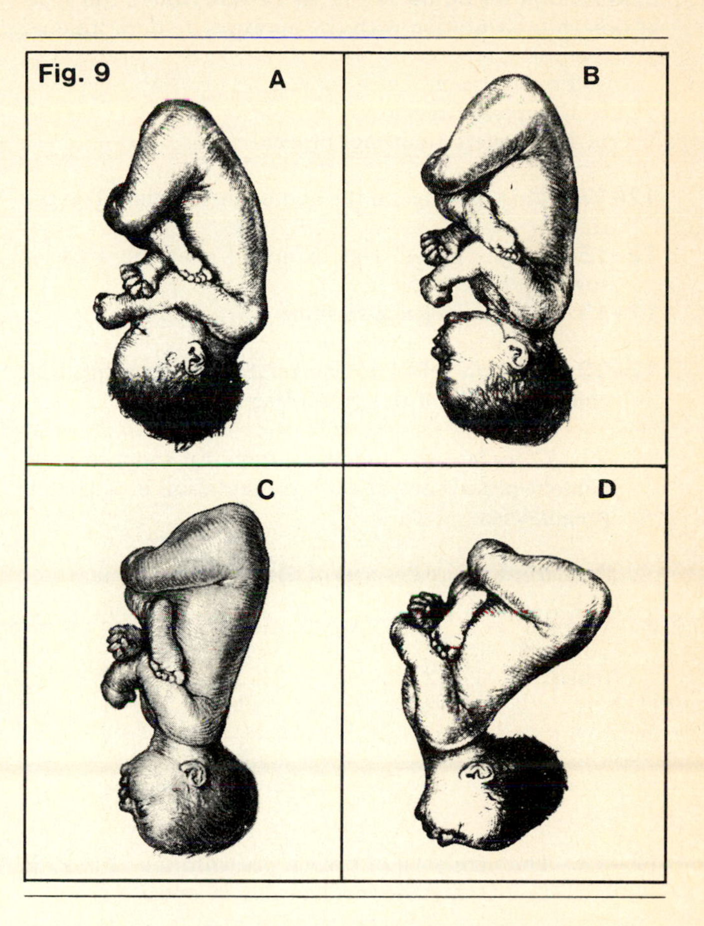

Instructions for Items 12–12 to 12–15: Match the type of cephalic presentation with the appropriate description.

a. Face presentation
b. Vertex presentation
c. Brow presentation
d. Sinciput presentation

12–12. Occipital fontanel presenting
12–13. Head in extreme extension
12–14. Head in partial extension
12–15. Anterior fontanel presenting

12–16. Sinciput and brow presentations almost always convert to face or vertex presentations during labor.

a. True
b. False

Instructions for Items 12-17 to 12-19: Match the type of breech presentation with the appropriate description.

a. Frank breech
b. Complete breech
c. Incomplete (footling) breech

12-17. Thighs flexed on the abdomen, legs flexed on the thigh
12-18. Thighs flexed, legs extended over the anterior surface of the body
12-19. Feet or knees lowermost

12-20. Position refers to the relation of an arbitrarily chosen portion of the presenting fetal part to ______.

12-21. Complete the following table by supplying the percent occurrence of each presentation in singleton pregnancies.

Presentation	Percent of Singleton Pregnancies
Vertex	______ (a)
Breech	______ (b)
Face	______ (c)
Shoulder	______ (d)

12-22. The incidence of breech presentation at term is ______ the incidence at 34 weeks.

a. Greater than
b. The same as
c. Less than

12-23. Which of the following statements related to fetal presentation is correct?

a. The podalic pole of the fetus is bulkier than the cephalic pole.
b. At 32 weeks, the fetus starts becoming less crowded by the uterine walls.
c. At about 32 weeks, the fetal lie becomes more dependent upon the piriform shape of the uterus.
d. Fetal attitude may prevent it from turning in utero.
e. The cephalic pole in hydrocephalic fetuses is larger than the podalic pole.

12-24. Which of the following methods may be used to determine the position and presentation of the fetus?

a. Ultrasonography
b. X-ray
c. Abdominal palpation
d. Vaginal palpation
e. Auscultation

Instructions for Items 12-25 to 12-28: Match the maneuver of Leopold with its proper description.

a. First maneuver
b. Second maneuver
c. Third maneuver
d. Fourth maneuver

12-25. Examiner faces patient's head, determines engagement, lie, position
12-26. Examiner faces patient's head, determines position/orientation
12-27. Examiner faces patient's head, determines fetal pole, lie, presentation
12-28. Examiner faces patient's feet, determines engagement, presentation

12-29. What information can be obtained using the maneuvers of Leopold?

a. Fetal descent
b. Fetal position
c. Fetal presentation
d. Estimation of fetal size

12-30. The fetal cephalic suture felt during vaginal examination that provides information of primary importance is the ______.

12-31. Which statements about auscultation in relation to fetal position and presentation is correct?

a. Auscultation by itself provides very reliable information about fetal position.
b. Fetal heart sounds are heard best through the fetal thorax in a face presentation.
c. In a cephalic presentation, fetal heart sounds are best heard midway between the maternal umbilicus and the anterior superior spine of the ilium.
d. In the occiput anterior position, heart sounds are best heard in the maternal flank.

12-32. In light of the safety of ultrasonography, there is no indication for the use of diagnostic x-rays in determining fetal position or presentation.

a. True
b. False

13. PRENATAL CARE

13–1. Which of the following statements about prenatal care is correct?

a. The goal is delivery of a healthy baby without impairing the health of the mother.
b. Bad prenatal care may be worse than no care at all.
c. Prenatal care should be a continuation of comprehensive health care prior to pregnancy.

13–2. Prenatal care is a special kind of medical treatment for the pathophysiologic changes in maternal physiology that are engendered by pregnancy.

a. True
b. False

Instructions for Items 13–3 to 13–9: Match the terms with their definitions.

a. Nulligravida
b. Gravida
c. Nullipara
d. Primipara
e. Multipara
f. Parturient
g. Puerpera

13–3. A woman delivered once of a fetus or fetuses who reached the state of viability
13–4. A woman who is or has been pregnant
13–5. A woman who has never completed a pregnancy beyond an abortion
13–6. A woman who has just given birth
13–7. A woman in labor
13–8. A woman who has completed two or more pregnancies to the stage of viability
13–9. A woman who has never been pregnant.

13–10. A woman who was delivered of one set of twins and has had no other pregnancies would be defined as a ______________________.

13–11. A woman whose obstetric history is described by the digits 4-0-1-3 has how many living children?

a. 4
b. 0
c. 1
d. 3

13–12. The mean duration of a normal pregnancy from the 1st day of the last normal menstrual period is about

a. 250 days
b. 260 days
c. 270 days
d. 280 days
e. 290 days

13–13. According to Naegele's rule, if a pregnant woman's last menstrual period began on June 3, her expected date of delivery would be ______________.

13–14. Gestational age is synonymous with

a. Ovulatory age
b. Menstrual age
c. Fertilization age

13–15. Clinically, the most useful and appropriate unit of measure for a pregnancy is the

a. Trimester
b. Months of gestation completed
c. Weeks of gestation completed

13–16. The goals of the initial comprehensive obstetric evaluation include

a. Defining the health status of the mother
b. Defining the health status of the fetus
c. Determining the gestational age of the fetus
d. Initiating a plan for continuing obstetric care

13–17. Which of the following contributes to difficulties in determining gestational age?

a. Menstrual cycle significantly longer than 30 days
b. Irregular menstrual cycles
c. Use of steroidal contraceptives
d. Presence of an intrauterine device

13–18. Which of the following are standard procedures at the initial prenatal obstetric examination?

a. Obtaining specimens for cervical cytology
b. Obtaining urethral culture
c. Performing colposcopy
d. Obtaining cervical culture for gonorrhea
e. Biopsying suspected Nabothian cysts

13–19. Which of the following types of vaginal secretions is normal in pregnancy?

a. Foamy yellow liquid
b. Curdlike discharge
c. White mucoid discharge
d. Frothy, red tinged discharge

13–20. Characterization of the bony architecture of the pelvis is the most important aspect of the internal examination in pregnancy.

a. True
b. False

13–21. Between 18 and 32 weeks, what is the relationship between the gestational age of the fetus and the height of the uterine fundus?

13–22. During the prenatal examination, carious teeth should be identified but dental repair should be postponed as it is dangerous during pregnancy.

a. True
b. False

13–23. List the ten danger signs that a pregnant woman should be warned to report immediately.

13–24. Factors which may warrant classification of a pregnancy as "high risk" include

a. Preexisting medical illness
b. Previous poor pregnancy outcome
c. Previous placental accidents or maternal hemorrhage
d. Evidence of maternal malnutrition

Instructions for Items 13–25 to 13–27: Match the appropriate interval of prenatal visits with the phase of pregnancy.

a. Every week
b. Every 2 weeks
c. Every 4 weeks
d. Every 6 weeks

13–25. Weeks 1 to 28
13–26. Weeks 28 to 36
13–27. Weeks 36 through delivery

13–28. Which of the following statements about findings during routine prenatal return visits is correct?

a. Using a DeLee fetal stethoscope, fetal heart sounds are first audible in essentially all pregnancies between 16 and 19 weeks' gestation.
b. A common cause of error in fundal height measurement is a full maternal bladder.
c. Fundal height measurements correlate exactly with gestational age from the time the fundus is palpable until delivery.
d. The time of first reported fetal movement can aid in the accuracy of gestational age determinations.
e. An accurate date for the LMP and serially appropriate fundal heights may firmly establish gestational age.

13–29. Which of the following should be routinely monitored at prenatal visits?

a. Fetal movement
b. Presenting part
c. Amount of amnionic fluid
d. Fetal heart rate
e. Size of fetus

13–30. Which maternal physical signs are monitored at every prenatal visit?

a. Blood pressure
b. Weight
c. Fundal height
d. Cervical dilation
e. Measurement of bony pelvis

13–31. Which of the following laboratory tests should be repeated at every prenatal visit?

a. Hematocrit
b. Serologic test for syphilis
c. Cervical culture for gonorrhea
d. Urine test for protein
e. Urine test for glucose

13–32. Rigid caloric restriction during pregnancy is necessary to minimize the risk of preeclampsia.

a. True
b. False

13–33. The neonatal mortality rate for low birth weight infants (less than 2500 g) is approximately ______________ times as high as for infants weighing more than 2500 g.

13–34. The nutritional status of the expectant mother is more likely to be compromised in which of the following circumstances?

a. She is less than 16 years old.
b. She is economically deprived.
c. She is pregnant for the third time within 2 years.
d. She smokes, drinks, or uses hard drugs.
e. She is underweight at the onset of pregnancy.
f. Her weight gain for any month during the second and third trimesters is less than 2 pounds.

13–35. Which of the following statements about weight gain in pregnancy is correct?

a. During a normal pregnancy with a single fetus, there is a physiologic basis for a weight gain of at least 20 pounds.
b. Birth weight is influenced by total maternal caloric intake.
c. A balanced diet is the most appropriate way for a pregnant woman to obtain needed calories.
d. Birth weight parallels maternal weight gain.

13–36. The recommended daily caloric increase throughout pregnancy is ______________ kcal.

13–37. Which of the following statements about protein requirements in pregnancy is correct?

a. When insufficient calories are available, protein may be metabolized rather than being spared for fetal growth and development.
b. An additional 30 grams of protein above the normal nonpregnant requirement is recommended during pregnancy.
c. Milk and milk products are the ideal sources for additional protein in all pregnant women.
d. Protein from animal or vegetable sources is equally satisfactory as a source of protein during pregnancy.

13–38. List the minerals that should be added to the diet of a pregnant woman who consumes sufficient calories for appropriate weight gain.

13–39. Which of the following statements about iron ingestion in pregnancy is correct?

a. Total average iron requirements during the latter part of pregnancy are 7 mg per day.
b. The majority of women have sufficient iron stores for the increased requirements of pregnancy.
c. Dietary iron can usually adequately supplement any deficient iron stores.
d. Thirty mg of iron as a simple salt is the minimum daily supplement recommended.
e. Calcium and magnesium contained in some vitamin-mineral supplements can impair the absorption of iron.

13–40. Iron supplementation during pregnancy

a. Is not necessary during the first 4 months
b. Can cause congenital malformations and impaired fetal well-being
c. Can exacerbate first trimester nausea and vomiting
d. Should be taken at night to minimize any adverse gastrointestinal reactions

13–41. Which of the following statements about calcium in pregnancy is correct?

a. Calcium supplementation in pregnancy is necessary in women over 30 to avoid the possibility of osteomalacia.
b. Maternal calcium is readily mobilized as needed for fetal growth.
c. There is increased absorption of calcium through the intestine in pregnancy.
d. The amount of calcium retained in pregnancy represents 25 percent of total maternal calcium.

13–42. Which of the following statements about zinc in pregnancy is correct?

a. Severe zinc deficiency may lead to impaired wound healing.
b. Profound zinc deficiency may lead to acrodermatitis enteropathica.
c. Zinc in plasma is mainly in the ionized, unbound form.
d. There is no strong evidence that zinc supplementation has any material or fetal benefits.
e. Low maternal zinc levels lead to babies who are small for gestational age.

13–43. Which of the following statements about dietary supplementation during pregnancy is correct?

a. Phosphorus is commonly inadequate in western diets.
b. Severe maternal iodine deficiency in expectant mothers predisposes the fetus to cretinism.
c. Fetal goiter may result from maternal ingestion of large amounts of seaweed or iodine.
d. Magnesium deficiency as a consequence of pregnancy alone occurs in about 25 percent of women.
e. Hypokalemia develops in the same ways in pregnant and in nonpregnant women.

13–44. Sodium restriction in pregnancy reduces the incidence of preeclampsia.

a. True
b. False

13–45. Which of the following statements concerning fluoride supplementation in pregnancy is correct?

a. Supplemental fluoride taken by the lactating mother increases the fluoride concentration in her milk.
b. Supplemental fluoride increases fetal bone density.
c. Offspring of mothers who ingest sodium fluoride during pregnancy have fewer caries.

13–46. There is abundant evidence that the usual vitamin supplements are of significant benefit to the fetus but of little benefit to the mother.

a. True
b. False

13–47. Which of the following statements about folic acid supplementation in pregnancy is correct?

a. Folic acid supply is more likely to be inadequate when pregnancy is complicated by prolonged vomiting or multiple fetuses.
b. Administration of folic acid during pregnancy can reduce the incidence of placental abruption and preeclampsia.
c. One mg of folic acid orally per day should provide sufficient supplementation when needed.

13–48. Which of the following statements about vitamin B_{12} in pregnancy is correct?

a. Vitamin B_{12} levels in maternal plasma decrease variably in normal pregnancies.
b. Strict vegetarians may give birth to infants whose vitamin B_{12} stores are low.
c. The breast milk of a vegetarian mother contains little vitamin B_{12}.
d. Excessive ingestion of vitamin C can lead to a functional deficiency of vitamin B_{12}.

13–49. Vitamin B_6

a. Deficiency induces excessive excretion of xanthurenic acid after ingestion of a trytophan load
b. Deficiency leads to a lowering of the biologic activity of endogenous insulin
c. Ingestion in large excess can lead to nervous system dysfunction
d. Requirements in pregnancy are twice those for nonpregnant women

13–50. Large doses of vitamin C, ingested by the pregnant woman for the prevention of colds, have been shown to have no deleterious effects on the fetus.

a. True
b. False

Instructions for Items 13–51 to 13–57: Match the following circumstances involving vitamins with the appropriate associated abnormal or pathologic conditions.

a. Vitamin C excess
b. Iodine deficiency
c. Iodine excess
d. Folic acid deficiency
e. Zinc deficiency
f. Vitamin D deficiency
g. Vitamin B_{12} deficiency
h. Vitamin B_6 excess

13–51. Fetal cretinism
13–52. Hypersegmented neutrophils
13–53. Acrodermatitis enteropathica
13–54. Fetal goiter
13–55. Scurvy
13–56. Megaloblastic anemia
13–57. Progressive sensory ataxia

13–58. Which of the following nutritional recommendations should be made to pregnant women?

a. Eat certain foods regardless of food preferences.
b. Gain at least 20 pounds.
c. Take tablets of simple iron salts providing 30 to 60 mg of iron daily.
d. Do not add salt to food.

13–59. In general, it is not necessary for a pregnant woman to limit exercise, assuming she does not become excessively fatigued or risk injury to herself or the fetus.

a. True
b. False

13–60. Which of the following pregnancy complications may benefit from limitation of exercise?

a. Pregnancy-induced hypertension
b. Multiple fetuses
c. Intrauterine growth retardation
d. Breech presentation

13–61. Which of the following statements about employment during pregnancy is correct?

a. Severe physical strain should be avoided.
b. Work should not cause undue fatigue.
c. Adequate rest should be provided during the work day.
d. Women with repetitive complications of pregnancy should minimize physical work.

13–62. Which of the following statements about travel during pregnancy is correct?

a. Travel, especially in airplanes, should be avoided in pregnancy.
b. At least every 2 hours, the pregnant woman should walk about.
c. The greatest risk with international travel is the development of a pregnancy complication remote from adequate treatment facilities.

13–63. Which articles of clothing should be avoided in pregnancy?

a. Jeans
b. Constricting garters
c. Pantyhose
d. High-heeled shoes

13–64. All laxatives should be avoided by the pregnant woman.

a. True
b. False

13–65. Coitus should be avoided during pregnancy.

a. True
b. False

13–66. What limitations to douching in pregnancy should be emphasized?

a. Only hand bulb syringes should be used.
b. The douche bag should be not more than 2 feet above the level of the hips.
c. The nozzle should not be inserted more than 3 inches through the vulva.
d. The pregnant woman should only douche once a week.

13-67. Massage and ointments reduce the incidence of striae on the breast and abdomen.

a. True
b. False

13-68. Smoking during pregnancy is associated with an increased incidence of

a. Perinatal death
b. Maternal hypertension
c. Low birth weight infants
d. Diabetes in pregnancy

13-69. Which of the following have been implicated to explain the adverse effects of smoking during pregnancy?

a. Inactivation of fetal and maternal hemoglobin by carbon monoxide.
b. A vasoconstrictor action of nicotine which causes reduced perfusion of the placenta.
c. Reduced appetite and, in turn, reduced caloric intake in women who smoke.
d. Decreased plasma volume in women who smoke.

13-70. Fetal alcohol syndrome is associated with

a. Craniofacial anomalies
b. Anomalies of the limbs
c. Cardiovascular defects
d. Growth retardation
e. Impaired gross and fine motor function
f. Impaired speech

13-71. The chronic use of which of the following drugs is associated with harmful fetal effects such as intrauterine distress and low birth weight?

a. Marijuana
b. Opium derivatives
c. Barbiturates
d. Amphetamines

13-72. Which of the following immunizations are contraindicated during pregnancy

a. Influenza
b. Measles
c. Mumps
d. Typhoid
e. Rubella
f. Hepatitis A

Instructions for Items 13-73 to 13-76: Match the drug with its possible fetal effects if taken during pregnancy.

a. Diphenylhydantoin
b. Aspirin
c. Prostaglandin synthetase inhibitors

13-73. Deficient vitamin K coagulation factors
13-74. Platelet dysfunction
13-75. Premature closure of the ductus arteriosus
13-76. Fetal malformation

13-77. The placenta serves as an effective barrier to most drugs, even those that exert a systemic effect in the mother.

a. True
b. False

13-78. Which of the following statements about the nausea and vomiting of pregnancy is correct?

a. It only occurs in the morning.
b. It usually disappears by the 4th month.
c. The severity of vomiting is correlated with serum levels of chorionic gonadotropins.
d. Therapeutic abortion is frequently the only successful therapy for severe nausea (hyperemesis gravidarum).
e. Pregnancies with nausea and vomiting are more likely to have a favorable outcome.

13-79. Which of the following statements about backache in pregnancy is correct?

a. A lightweight maternity girdle may afford relief in mild cases.
b. Disc herniation is more frequent during pregnancy.
c. Back pain may be due to general relaxation of pelvic ligaments and motion in the lumbosacral joints.

13-80. Surgical correction of varicosities of the lower extremities is often necessary to provide relief during pregnancy.

a. True
b. False

13-81. Which of the following statements about hemorrhoids in pregnancy is correct?

a. Development of hemorrhoids is related to obstruction of venous return by the enlarging uterus.
b. Bleeding from hemorrhoidal veins may result in blood loss sufficient to cause iron deficiency anemia.
c. Hemorrhoids usually become asymptomatic after delivery.
d. Pain and swelling are usually relieved by stool softeners, warm soaks, and topical anesthetics.

13-82. Sodium hydroxide is the antacid of choice for the treatment of heartburn in pregnancy.

a. True
b. False

13–83. Pica results primarily from an unconscious response to subtle physiologic needs for trace elements.

a. True
b. False

13–84. Which of the following is more common early in pregnancy than late in pregnancy?

a. Backache
b. Fatigue
c. Heartburn
d. Headache
e. Hemorrhoids

13–85. Which of the following statements about vaginitis and vaginal discharge in pregnancy is correct?

a. Increased cervical mucus production in response to hyperestrogenemia is the most common cause of increased vaginal discharge in pregnancy.
b. *Trichomonas vaginalis* vaginitis may be treated with metronidazole.
c. *Candida albicans* vaginitis in pregnancy may be successfully treated with miconazole nitrate cream.
d. Candidiasis is likely to recur during pregnancy.

14. TECHNIQUES TO EVALUATE FETAL HEALTH

14–1. Which of the following factors have contributed to the relatively recent fall in the perinatal death rate?

a. Family planning programs
b. Legalized elective abortion
c. Better, more available antepartum care
d. Selective therapeutic abortion
e. Liberal hospitalization practices
f. Greater attention to evaluation of fetal well-being
g. Increased cesarean birth rate
h. Available, high quality neonatal care

14–2. Which of the following is a risk from amniocentesis?

a. Abortion
b. Rh isoimmunization
c. Placental hemorrhage
d. Trauma to the umbilical cord
e. Intrauterine fetal infection
f. Premature labor

14–3. Which of the following categories of disorders contain diseases diagnosable by amnionic fluid analysis?

a. Chromosomal anomalies
b. Skeletal disorders
c. Fetal infections
d. Central nervous system diseases
e. Hematologic disorders
f. Inborn errors of metabolism

14–4. Undesirable outcomes from amniocentesis may be minimized by

a. Performing the amniocentesis puncture suprapubically
b. Examining the newly delivered infant as soon as possible for evidence of trauma
c. Locating the placenta sonographically in any case where clinical examination is inadequate
d. Administering prophylactic anti-Rho(D) globulin to nonsensitized Rh(D) negative women

14–5. Which of the following factors increases the risk of fetal injury during amniocentesis?

a. Small volume of amnionic fluid
b. Thick amnionic fluid
c. Postterm pregnancy
d. Repeated taps
e. Use of a large (18-gauge) needle

14–6. In what circumstances should the fetal heart rate be closely monitored following amniocentesis?

14–7. The overall accuracy of prenatal diagnosis from amniocentesis performed near midpregnancy is approximately ________ percent.

a. 70
b. 80
c. 90
d. 95
e. 99

14–8. Which of the following statements about bloody taps obtained during amniocentesis is correct?

a. Erythrocytes may inhibit the replication in culture of fetal cells.
b. Small amounts of maternal blood can lead to falsely high levels of α-fetoprotein in amnionic fluid.
c. Blood in the amnionic fluid produces a lowered L/S ratio.
d. Amnionic fluid should be considered unsatisfactory for measurement of L/S ratios if the hematocrit of a spun sample exceeds 1 percent.

14–9. Surface-active phospholipids are produced in fetal lung alveoli by ________________.

14–10. In amnionic fluid, the concentration of lecithin relative to sphingomyelin begins to rise at ____________ weeks of gestation?

a. 28
b. 30
c. 32
d. 34
e. 36
f. 38

14–11. Which of the following statements about the L/S ratio in amnionic fluid is correct?

a. Slight variations in technique can significantly affect the accuracy of the results.
b. When the L/S ratio is 1.5 or below, a majority of infants develop respiratory distress.
c. An L/S ratio of less than 1.0 is incompatible with fetal survival.
d. An L/S ratio of 2.0 or greater precludes the development of respiratory distress.

14–12. When the L/S ratio is below 1.5, the death rate among newborns is approximately ____________ percent.

14–13. In which of the following situations is there a significant possibility that an infant may develop respiratory distress even if the L/S ratio is 2.0 or more?

a. Class A maternal diabetes
b. Class B maternal diabetes
c. Esophageal atresia
d. Erythroblastosis fetalis
e. Gestational age less than 36 weeks

14–14. The identification of which of the following in amnionic fluid suggests that respiratory distress syndrome is less likely to develop.

a. Phosphatidylglycerol
b. Lecithin
c. Sphingomyelin
d. Phosphatidylinositol

14–15. Which of the following tests is used to determine the presence of surfactant in amnionic fluid?

a. L/S ratio
b. Phosphatidylglycerol measurement
c. Foam stability test
d. Lumadex-FSI test
e. Fluorescent polarization
f. Amnionic fluid absorbence at 650 nm

14–16. In the foam stability test, a false-positive result is more common than a false-negative result.

a. True
b. False

14–17. Which of the following statements about amnionic fluid bilirubin is correct?

a. Hemolysis yields bilirubin, most of which remains unconjugated by the fetus.
b. Fetal bilirubin reaches the amnionic fluid by way of the fetal urine.
c. The amount of bilirubin in amnionic fluid normally falls during the last few weeks of pregnancy.
d. Amnionic fluid bilirubin is best measured by chemical means.

14–18. In which of the following cases is amnionic fluid bilirubin usually elevated?

a. Maternal hyperbilirubinemia
b. Maternal sickle cell anemia
c. Fetal hemolytic disease
d. Intrauterine growth retardation

14–19. Chromosomal analysis of fetal somatic cells is often of value in which of the following circumstances?

a. Pregnancy after three or more spontaneous abortions
b. Pregnancy in a woman over 35 years of age
c. A previous child or parent with a neural tube defect
d. Down syndrome in a close family member
e. A previous infant born with multiple major malformations

Instructions for Items 14–20 to 14–25: Match the chromosomal abnormality with its reported frequency.

a. 1/800 births
b. 1/950 female births
c. 1/1000 male births
d. 1/8000 births
e. 1/10,000 female births
f. 1/20,000 births

14–20. Trisomy 13
14–21. Trisomy 18

14–22. Trisomy 21
14–23. XXY
14–24. XXX
14–25. XO

14–26. Which of the following differentiates amnionic fluid from maternal urine?

a. Crystallization of fluid when dried on a glass slide
b. Color of fluid
c. Presence of glucose
d. Presence of protein
e. Odor of fluid

14–27. Cytogenetic studies are recommended for women only after the age of 40.

a. True
b. False

14–28. In the case of X-linked recessive diseases for which no specific prenatal diagnostic test is available, sex identification is of no prognostic value.

a. True
b. False

14–29. At 15 to 18 weeks' gestation, which of the following methods may be used to accurately determine fetal sex?

a. Demonstration of Barr body
b. Y chromosome staining
c. Testosterone levels in amnionic fluid
d. FSH levels amnionic fluid

14–30. Approximately how many recessively inherited X-linked or autosomal metabolic disorders are detectable through amniocentesis?

a. 25
b. 50
c. 75
d. 100
e. 200

14–31. In which of the following conditions can an affected fetus be diagnosed in utero?

a. Diabetes
b. β-thalassemia
c. Hemoglobinopathy
d. Hyperthyroidism

14–32. Which of the following statements about α-fetoprotein is correct?

a. The placenta is the major site of α-fetoprotein synthesis.
b. It is the major protein in the serum of the embryo and early fetus.
c. The amnionic fluid concentration of α-fetoprotein is highest around the 13th week of gestation.
d. The concentration of α-fetoprotein in fetal serum is greater than in the amnionic fluid.
e. The levels of α-fetoprotein in amnionic fluid and in fetal serum normally decrease rapidly beginning at the 13th week of gestation.

14–33. Amnionic fluid α-fetoprotein levels are usually elevated in

a. Open neural tube defects
b. Congenital nephrosis
c. Bladder neck obstruction
d. Esophageal and duodenal atresia
e. Turner syndrome
f. Fetal death
g. Abdominal pregnancy
h. Down syndrome

14–34. Screening of maternal serum for elevated α-fetoprotein levels is indicated in which of the following situations?

a. A pregnant woman with a family history of neural tube defects.
b. A pregnant woman whose previous pregnancy resulted in an infant with spina bifida.
c. A pregnant woman who is over 40 years old.
d. A woman whose previous pregnancy resulted in an infant with congenital nephrosis.

Instructions for Items 14–35 to 14–38: Match the amnionic fluid component with the appropriate procedure.

a. Amnionic fluid supernatant
b. Amnionic fluid cell sample

14–35. Determination of genetic sex
14–36. Determination of fetal lung maturity
14–37. Detection of hemolytic disease of the newborn
14–38. Detection of fetal neural tube defects

14–39. The source of most cases of elevated amnionic fluid acetylcholinesterase is ______________.

14–40. What advantage does chorionic villus biopsy have over amniocentesis for obtaining fetal cells to use in genetic diagnosis?

14–41. Ultrasonography may be used to determine

a. The presence of intrauterine pregnancy
b. The presence of multiple fetuses
c. Gestational age
d. Abnormal amounts of amnionic fluid
e. Placental location
f. Placental abnormalities

14–42. Which of the following statements about fetal motion as detected by real time ultrasonography is correct?

a. Fetal heart beat has been demonstrated by 7 weeks of gestation.
b. Fetal trunk movement has been demonstrated by 8 weeks of gestation.
c. Fetal limb movement has been demonstrated by 9 weeks of gestation.
d. Filling and emptying of the fetal bladder have been demonstrated.

14–43. For which of the following determinations is ultrasonography more precise than radiography?

a. Fetal age
b. Placental localization
c. Fetal size
d. Identification of hydatidiform mole

Instructions for Items 14–44 to 14–47: Match the procedure with its application.

a. Amnioscopy
b. Fetoscopy
c. Amniography
d. Fetography

14–44. Direct visualization of the fetus and placenta
14–45. Visualization of meconium-stained amnionic fluid
14–46. Identification of external fetal outline
14–47. Visualization of the fetal gastrointestinal tract

14–48. Which of the following contraindicate or complicate amnioscopy?

a. Inadvertent rupture of the membranes
b. Inaccessible cervix
c. Possibility of infection
d. Lack of cervical dilation

14–49. Which of the following has been proven to be a clinically useful tool for assessing fetal well-being?

a. Fetoscopy
b. Nuclear magnetic resonance
c. Human placental lactogen
d. Chorionic gonadotropin
e. Maternal plasma progesterone
f. Metabolic clearance of dehydroisoandrosterone sulfate

14–50. Which of the following statements about fetal movement is correct?

a. The number of fetal movements increases progressively until delivery.
b. The pattern of fetal movement may be exactly correlated with gestational age.
c. The absolute number of fetal movements per day is less important than the degree of change in the frequency of fetal movements.
d. A marked increase in movement is an indication of fetal well-being.
e. A sudden decrease in movement is a sign of possible loss of fetal well-being.

14–51. Which of the following does *not* describe a contraction stress test?

a. Usually takes 1 to 2 hours
b. Actual intrauterine pressure is measured
c. An ultrasound transducer is utilized
d. Maternal blood pressure is recorded
e. Oxytocin is administered intramuscularly

14–52. Which of the following conditions may contraindicate the use of oxytocin to perform a fetal contraction stress test?

a. Multiple fetuses
b. An L/S ratio less than 2
c. Previous classical cesarean section
d. Previous multiple pregnancy
e. Hydramnios
f. Threatened preterm labor
g. Placenta previa
h. Rupture of the membranes
i. Previous preterm labor

14–53. A contraction stress test is indicated at any time in the second or third trimester when the fetus is suspected of being in jeopardy.

a. True
b. False

Instructions for Items 14–54 to 14–58: Match the following interpretations for a contraction stress test with their best descriptions.

a. Positive
b. Negative
c. Suspicious
d. Hyperstimulation
e. Unsatisfactory

14–54. At least three contractions in 10 minutes, each lasting at least 40 seconds, are identified without late decelerations of the fetal heart rate.
14–55. If uterine contractions are more frequent than every 2 minutes, or last longer than 90 seconds, or persistent uterine hypertonus is suspected.

14–56. There is inconstant late deceleration that does not persist with subsequent contractions.
14–57. The frequency of contractions is less than three per 10 minutes or the tracing is poor.
14–58. There is consistent and persistent late deceleration of the fetal heart rate.

14–59. If a contraction stress test is negative, it is usually repeated.

a. Monthly
b. Biweekly
c. Weekly
d. Weekly for 2 weeks, than monthly

14–60. A negative contraction stress test is *not* always compatible with placental function sufficient to maintain the fetus alive for at least 1 week.

a. True
b. False

14–61. False-negative contraction stress tests occur about ______________ percent of the time.

14–62. A positive contraction stress test is sufficiently ominous to warrant interruption of pregnancy within 24 hours.

a. True
b. False

14–63. Fetal movement is typically accompanied by transient ______________ of the fetal heart rate.

a. Acceleration
b. Deceleration

14–64. A nonstress test is generally considered reactive when ____.

14–65. No test of fetal well-being provides complete reassurance.

a. True
b. False

14–66. Acoustic stimulation studies and acceleration of fetal heart rate in response to transabdominal amniocentesis are more sensitive predictors of fetal well-being than the nonstress test.

a. True
b. False

14–67. Which of the following factors can compromise fetal well-being?

a. Maternal disease
b. Intrinsic fetal disease
c. Cord compression
d. Placental disease
e. Analgesia and anesthesia given to the mother

14–68. The internal spiral electrode should *not* be attached to the

a. Face
b. Buttocks
c. Genitalia
d. Fontanels
e. Extremities

14–69. Which method of monitoring the fetal heart rate is most accurate?

a. Ultrasound Doppler principle
b. Internal spiral electrode
c. Phonocardiography
d. Fetal electrocardiogram

14–70. Which of the following statements about intrapartum fetal monitoring is correct?

a. Dependable monitoring requires electronic detecting and recording devices.
b. Internal monitoring of heart rate requires a spiral electrode to be propelled through the fetal skin.
c. Intrauterine pressure measurement equipment presents a potential risk to the placenta.
d. External monitoring of uterine pressure and fetal heart rate is less precise than internal monitoring.

14–71. Centrally located electronic display units assure optimal intrapartum fetal monitoring and maternal surveillance.

a. True
b. False

Instructions for Items 14–72 to 14–74: Match the baseline fetal heart rate with the appropriate description.

a. Marked bradycardia
b. Mild bradycardia
c. Normal
d. Mild tachycardia
e. Marked tachycardia

14–72. 120 to 160 beats per minute
14–73. <100 beats per minute
14–74. 161 to 180 beats per minute

14–75. Periodic fetal heart rate is defined as ________.

Instructions for Items 14–76 to 14–78: Match the fetal heart rate deceleration pattern listed below with the clinical cause with which it is best associated.

a. Early (Type I)
b. Late (Type II)
c. Variable

14-76. Cord compression
14-77. Uteroplacental insufficiency
14-78. Compression of fetal head

Instructions for Items 14-79 to 14-84: Match the type of deceleration with the appropriate description.

a. Early (Type I)
b. Late (Type II)
c. Variable

14-79. Associated with vagus nerve stimulation
14-80. Corrected by administering atropine to the mother
14-81. A change in maternal position may be helpful
14-82. Potentially dangerous for the fetus
14-83. Slowing of heart at the beginning of a contraction
14-84. Slowing of heart as contraction peaks

14-85. Which of the following may result in the absence of beat-to-beat variability in fetal heart rate?

a. Prematurity
b. Fetal sleep state
c. Morphine
d. Magnesium sulfate
e. Meperidine

14-86. Which of the following statements about fetal heart rate patterns is correct?

a. A sinusoidal pattern may be due to maternal medication.
b. Mild bradycardia without acceleration or deceleration is usually associated with fetal distress.
c. Persistent tachycardia without deceleration may be due to hypoxia.
d. Fetal bradycardia may be associated with maternal hypothermia.
e. Distinguishing fetal from maternal heart rate is often difficult.
f. Fetal arrhythmias must be corrected to a normal rate and rhythm in order to assure fetal well-being.

Instructions for Items 14-87 to 14-89: Match the fetal heart rate pattern with the appropriate statement.

a. Sinusoidal
b. Persistent fetal tachycardia
c. Mild persistent fetal bradycardia
d. Severe persistent fetal bradycardia

14-87. Identified in severely anemic fetuses
14-88. Present with congenital fetal heart block
14-89. Response to maternal febrile illness

14-90. Which of the following is an integral part of fetal blood sampling?

a. Ruptured membranes
b. Ethyl Chloride spray
c. Skin incision
d. Heparinized capillary tube

Instructions for Items 14-91 to 14-93: Match the confirmed fetal blood pH with the appropriate management.

a. Observation of labor
b. Repeat pH determination in less than 30 minutes
c. Immediate delivery (abdominal or vaginal)

14-91. pH 7.10
14-92. pH 7.20
14-93. pH 7.30

14-94. Which of the following statements about fetal blood pH is correct?

a. A fall in pH is an early indication of hypoxia.
b. Fetal blood pH is appreciably influenced by maternal pH.
c. Fetal blood pH is a better indication of hypoxia than Po_2.
d. Continuous transcutaneous monitoring of fetal oxygen is a better predictor of fetal distress than pH.

14-95. What are potential direct dangers of amniotomy?

a. Fetal trauma
b. Infection
c. Cord prolapse
d. Precipitous loss of amnionic fluid
e. Hemorrhage

14-96. Which of the following is a potential danger from internal fetal monitoring?

a. Early amniotomy
b. Fetal trauma
c. Placental trauma
d. Fetal infection

14-97. External monitoring techniques are without known direct or indirect risk to mother and fetus.

a. True
b. False

14-98. In which conditions can bleeding from the site of fetal blood sampling be particularly troublesome?

a. Diabetes
b. Hypertension
c. Delivery by vacuum extractor
d. Deficiency of vitamin K-dependent coagulation factors
e. Hemophilia

14–99. Systematic clinical monitoring has in no case been shown to be as effective as electronic monitoring for ensuring fetal well-being.

a. True
b. False

15. PHYSIOLOGY OF LABOR

15–1. Oxytocin

a. Serves an active role in the initiation of labor
b. Is important in placental expulsion
c. Is important in decreasing postpartum blood loss
d. Causes postpartum contraction of the uterus
e. May act to effect milk letdown in lactating women

15–2. Which of the following argue against an active role for oxytocin in the spontaneous onset of labor?

a. Pregnancy has been reported in women with diabetes insipidus.
b. Blood levels of oxytocin do not increase until the second stage of labor.
c. Oxytocin levels in the urine of women in labor are not increased.
d. Oxytocin levels in the umbilical cord increase before the onset of labor.
e. Oxytocin treatment does not result in the development of gap junctions in the myometrium.

15–3. Oxytocin ______________ cross the placenta.

a. Does
b. Does not

15–4. Oxytocin levels remain elevated in the blood of neonates for several days.

a. True
b. False

15–5. Progesterone levels in maternal blood decrease before the initiation of labor.

a. True
b. False

15–6. When during gestation will the administration of prostaglandins to the mother initiate myometrial contractions?

a. First trimester
b. Second trimester
c. Early third trimester
d. Late third trimester

15–7. Which of the following statements about labor in sheep is correct?

a. The sheep is the experimental animal in which the biomolecular events of parturition have been defined most clearly.
b. The signal for the initiation of labor clearly comes from the fetus.
c. Intact fetal hypothalamus or pituitary glands are not necessary for the initiation of labor.
d. The earliest trigger for labor is a sharp increase in fetal cortisol production.
e. Infusion of ACTH causes premature parturition.

15–8. Which of the following statements about fetal anencephaly is correct?

a. There is an association between anencephaly and prolonged gestation.
b. Adrenal glands in an anencephalic fetus are larger than in a normal fetus.
c. The fetal zone accounts for most of the mass of the human fetal adrenal.

15–9. In the human, there is a clear-cut increase in fetal cortisol concentration before the onset of parturition.

a. True
b. False

15–10. Which of the following statements about prostaglandins and labor is correct?

a. Prostaglandins induce cervical softening and effacement.
b. Ingestion of prostaglandin synthetase inhibitors by pregnant women lengthens the time between induction and abortion in pregnancies terminated by hypertonic saline instillation.
c. Inhibitors of prostaglandin synthetase can suppress preterm labor.
d. Prostaglandin levels in amnionic fluid and maternal plasma are significantly increased during labor.

15–11. The basis of the Organ Communication System model is that the fetus signals its mother in a way that promotes accelerated formation of ______________.

15-12. Which of the following statements related to the Organ Communication System model is correct?

a. The fetus is in communication with the mother by means of the fetal membranes.
b. Premature onset of labor may be initiated by rupture, stripping, or infection of the fetal membranes.
c. Prostaglandin biosynthesis and metabolism in the fetal membranes is similar to that in other fetal tissues.
d. The only prostaglandin synthesized in the uterine decidua vera is PGE_2.

15-13. PGE_2 is ______________ (1) in the amnion and ______________ (2) in the chorion.

a. Synthesized and not metabolized
b. Synthesized and metabolized
c. Neither synthesized nor metabolized

15-14. The obligate precursor of prostaglandins of the 2-series is ______________________________.

15-15. PGDH (15-hydroxyprostaglandin dehydrogenase)

a. Catalyzes the rate-limiting step in the inactivation of prostaglandins
b. Is regulated by the concentration of phosphatidylinositol in fetal membranes
c. Is inhibited by arachidonic acid
d. Only acts on PGE_2

15-16. Which ion serves an important role in the regulation of arachidonic acid release?

15-17. Fetal kidney function and fetal urine formation appear to be important in the initiation and maintenance of labor.

a. True
b. False

Instructions for Items 15-18 to 15-19: Match the state of the uterus with the appropriate event involving calcium.

a. Uterine contraction
b. Uterine relaxation

15-18. Release of calcium from sarcoplasmic reticulum
15-19. ATP-dependent translocation of calcium to a stored form

15-20. What is the function of the myometrial extracellular matrix?

15-21. The function of gap junctions is to ____________.

15-22. Which of the following statements about myometrial gap junctions is correct?

a. Gap junctions are present in the myometrium throughout pregnancy.
b. The number of gap junctions increases during labor.
c. Gap junctions persist for 4 to 6 weeks postpartum.
d. Gap junctions are not present if labor is induced or premature.
e. Progesterone prevents the formation of gap junctions.
f. All prostanoids stimulate gap junction formation.
g. Estrogen promotes the formation of gap junctions.

15-23. Which of the following statements about uterine smooth muscle contraction is correct?

a. The protein of primary importance in muscle contraction is myosin.
b. The "head" portion of the myosin molecule controls its interaction with actin.
c. Calcium ion is required for muscle contraction.
d. The interaction of actin and myosin requires the dephosphorylation of myosin light chains.
e. Contraction is initiated through the interaction of phosphorylated myosin and actin.

15-24. The association of the calcium-dependent regulatory protein ______________ with myosin light chain kinase is mandatory for enzyme activity.

15-25. Cervical ripening is associated with which of the following events?

a. Collagen breakdown
b. Smooth muscle hypertrophy
c. Alteration in the relative amounts of glycosaminoglycans
d. Randomization of smooth muscle bundles
e. Altered capacity of the tissue to retain water

15-26. Which of the following prostanoids act to induce the maturational changes of cervical ripening?

a. PGE_2
b. $PGF_{2\alpha}$
c. Prostacyclin

15-27. The hormone that appears to be most closely related to accelerated prostaglandin synthesis is

a. Estrogen
b. Progesterone
c. Relaxin

15–28. Complete the following table which describes the stages of labor.

Stage	Begins When:	Ends When:
First	______ (a)	______ (b)
Second	______ (c)	______ (d)
Third	______ (e)	______ (f)

Instructions for Items 15–29 to 15–30: Match the stage of labor with the appropriate events.

a. Prelabor
b. Latent phase

15–29. Infrequent, irregular uterine contractions; precedes labor by several hours.

15–30. Increased uterine activity; precedes labor by several weeks

15–31. The time immediately after delivery of the placenta when uterine contractions are assisting hemostasis by contracting about the spiral arteries (arterioles) beneath the placental bed is defined as the ______________________________.

15–32. Ripening of the cervix occurs during the ______________ of labor.

a. Prelabor phase
b. First stage
c. Second stage
d. Third stage
e. Fourth stage

15–33. Which of the following statements about "lightening" is correct?

a. Change in abdominal shape may occur several weeks before the onset of labor.
b. Fundal height decreases at this time.
c. It is described by the mother as "the baby dropped."
d. It is due to fetal descent and development of the lower uterine segment.
e. It is due to an increase in the volume of amnionic fluid.

Instructions for Items 15–34 to 15–35: Match the type of labor with the appropriate description.

a. True labor
b. False labor

15–34. Discomfort mostly in lower abdomen and groin
15–35. Discomfort begins in the fundal region and radiates to the lower back

15–36. False labor

a. Is more common in nulliparous women
b. May proceed directly to true labor
c. May occur at any time during pregnancy
d. Contributes to cervical dilation
e. Is the only time infrequent, short-lived, yet uncomfortable contractions occur

15–37. Discharge of a small amount of blood-tinged mucus from the vagina prior to labor is called _____.

15–38. Which of the following statements about uterine contractions is correct?

a. The cause of the pain of uterine contractions during labor is unclear.
b. Uterine contractions are involuntary.
c. Uterine contractions are unaffected by epidural anesthesia.
d. Uterine contractions in paraplegic women are painless.
e. Pacemaker sites for contractions appear to be in the lower uterine segment.

15–39. Enhancement of myometrial activity by manual stretching of the cervix is referred to as the ________.

15–40. Uterine contractions

a. Are enhanced by cervical stretching
b. Occur about 1 minute apart during the second stage of labor
c. Average about 1 minute in length during the active phase of labor
d. Vary in intensity

15–41. Periods of uterine relaxation between contractions are necessary to prevent development of fetal hypoxia.

a. True
b. False

15–42. During labor, the upper uterine segment ________ (1) and the lower uterine segment ______ (2).

a. Thins
b. Thickens

Instructions for Items 15–43 to 15–50: Match the segment of the uterus with the appropriate characteristics.

a. Upper uterine segment
b. Lower uterine segment

15–43. Develops gradually during pregnancy
15–44. Actively contracts
15–45. Retracts during labor
15–46. Distends during labor
15–47. Myometrial fibers progressively shorten during labor

15-48. Myometrial fibers progressively lengthen during labor
15-49. Uterine corpus
15-50. Uterine isthmus

15-51. In cases of obstructed labor, the ring marking the boundary between the upper and lower uterine segments becomes very prominent. In extreme cases it is termed the ______________.

15-52. In normal labor, the uterine contractions in the lower uterine segment are shorter and less intense than the contractions in the upper uterine segment.

a. True
b. False

15-53. During early labor, each contraction ______ (1) the horizontal diameter of the uterus and ______ (2) the uterine length.

a. Increases
b. Decreases

15-54. A voluntary increase in intraabdominal pressure—"pushing"—is useful during which stage of labor?

a. First stage
b. Second stage
c. Third stage
d. Fourth stage

15-55. The work involved in labor is close to the functional capacity of the normal woman.

a. True
b. False

15-56. The process by which the cervical canal shortens and the internal os is drawn up to become part of the lower uterine segment is known as ______.

15-57. Which of the following statements about labor is correct?

a. The cervix must dilate to 10 cm to allow the head of the average term fetus to pass.
b. Early rupture of the fetal membranes invariably retards cervical dilation.
c. More fetal descent occurs during cervical effacement than during dilation.
d. During the second stage of labor, descent of the fetal presenting part may be very rapid in multiparas.

15-58. What two elements are considered by Friedman to be most useful in assessing the progression of labor?

Instructions for Items 15-59 to 15-62: Match the phase of cervical dilation with the appropriate statement.

a. Latent phase
b. Active phase

15-59. May be prolonged by sedation
15-60. Subdivided into an acceleration phase, phase of maximum slope, and deceleration phase
15-61. Duration has little bearing on the subsequent course of labor
15-62. Cervical dilation completed

15-63. According to Friedman, the acceleration phase is related to ______ (1), the maximum slope is related to ______ (2), and the deceleration phase is related to ______ (3).

a. Fetopelvic relationships
b. The outcome of labor
c. The "efficiency of the machine"

15-64. Engagement always precedes the onset of labor.

a. True
b. False

Instructions for Items 15-65 to 15-69: Match the functional division of labor according to Friedman with the appropriate description.

a. Preparatory
b. Dilational
c. Pelvic

15-65. Changes occur in ground substance of the cervix
15-66. Dilation is at most rapid rate
15-67. Sensitive to sedation and anesthesia
15-68. Begins with deceleration phase of cervical dilation
15-69. Includes cardinal movements of labor

15-70. If the fetal membranes remain intact until the completion of delivery, the portion covering the head of the newborn is referred to as the ______.

15-71. Place the components of the pelvic floor in correct order (from the inside proceeding outward).

a. Internal pelvic fascia
b. Subcutaneous tissue
c. Skin
d. Levator ani and coccygeus muscles
e. Subperitoneal connective tissue
f. Peritoneum
g. Superficial muscles and fascia
h. External pelvic fascia

15–72. Which of the following statements about the levator ani and its upper and lower fascial coverings is correct?

a. It fills the entire pelvic floor.
b. It consists of pelvic and iliac portions.
c. It encircles both the rectum and vagina.
d. It remains unchanged in pregnancy.
e. Contraction of the muscle acts to close the vagina.

15–73. Which of the following structures are part of the urogenital diaphragm?

a. Three fascial layers
b. Pubic vessels and nerves
c. Sphincter ani
d. Rami of clitoris
e. Bulbocavernosus muscle
f. Ischiocavernosus muscle

15–74. What is the principal change in the pelvic floor as a result of labor?

15–75. Placental separation occurs as a result of ______.

15–76. Which of the following statements about placental separation is correct?

a. The formation of a hematoma is usually the cause of placental separation.
b. The entire decidua is cast off with the placenta.
c. The membranes usually remain in situ until the separation of the placenta is nearly complete.
d. Women frequently cannot expel the placenta spontaneously.

Instructions for Items 15–77 to 15–80: Match the mechanism of placental extrusion with the appropriate statement.

a. Mechanism of Schultze (central placental expulsion)
b. Mechanism of Duncan (peripheral placental expulsion)

15–77. Most common type of placental separation
15–78. Maternal surface appears first
15–79. Fetal surface appears first
15–80. Blood does not escape externally until after placental extrusion

16. MECHANISM OF NORMAL LABOR IN THE OCCIPUT PRESENTATION

16–1. Occiput (vertex) presentations occur in about ______________ percent of all labors.

16–2. Which of the following statements about the diagnosis of occiput presentation is correct?

a. Presentation is usually first determined by abdominal examination and confirmed by vaginal exam.
b. The vertex usually enters the pelvis with the sagittal suture in the anteroposterior pelvic diameter.
c. With the fetus in the left occiput transverse (LOT) position, the fetal back is palpable in the maternal left flank.
d. In the LOT position, the anterior fontanel is in the maternal right.
e. In the LOT position, the fetal heart tones are best heard on the maternal right.

16–3. In the occiput anterior positions (LOA or ROA), the mechanism of labor is usually similar to that in the transverse positions (LOT or ROT).

a. True
b. False

16–4. Which of the following statements about the occiput posterior positions is correct?

a. Occiput posterior positions occur in approximately 40 percent of pregnancies.
b. The right occiput posterior position (ROP) is more common than the left (LOP).
c. Posterior positions are associated with a narrow forepelvis.
d. In the ROP position, the small fontanel is felt opposite the right sacroiliac synchondrosis.

16–5. Place the following cardinal movements of labor in their proper chronologic sequence.

a. Extension
b. Internal rotation
c. Flexion
d. Descent
e. Engagement
f. External rotation
g. Expulsion

16–6. Which of the following statements about the cardinal movements of labor in the occiput presentation is correct?

a. The cardinal movements of labor occur as the fetal head adapts and accommodates to the diameters of the maternal pelvis during labor.
b. The cardinal movements of labor occur separately and independently in chronologic sequence.
c. The cardinal movements of labor are independent of descent of the presenting part.
d. The cardinal movements of labor occur concomitantly with modification of the habitus of the fetus under the influence of uterine contractions.
e. As part of labor, the fetus straightens.
f. As labor progresses, the extremities become more closely applied to the body.

16–7. In most multiparous women, engagement of the fetal head usually takes place after the start of labor.

a. True
b. False

16–8. Lateral deflection of the fetal head, where the sagittal suture is deflected either posteriorly or anteriorly, is termed ________________.

16–9. If the sagittal suture approaches the sacral promontory, it is termed ____________ asynclitism.

a. Anterior
b. Posterior

16–10. Moderate degrees of asynclitism are common in normal labor.

a. True
b. False

16–11. Descent is brought about by which of the following forces?

a. Pressure of the amnionic fluid
b. Direct pressure of the fundus upon the breech
c. Contraction of the abdominal muscles
d. Extension and straightening of the fetal body

16–12. As flexion occurs, the shorter suboccipitobregmatic diameter is substituted for the longer ____________ diameter.

16–13. Internal rotation is usually not accomplished until the head has reached the level of the ________.

16–14. Which of the following statements about the cardinal movements of labor in the occiput anterior position is correct?

a. Extension brings the base of the occiput into direct contact with the inferior margin of the symphysis pubis.
b. Immediately after its birth, the head drops downward.
c. The delivered head returns to the oblique position.
d. Restitution is followed by completion of external rotation to the transverse position.
e. The posterior shoulder is delivered before the anterior shoulder.

16–15. Transverse arrest and persistent occiput posterior position represent deviations from the normal mechanism of labor.

a. True
b. False

16–16. Which of the following statements about changes in the shape of the fetal head is correct?

a. Swelling of the fetal scalp that develops during labor is known as caput succedaneum.
b. Caput may be extensive enough to prevent differentiation of anatomic landmarks on the fetal head.
c. In molding, the margins of the occipital bone may be pushed under those of the parietal bone.
d. Molding may account for a diminution in the biparietal diameter.

17. CONDUCT OF NORMAL LABOR AND DELIVERY

17–1. Which of the following are elements of natural childbirth?

a. Elimination of fear
b. Elimination of pain
c. Antepartum education
d. Exercises to promote relaxation
e. Elimination of anesthetics

Instructions for Items 17–2 to 17–6: Select the characteristics of the contractions of true or false labor.

a. True labor
b. False labor

17–2. Occur at irregular intervals
17–3. Cervix dilates

17–4. Not stopped by sedation
17–5. Intensity remains the same
17–6. Discomfort mostly in the lower abdomen

17–7. A woman should be told to be sure she is in true labor before reporting to her health care provider.

a. True
b. False

17–8. Questions that should be a routine part of the basic admission procedures for a woman in labor include

a. Frequency of uterine contractions
b. Intensity of uterine contractions
c. Time when uterine contractions became uncomfortable
d. Degree and quality of uterine contraction discomfort
e. Whether fluid has leaked from the vagina
f. Whether there has been bleeding from the vagina

17–9. The best way to ascertain the significance of vaginal bleeding in late pregnancy is a pelvic examination at the time of admission to the labor area.

a. True
b. False

17–10. Which statements about the initial vaginal examination during labor are correct?

a. If bleeding greater than a bloody show is present, the examination must be done with a sterile speculum.
b. A sterile speculum examination always precedes the digital examination.
c. The cervix is examined for softness, position, dilation, and effacement.
d. The presenting part and station should be ascertained.
e. X-ray pelvimetry to evaluate pelvic architecture should be obtained as early in labor as possible.
f. Distensibility of the vagina and firmness of the perineum should be assessed.

17–11. If the cervix is one-fourth of its original length, it is ______________ effaced.

a. 25 percent
b. 50 percent
c. 75 percent
d. 100 percent

17–12. The cervix is fully dilated when it has opened about ______________ cm.

a. 8
b. 9
c. 10
d. 11

17–13. Which of the possible positions of the cervix is suggestive of premature labor?

a. Anterior
b. Midposition
c. Posterior

17–14. Which of the following statements about the evaluation of station is correct?

a. It identifies the level of the presenting part in the birth canal.
b. If the presenting part is at the level of the ischial spines, it is at 0 station.
c. Progressive dilation of the cervix without a change of station implies fetopelvic disproportion.
d. If the vertex is at 0 station, it is certain that engagement of the fetal head has occurred.

17–15. If the presenting part is located two-thirds of the distance from the plane of the pelvic inlet to the midplane of the pelvis, its station is said to be

a. −3
b. −2
c. −1
d. 0
e. +1
f. +2
g. +3

17–16. Which of the following make rupture of the membranes a significant occurrence?

a. Risk of infection
b. Imminent onset of labor
c. Risk of cord prolapse
d. Risk of maternal hypovolemia

17–17. The normal pH of vaginal fluid is about ______________ (1), whereas that of amnionic fluid is usually ______________ (2).

17–18. Which of the following statements about rupture of the membranes is correct?

a. No test for detection of rupture of the membranes is completely reliable.
b. Amnionic fluid is more acidic than vaginal secretions.
c. Nitrazine paper turns blue if in contact with amnionic fluid.
d. The nitrazine test may provide a falsely positive reading if there is excessive bloody show.

17–19. Which of the following statements about the care of a woman in labor is correct?

a. Shaving of the perineum is necessary for hygiene.
b. For the fetus, rectal examinations are considerably safer than vaginal examinations.
c. Enemas are recommended to stimulate labor.
d. The hematocrit or hemoglobin concentration should be rechecked on admission.

17-20. Since the average duration of the first stage of labor is 8 hours in the nullipara and 5 hours in the multipara, a woman in the first stage of labor may be given reasonably accurate assurances as to the time of delivery.

a. True
b. False

17-21. Which of the following statements about monitoring fetal heart rate during labor is correct?

a. All women must be electronically monitored during labor.
b. Ominous fetal heart rates are best heard during the maximal intensity of a contraction.
c. Fetal distress is suspected if the fetal heart rate is less than 120 beats per minute.
d. Maternal tachycardia may be misinterpreted as a normal fetal heart rate.

17-22. Which statements about the management of labor are correct?

a. Intensity of uterine contractions may be gauged manually.
b. Trained labor room personnel can provide care that may lead to outcomes as good as with electronic monitoring.
c. The patient must not be allowed to lie in the supine position.
d. After the initial examination, the next vaginal examination should be performed when the patient feels the urge to push.
e. Maternal vital signs may vary relative to a contraction.

17-23. Which of the following contribute to the decision to administer analgesia in labor?

a. Degree of discomfort
b. Amount of cervical dilation
c. Pattern of labor
d. Estimated interval of time until delivery

17-24. Which of the following statements about amniotomy is correct?

a. Amniotomy will significantly shorten the first stage of labor.
b. Amniotomy is beneficial to the fetus.
c. Aseptic technique is required.
d. Care must be taken not to dislodge the fetal head from the pelvis.
e. Amniotomy is hazardous to maternal health.

17-25. Which of the following statements about nutrition in labor is correct?

a. Gastric emptying time is reduced during labor.
b. Intravenous fluids should be initiated upon admission to the hospital.
c. Fluids should be minimized in order to reduce urine production.
d. Food and oral fluids should be withheld during active labor.

17-26. Which of the following statements about urinary bladder function in labor is correct?

a. Bladder distention can obstruct labor.
b. A woman in labor is unable to void without catheterization.
c. All women should have an indwelling bladder catheter.
d. Bladder hypotonia and infection may be sequelae of overdistention.

17-27. How may the second stage of labor be characterized?

a. Full dilation of the cervix
b. Urge to defecate
c. Contractions lasting about 90 seconds
d. No more than 1 minute of myometrial relaxation between contractions

17-28. For all term singleton pregnancies, the second stage of labor lasts between 20 and 50 minutes.

a. True
b. False

17-29. Which of the following statements about fetal heart rate in the second stage of labor is correct?

a. The fetal heart rate should be identified more frequently than during the first stage.
b. Slowing of the fetal heart rate is due solely to fetal head compression.
c. Reduction of uterine volume due to fetal descent may trigger premature placental separation.
d. Blood flow through the umbilical cord may be compromised as loops of cord tighten around the fetus.
e. Failure of the fetal heart rate to recover between uterine contractions is abnormal.

17-30. During the second state of labor,

a. The desire to bear down is reflex and spontaneous
b. The woman should be coached to "push" as much as possible regardless of the duration of the contraction
c. Expulsion of feces indicates imminent delivery
d. The mother should be informed of the progress of labor

17–31. The most common position used for vaginal delivery is the ________________.

17–32. Leg cramping during delivery may occur as a result of pressure on pelvic nerves, and requires no action beyond reassurance to the mother.

a. True
b. False

17–33. Which of the following measures assures a noninfected outcome after vaginal delivery?

a. Use of scrub suit, mask, and hat
b. Perineal scrubbing
c. Sterile drapes
d. Sterile gloves
e. Careful hand washing

17–34. The encirclement of the largest diameter of the fetal head by the vulvar ring is known as ________.

17–35. Which statements about the delivery of the fetal head are correct?

a. The vulvovaginal opening may become smaller between contractions.
b. As the perineum thins, the anterior wall of the rectum may become visible through the anus.
c. A properly timed episiotomy can prevent the long-term sequelae of pelvic relaxation.

17–36. The obstetric maneuver by which the physician facilitates delivery of the head is called the ________.

17–37. What should always be done prior to delivery of the fetal shoulders?

a. Wipe face
b. Aspirate nares
c. Aspirate mouth
d. Check for nuchal cord

17–38. Which of the following statements about the delivery of the fetal shoulders is correct?

a. In most cases the shoulders are born spontaneously.
b. Any traction should be directed in the long axis of the fetus.
c. Delivery of the shoulders occurs when they are in the transverse diameter of the pelvis.
d. Hooking a finger in the axillae should be done to deliver the anterior shoulder only.
e. Gushing of amnionic fluid tinged with blood after delivery of the infant is an ominous sign.

17–39. Direct causes of fetal nerve injury during delivery include

a. Traction in the axillae
b. Oblique traction to the fetal head
c. Pressure on the uterine fundus
d. Poorly timed episiotomy

17–40. Which of the following statements about the management of the placenta and umbilical cord at delivery is correct?

a. Nuchal cord occurs in about 55 percent of cases.
b. If a nuchal cord cannot be slipped over the baby's head, it may be clamped and cut provided the infant is delivered promptly thereafter.
c. After delivery of the baby, the cord should usually be clamped within about 1 cm of the baby's abdomen.
d. If the infant is placed at the level of the vaginal introitus or below before the cord is clamped, blood will be shifted from the placenta to the infant (infant transfusion).
e. Infant transfusion should be avoided as the circulatory overload is always dangerous to the infant.
f. Neonatal hyperbilirubinemia may result from infant transfusion.

17–41. Which of the following is a sign of placental separation?

a. The uterus becomes globular and usually firmer.
b. A sudden gush of blood occurs in many cases.
c. A sudden transient drop in maternal blood pressure and rise in pulse rate occurs.
d. The uterus rises in the abdomen.
e. The umbilical cord protrudes farther out of the vaginal opening.
f. A significant decrease in uterine pain occurs.

17–42. Which of the following is a correct statement about the management of the third stage of labor?

a. Signs of placental separation usually appear within 1 to 5 minutes after delivery of the baby.
b. As long as the uterus remains firm and there is no unusual bleeding, watchful waiting for spontaneous placental separation is usually acceptable practice.
c. During placental separation and delivery, abdominal palpation of the uterus is indicated to be sure that the uterus is contracting and remaining firm.
d. Placental expulsion should be hastened by traction on the umbilical cord.
e. The placenta and membranes should be examined immediately after their delivery to ascertain their completeness.

17–43. Attempts to express the placenta prior to placental separation may result in ________________.

17–44. If there is brisk bleeding and the placenta cannot be expressed, manual removal is indicated.

a. True
b. False

17–45. Routine manual removal of the placenta has proven safe only under which of the following circumstances?

a. A minimal number of vaginal examinations during labor
b. A multiparous patient
c. A properly prepared and draped perineum
d. A delivery uncomplicated by bacterial contamination of the genital tract
e. Satisfactory anesthesia

17–46. Following delivery of the placenta, which of the following should occur?

a. Inspection of the placenta, membranes, and cord
b. Administration of oxytocics
c. Frequent monitoring for uterine atony
d. Frequent inspection of the perineum for excessive bleeding

17–47. The primary mechanism by which hemostasis is achieved at the placental site is ________________.

17–48. Which of the following is an oxytocic commonly used in the third or fourth stage of labor?

a. Oxytocin
b. Ergonovine maleate
c. Epinephrine
d. Methylergonovine maleate

17–49. Which of the following statements about oxytocin is correct?

a. It is a naturally occurring decapeptide.
b. The half-life for intravenously infused oxytocin is about 3 minutes.
c. Oxytocin may cause postpartum uterine rupture.
d. It is effective if given by mouth, intravenously, or intramuscularly.
e. If given as a large intravenous bolus, it may cause maternal hypotension.
f. It may cause water intoxication if administered in a large volume of electrolyte-free IV solution.

17–50. Which of the following are characteristics of ergonovine and methylergonovine?

a. They stimulate myometrial contractions.
b. They can be administered intravenously, intramuscularly, or orally.
c. Parenteral administration can initiate transient hypertension.
d. They are dangerous to the fetus if administered before delivery.
e. The effects of these drugs may persist for hours.

17–51. What is a potential danger of oxytocin administration prior to delivery of the placenta?

Instructions for Items 17–52 to 17–55: Match the degree of laceration with the affected anatomy.

a. First degree
b. Second degree
c. Third degree
d. Fourth degree

17–52. Fascia and muscles of the perineal body
17–53. Anal sphincter
17–54. Vaginal mucous membrane and perineal skin
17–55. Rectal mucosa

17–56. Episiotomy

a. Substitutes a neat, straight surgical incision for a ragged laceration of the perineum and vagina
b. Is easier to repair, heals better, and is less painful than a birth canal laceration
c. Provides additional room for difficult deliveries (large babies, forceps deliveries, the breech)
d. Is commonly performed when the head is visible to a diameter of 3 to 4 cm during a contraction
e. Is commonly repaired after delivery of the placenta

Instructions for Items 17–57 to 17–63: Match the statement to the type of episiotomy with which it is best associated.

a. Median (midline)
b. Mediolateral

17–57. Less painful in puerperium
17–58. Blood loss greater
17–59. Extension through the anal sphincter is uncommon
17–60. Faulty healing is rare
17–61. Possibility of a fourth degree extension greater with forceps delivery
17–62. More difficult to repair
17–63. Type most frequently performed

17–64. What are the two essentials for success in episiotomy repair?

17–65. Which of the following are helpful measures in caring for the routine adjunctive second degree episiotomy?

a. Prophylactic antibiotics
b. Enemas
c. Stool softeners
d. Ice packs
e. Heat lamp
f. Local anesthetics

17–66. What are the conditions that may cause persistent severe pain after episiotomy?

18. ANALGESIA AND ANESTHESIA

18–1. Which of the following distinguishes obstetric from surgical anesthesia?

a. Number of patients to consider
b. Absolute necessity of utilizing anesthesia
c. Duration of anesthesia
d. Preoperative time to prepare the patient

18–2. Which of the following statements about the general principles of obstetric analgesia and anesthesia is correct?

a. The proper psychological management of the mother throughout the antepartum period and labor is of great importance in successful analgesia.
b. Maintenance of satisfactory fetal oxygenation is essential for safe obstetric pain relief.
c. Obstetric pain relief requires close supervision of the laboring woman.
d. Whatever agents are used must have little or no deleterious effect upon uterine contractions or maternal voluntary expulsive forces.
e. Constant attention to the status of both mother and unborn child are basic to safe obstetric analgesia and anesthesia.

18–3. Which of the following statements about meperidine for analgesia is correct?

a. A dose of 50 to 100 mg is recommended.
b. Intramuscular doses may be administered every 3 to 4 hours.
c. Larger doses administered less frequently are preferable to small doses given more often.
d. Maximal analgesia occurs 45 minutes after an intravenous dose.
e. Meperidine in doses utilized for analgesia may prolong labor by decreasing the effectiveness of uterine contractions.

18–4. Which of the narcotics and tranquilizers used for analgesia during labor do not reach the fetus?

18–5. What is the drug of choice for treating narcotic depression in the newborn?

a. Naloxone hydrochloride (Narcan)
b. Levallorphan (Lorfan)
c. Nalorphine (Nalline)
d. Phenergan

18–6. Which of the following statements about Narcan (naloxone hydrochloride) is correct?

a. It displaces the narcotic from receptors in the central nervous system.
b. It does not inhibit the analgesic effects of narcotics.
c. It does not inhibit narcotic-related euphoria.
d. It may precipitate withdrawal symptoms in the physically dependent.
e. An intravenous dose acts within 2 minutes.
f. A single dose is sufficient to treat either mother or newborn.

18–7. Which of the following statements about general anesthesia is correct?

a. The placenta is a selective barrier for some anesthetic agents.
b. Fasting before anesthesia is an effective safeguard against aspiration.
c. Endotracheal intubation minimizes the risk of aspiration.
d. The concentration of inhalation anesthetic increases more rapidly in the lungs of pregnant women than in nonpregnant women.

18–8. Nitrous oxide

a. May be used during both labor and delivery
b. Provides true anesthesia
c. Does not interfere with uterine contractions
d. Should not be used in concentrations higher than 70 percent
e. Use requires the close supervision of qualified personnel

18–9. Which of the following volatile anesthetics does not cross the placenta and potentially cause fetal narcosis?

a. Ether
b. Halothane (Fluothane)
c. Methoxyflurane (Penthrane)
d. Enflurane (Ethrane)

Instructions for Items 18–10 to 18–12: Match the volatile anesthetic with the appropriate description.

a. Ether
b. Halothane
c. Methoxyflurane
d. Enflurane

18–10. Causes uterine relaxation
18–11. Nephrotoxic
18–12. Hypotensive effect

18–13. Which of the following is an advantage of intravenous thiopental?

a. Rapid induction
b. Allows for ample oxygenation
c. Controllability
d. Minimal association with postpartum bleeding
e. Prompt recovery without vomiting

18–14. Thiopental

a. Is an excellent analgesic agent
b. Is best used as the sole anesthetic agent
c. Is commonly used to induce general anesthesia
d. Is commonly used in conjunction with succinylcholine and nitrous oxide

18–15. General anesthesia always causes appreciable respiratory depression in the newborn infant.

a. True
b. False

18–16. Ketamine

a. Produces appreciable anesthesia when administered intravenously
b. May accentuate maternal hypertension
c. May cause unpleasant delirium and hallucinations
d. May cause respiratory depression in the newborn

18–17. The *most* common cause of anesthetic death in obstetrics is ______________________________.

18–18. Which of the following statements about the prevention of aspiration during general anesthesia is correct?

a. Fasting for 12 hours will rid the stomach of acidic liquid.
b. Ingestion of antacids before induction of anesthesia can reduce the acidity of gastric juice.
c. Emptying the stomach by use of a nasogastric tube is totally effective.
d. Intubation should be performed in the supine position.
e. Extubation should be performed with the patient awake and in the lateral recumbent position.

18–19. Aspiration of strongly acidic gastric juice is probably more common than aspiration of gastric contents containing particulate matter.

a. True
b. False

18–20. Which of the following statements about aspiration pneumonitis is correct?

a. If the pH of aspirated fluid is below 2.5, severe chemical pneumonitis is more likely to ensue.
b. The right lower lobe of the lung is most often involved.
c. The woman who aspirates always develops respiratory distress immediately.
d. Roentgenographic changes occur early in aspiration pneumonitis.
e. Chest x-ray alone should not be used to exclude aspiration pneumonitis.

18–21. Which of the following is of *proven* benefit in the treatment of aspiration pneumonitis?

a. Suction of the pharynx and trachea
b. Saline lavage
c. Steroids
d. Oxygen
e. Antibiotics

18–22. Which of the following statements about anesthetic gas exposure and pregnancy outcome is correct?

a. The embryo and fetus may be exposed to some danger if the pregnant woman works in an operating room.
b. The congenital malformation rate is markedly higher in children of women who work in operating rooms.
c. The midtrimester abortion rate is markedly higher for women who work in an operating room.
d. Women chronically exposed to anesthetic gases should be advised to stop working as soon as pregnancy is confirmed.

18–23. Which of the following statements about the innervation of the uterus is correct?

a. Visceral sensory fibers from the uterus, cervix, and upper vagina travel to the pelvic plexus via Frankenhaüser's ganglion.
b. Sensory fibers enter the spinal cord in association with the 10th, 11th, and 12th thoracic and 1st lumbar nerves.
c. Motor pathways to the uterus leave the spinal cord at the level of the seventh and eighth thoracic vertebrae.
d. Only sensory blocks that do not block motor pathways should be used for analgesia during labor.

18–24. The pudendal nerve provides sensory innervation for the

a. Perineum
b. Anus
c. Medial and inferior parts of the vulva and clitoris
d. Superior parts of the vulva and clitoris
e. Upper vagina

18–25. The sensory nerve fibers of the pudendal nerve are derived from the ventral branches of the _______________ nerves.

18–26. Which of the following statements about central nervous system toxicity induced by agents used to produce local or regional anesthesia and analgesia is correct?

a. Symptoms are limited to convulsions and loss of consciousness.
b. Immediate management includes airway control (with intubation if needed) and oxygenation.
c. Succinylcholine may be used to abolish peripheral neural manifestations.
d. Thiopental may be used as a central inhibitor of convulsions.
e. Diazepam may be used as a central inhibitor of convulsions.
f. Rapid fluid administration, intravenous ephedrine, and placement on the left side are useful to treat hypotension associated with CNS toxicity reactions.
g. In cases of convulsions, the fetus should be delivered immediately by cesarean section.

18–27. Local infiltration of the genital tract with anesthetics is useful

a. For analgesia during labor
b. Before episiotomy and delivery
c. After delivery for episiotomy repair
d. For inspection of the genital tract after delivery
e. For its relative safety
f. For its immediate effectiveness

18–28. Which of the following statements about pudendal block is correct?

a. After needle placement, aspiration is always attempted to avoid intravenous injection of local anesthetic.
b. Injection is made at the site where the pudendal nerve passes adjacent to the sacrospinous ligament.
c. Pudendal block is usually effective within 3 to 4 minutes.
d. An anesthetic with high tissue penetration and rapid action should be utilized.
e. Before pudendal block, it is useful to infiltrate the site where episiotomy will be made.

18–29. For which types of delivery is pudendal block likely to provide adequate anesthesia?

a. Cesarean section
b. Midforceps delivery
c. Low forceps delivery
d. Spontaneous delivery

18–30. Which of the following are possible complications of pudendal block?

a. Infection
b. Hematoma formation
c. Convulsions
d. Fetal distress
e. Protracted labor

18–31. Paracervical block

a. Is useful to relieve the pain of uterine contractions
b. May need to be repeated during labor
c. Is useful for delivery
d. May cause fetal bradycardia

18–32. Which of the following statements about the use of spinal anesthesia is correct?

a. Spinal block involves the injection of local anesthetic into the subarachnoid space.
b. For vaginal and cesarean deliveries, block at the level of tenth thoracic dermatome (T10) is appropriate.
c. For vaginal deliveries, the anesthetic should not be administered until the cervix is fully dilated and all other requirements for delivery are completed.
d. A somewhat larger dose of anesthetic is utilized for cesarean deliveries than for vaginal deliveries.
e. Spinal block may be utilized for pain relief during labor.

18–33. Which of the following are possible complications of spinal anesthesia?

a. Hypotension
b. Respiratory paralysis
c. Anxiety
d. Headache
e. Bladder dysfunction
f. Meningitis

18–34. Which of the following is effective in the prophylaxis and treatment of maternal hypotension following spinal anesthesia?

a. Uterine displacement
b. Hydration with balanced salt solution
c. Intravenous injection of ephedrine
d. Use of a small-gauge needle to administer the anesthetic

18–35. The most common cause of complete spinal blockade with respiratory paralysis is _______________.

18–36. Which of the following is useful in supplementing a spinal anesthetic that is providing inadequate analgesia?

a. Nitrous oxide
b. Morphine
c. Meperidine
d. Fentanyl

18–37. Spinal headaches are caused by _______________.

18–38. Which of the following is a *proven* preventive or treatment measure for spinal headaches?

a. Use of a small-gauge needle
b. A single puncture to administer the anesthetic
c. Supine position
d. Hyperhydration
e. Blood patch
f. Saline patch
g. Abdominal binder

18–39. Hypertension from ergot medication is most common in women who have received spinal or epidural block.

a. True
b. False

18–40. List the *major* maternal contraindications to spinal anesthesia.

18–41. Which of the following statements about epidural (peridural) block is correct?

a. Epidural block may be used to provide both analgesia and anesthesia for labor and anesthesia for delivery.
b. Block from T10 to S5 is indicated for analgesia and anesthesia in vaginal delivery.
c. Block from T8 to S1 is indicated for anesthesia in abdominal delivery.
d. The spread of epidural anesthesia depends only on the location of the injection site.
e. Epidural block is usually made through a thoracic level injection.

18–42. Which of the following is a potential complication of epidural anesthesia?

a. Inadvertent spinal anesthesia
b. Ineffective anesthesia
c. Hypotension
d. Central nervous system stimulation
e. Depression of uterine activity

18–43. There is likely to be an increased incidence of midforceps deliveries in patients given epidural anesthesia.

a. True
b. False

18–44. List the *major* maternal contraindications to the use of epidural block.

18–45. The Lamaze-prepared woman never needs either conduction anesthesia or narcotic analgesia.

a. True
b. False

19. THE PUERPERIUM

19–1. The puerperium is commonly defined as the time from the birth of an infant to the beginning of the first postpartum menstrual period.

a. True
b. False

Instructions for Items 19–2 to 19–7: Match the time after delivery with the appropriate events.

a. Just after delivery
b. 1 day after delivery
c. 2 days after delivery
d. 3 to 5 days after delivery
e. 1 week after delivery
f. 2 weeks after delivery
g. 3 weeks after delivery
h. 4 weeks after delivery
i. 6 weeks after delivery

19–2. The fundus of the uterus is about midway between the umbilicus and the symphysis
19–3. The uterus has descended into the true pelvis
19–4. The uterus has regained its nonpregnant size
19–5. The uterus weighs about 1 kg
19–6. The uterus weighs about 500 g
19–7. The uterus weighs about 300 g

19–8. Which of the following statements about involution of the uterus is correct?

a. Immediately after expulsion of the placenta, the fundus is palpable just above the pubic symphysis.
b. The uterus reaches its nonpregnant weight within 2 weeks.
c. Due to involution, the uterus at 1 week postpartum weighs one-half what it did just after delivery.
d. The connective tissue framework of the uterus undergoes rapid involution after delivery.

19-9. During involution, the total number of myometrial cells ________ (1) and the size of an individual myometrial cell ________ (2).

a. Increases
b. Remains the same
c. Decreases

19-10. How long does it take for the entire endometrium to be regenerated after delivery?

a. 1 week
b. 2 weeks
c. 3 weeks
d. 4 weeks
e. 6 weeks

19-11. Incomplete extrusion of the placental site may result in what clinical problem?

19-12. Which of the following statements about involution of the placental site is correct?

a. The process may take up to 6 weeks.
b. An intermediate step in involution is thrombus formation.
c. The final step in involution is absorption in situ.
d. Each pregnancy leaves a fibrous scar in the endometrium.

19-13. During the puerperium, the blood vessels leading to and from the uterus as well as the vessels within the uterus return to their prepregnant state, such that no vestiges of a previous pregnancy can be identified.

a. True
b. False

19-14. Which of the following return to their prepregnant condition (size or appearance) after delivery?

a. Cervix
b. Lower uterine segment
c. Vagina
d. Hymen
e. Abdominal wall

19-15. Which of the following statements about the puerperal abdominal wall is correct?

a. It takes several weeks for the abdominal wall to return to normal.
b. Exercise does not aid the recovery of the abdominal wall.
c. Striae may be eliminated with hormonal salves.
d. Diastasis recti may persist.

19-16. Which of the following statements about the urinary tract during the puerperium is correct?

a. The postpartum bladder is often hyperemic and edematous.
b. The puerperal bladder has an increased capacity.
c. After an uncomplicated delivery, the puerperal urinary tract is at relatively low risk for the development of infection.
d. Physiologic and anatomic changes occurring in an uncomplicated pregnancy are not permanent.

19-17. Which of the following statements about breast development is correct?

a. Mammary gland anlagen are contained in the ectodermal ridges that form on the ventral surface of the embryo.
b. Normally only one pair of breast buds develops.
c. The fetal mammary buds begin to grow and divide near term.
d. Thelarche is due to progesterone stimulation.
e. The constituents of milk are synthesized in the alveolar epithelium.

19-18. Colostrum has more ________ than mature milk.

a. Protein
b. Fat
c. Sugar
d. Minerals

19-19. Which of the following statements about colostrum is correct?

a. Colostrum is secreted during the first 2 postpartum days.
b. Colostrum contains immunoglobulin A which may help protect the newborn against enteric infection.
c. Colostrum contains no vitamins.
d. The colostrum corpuscles are large fat globules of uncertain origin.

19-20. Which of the following statements about human milk is correct?

a. Milk is isotonic with plasma.
b. Most proteins in milk are not found elsewhere.
c. All vitamins except vitamin K are present in human milk.
d. Increasing maternal iron stores increases the amount of iron in breast milk.
e. The mammary gland concentrates iodine, which appears in breast milk.

19–21. Which of the following appear to help stimulate growth and development of the milk-secreting apparatus of the mammary gland?

a. Estrogen
b. Progesterone
c. Cortisol
d. Prolactin
e. Insulin
f. Placental lactogen

19–22. A decrease in the level of which two hormones serves to initiate lactation?

19–23. Which of the following statements concerning lactation is correct?

a. Prolactin is essential for lactation.
b. Suckling triggers a rise in prolactin.
c. Suckling stimulates the neurohypophysis to release oxytocin.
d. Expression of milk is due to contractions of myoepithelial cells in the breast alveoli.
e. Milk letdown may be inhibited by stress.

19–24. Which statements concerning breast milk and immunology are correct?

a. The antibodies present in human colostrum and milk are poorly absorbed from the infant's gut.
b. The predominant immunoglobulin in milk is IgA.
c. Breast milk contains IgA against *E. coli.*
d. Human milk has T but no B lymphocytes.
e. There are greater amounts of protective factors in the milk of older women.

19–25. Which of the following statements about breast feeding is correct?

a. The frequency of breast feeding among women in the United States is greater now than 25 years ago.
b. Nursing accelerates uterine involution.
c. If a woman's milk supply is insufficient at first, even with suckling it will not become sufficient later.
d. Drugs are secreted in milk at higher concentration than they are present in maternal plasma.

19–26. What factors are associated with more severe afterpains?

a. Primiparity
b. Retained placental fragments
c. Breast feeding
d. Forceps delivery
e. Blood clots in the uterus

19–27. Which of the following are contained in lochia?

a. Erythrocytes
b. Microorganisms
c. Shreds of decidua
d. Epithelial cells

19–28. Which of the following statements about lochia is correct?

a. Lochia rubra precedes lochia alba.
b. Foul-smelling lochia proves that infection is present.
c. Women who receive methylergonovine maleate are likely to lose less blood postpartum.
d. The amount of lochia is the same in women who received methylergonovine maleate in the immediate puerperium and those who did not.
e. Lochia rubra that lasts longer than 2 weeks is abnormal.

19–29. Which of the following statements about urine production in the puerperium is correct?

a. Postpartum diuresis occurs even if intravenous fluids were not vigorously infused intrapartum.
b. Preeclampsia may be the cause of increased postpartum diuresis.
c. Marked glycosuria is not uncommon in the puerperium.
d. Acetone in the urine is abnormal even after a long labor.

19–30. Which of the following statements about clinical aspects of the puerperium is correct?

a. Breast fever, a commonly occurring physiologic temperature elevation beginning on the 3rd or 4th day of lactation, often lasts 3 to 4 days.
b. A rise in temperature in the puerperium usually implies a maternal infection, most likely somewhere in the genitourinary tract.
c. Afterpains usually decrease in intensity by the 3rd day after delivery.
d. Puerperal diuresis is common in the 2nd to 5th postpartum days.
e. A blood leukocyte count in the puerperium of greater than 12,000 per microliter is always indicative of maternal infection.

19–31. Which are normal findings in the blood during the 1st postpartum week?

a. Leukocytosis
b. Relative lymphopenia
c. Marked anemia
d. Elevated sedimentation rate
e. Decreased fibrinogen

19–32. There is significant weight loss during the puerperium that cannot be attributed to the involution of the uterus and normal blood loss.

a. True
b. False

19–33. Which of the following statements about the care of the mother immediately postpartum is correct?

a. As long as the fundus is firm, there is no danger of postpartum hemorrhage.
b. Progressive uterine enlargement may be an indication of bleeding.
c. During the immediate postpartum period, the vulva should be cleansed after each bowel movement and before any local treatment or examination.
d. The episiotomy should be nearly asymptomatic by the end of the 3rd week.
e. Perineal discomfort at the episiotomy site that is unresponsive to local analgesics may indicate that a hematoma has formed.

19–34. The presence of which factors involved in postpartum depression warrant immediate psychiatric intervention?

a. Emotional letdown
b. Pain
c. Fatigue
d. Anxiety
e. Fears of loss of attractiveness

19–35. What are the benefits of early postpartum ambulation?

a. The patient feels better.
b. There is less constipation.
c. There is less chance of pulmonary emboli.
d. There is improved lactation.

19–36. Which of the following statements about the abdominal wall during the puerperium is correct?

a. An abdominal binder is usually unnecessary.
b. A girdle should be worn to help in involution.
c. Abdominal wall exercises may be started at any time after a vaginal delivery.
d. Abdominal wall exercises after cesarean section should be started after the 6-week check-up.

19–37. Which of the following dietary considerations should apply to the postpartum woman?

a. Nothing should be given by mouth for the first 12 hours.
b. Only liquids should be administered for the first 2 days.
c. Fluids should be restricted for women who do not nurse.
d. As compared to the diet of the pregnant woman, the diet of the lactating woman should be increased in calories and protein.

19–38. Which of the following factors lead to bladder overdistention during the puerperium?

a. Intravenous fluid administration
b. Cessation of oxytocin administration
c. Anesthesia
d. Pain in the pelvic region

19–39. If the bladder becomes palpable suprapubically, catheterization is indicated.

a. True
b. Falses

19–40. Which of the following may normally be expected postpartum?

a. Constipation
b. Nipple irritation
c. Nausea
d. Urinary urgency

19–41. The postpartum hospital stay does not normally exceed ______________ days.

a. 1
b. 2
c. 3
d. 4

19–42. Which statements about the return of ovulation and menstruation is correct?

a. In the nonnursing woman, menstruation usually returns within 6 to 8 weeks.
b. In lactating women, the first period occurs after the cessation of nursing.
c. Ovulation may be reestablished within 2 weeks of birth.
d. Pregnancy can occur while a woman is nursing.
e. Amenorrhea during lactation is due to lack of pituitary gonadotropin stimulation of the ovary.

19–43. Which of the following activities should be curtailed until 6 weeks postpartum?

a. Bathing
b. Household work
c. Driving
d. Coitus
e. Contraception

20. THE NEWBORN INFANT

20–1. Except for cases of hypoxic stress in utero, the infant makes its first respiratory efforts after delivery.

a. True
b. False

20–2. Which of the following statements about the initiation of air breathing is correct?

a. Soon after birth, the infant changes from an initial shallow-breathing pattern to a pattern of deeper, regular inhalations.
b. The initial breaths are especially difficult because they involve the inflation of a collapsed structure.
c. Residual alveolar fluid is cleared primarily by the pulmonary circulation and lymphatics.
d. Transient tachypnea of the newborn results from a delay in the removal of amnionic fluid from lung alveoli.
e. High negative intrathoracic pressures are required to bring about the initial entry of air into the fluid-filled alveoli.

20–3. By about the ______________ breath, the pressure-volume changes with each respiration in the normal mature infant are similar to those of the normal adult.

20–4. Closure of the ductus arteriosus is associated with the ______________ in pulmonary arterial pressure after birth.

a. Fall
b. Rise

20–5. What condition develops if there is a lack of sufficient pulmonary surfactant at the time of delivery?

20–6. Which of the following may stimulate the infant to initiate respiration?

a. Physical stimulation
b. Compression of the fetal thorax incident to delivery
c. Oxygen deprivation
d. Carbon dioxide accumulation

20–7. Babies born by cesarean section tend to have ______________ fluid in their lungs than babies born by vaginal delivery.

a. More
b. Less

20–8. Steps in the immediate care of the newborn infant include

a. Wiping the face
b. Suctioning the mouth and nares
c. Clamping and cutting the cord
d. Giving a sponge bath
e. Placing in an incubator with the head elevated

20–9. Which of the following are determinants of fetal well-being that should be considered prior to and during delivery?

a. Maternal health
b. Gestational age
c. Duration of labor
d. Duration of rupture of membranes
e. Analgesia administered to the mother
f. Duration and kind of maternal anesthesia
g. Difficulties encountered in delivery

20–10. What two methods are best utilized to determine the newborn's heart rate?

20–11. What is the minimal acceptable heart rate in the newborn?

a. 60
b. 80
c. 100
d. 120

20–12. Suctioning of the mouth and pharynx of the newborn should be performed in cases of bradycardia or infrequent respirations.

a. True
b. False

20–13. Which of the following is an effective method to stimulate breathing in the newborn?

a. Tubbing
b. Jackknifing
c. Rubbing of back
d. Slapping the soles of the feet
e. Dilation of sphincters

20–14. Which of the following may be causes of failure to establish effective respirations?

a. Fetal hypoxemia
b. Drugs given to the mother
c. Fetal immaturity
d. Upper airway obstruction
e. Pneumothorax
f. Lung abnormalities
g. Meconium aspiration
h. CNS injury

20–15. List the five signs that are used to determine the Apgar score.

20–16. Which of the following statements about the Apgar score is correct?

a. It is used to evaluate the infant at 1 and 5 minutes.
b. The maximum score that can be obtained is 10.
c. The initial Apgar score should always be determined before initiating resuscitation.
d. A low Apgar score at 5 minutes is associated with increased risk of infant mortality and morbidity.

20–17. An infant whose heart rate is 90, whose respiratory efforts are slow and irregular, who moves actively, grimaces when stimulated, and is completely pink in color would receive an Apgar score of ______.

20–18. The Apgar score of an infant who is defined as mildly to moderately depressed would be__________.

20–19. List the seven common errors in the resuscitation of the newborn.

20–20. List the four critically important components to successful newborn resuscitation.

20–21. It is not necessary to equip the site of every delivery for resuscitation as long as the necessary equipment and personnel are available within 5 minutes.

a. True
b. False

20–22. Which of the following statements about events surrounding ventilation by face mask is correct?

a. Persistent inadequate respirations lead to bradycardia and hypotonia.
b. Oxygen should be administered by mask as soon as inadequate respirations are identified.
c. The greater the pressure used through the mask, the better the infant will respond.
d. Mask ventilation should be continued for at least 30 minutes before endotracheal intubation is attempted.

20–23. Which of the following statements about the process of endotracheal intubation is correct?

a. The infant should be supine with the head level.
b. The laryngoscope is introduced through the left side of the mouth.
c. Elevation of the laryngoscope tip will expose the vocal cords.
d. The endotracheal tube is inserted through the vocal cords until the shoulder of the tube reaches the glottis.
e. The laryngoscope should be left in place as long as the endotracheal tube is being utilized.

20–24. The sources of oxygen that should be used with an endotracheal tube are __________ and __________.

Instructions for Items 20–25 to 20–27: Match the complications of endotracheal intubation with the appropriate cause.

a. Excessive positive pressure
b. Esophageal placement of endotracheal tube

20–25. Pneumothorax
20–26. Stomach expansion
20–27. Pneumomediastinum

20–28. Which of the following statements about the use of sodium bicarbonate in infant resuscitation is correct?

a. The correct dose is 1 mEq/kg.
b. Sodium bicarbonate is administered through the umbilical vein.
c. It should be used in cases of hypoxia where positive pressure oxygen does not bring a prompt response.
d. The dose of sodium bicarbonate may be repeated.
e. Effective ventilation must be continued to prevent respiratory acidosis.

20–29. A drug that can be used to correct respiratory depression caused by meperidine or other opioids is ______________________________.

20–30. Which of the following causes hypovolemia in the newborn?

a. Sepsis
b. Fetal to maternal hemorrhage
c. Placental trauma
d. Pooling of blood in the placenta due to cord compression
e. Twin-to-twin transfusion

20–31. External cardiac massage is indicated if cardiac activity was present just before birth and stops thereafter or if the heart stops after birth.

a. True
b. False

20–32. Which of the following statements about cardiac massage for resuscitation of the newborn is correct?

a. Adequate ventilation must also be established.
b. External cardiac massage is effected using two fingers to the anterior chest wall in the lower midline.
c. The rate of massage should be about 80 per minute.
d. Ten chest compressions should be alternated with each lung inflation.
e. A delay in cardiac massage may have fatal consequences.

20–33. In the resuscitation of the neonate, epinephrine should first be administered intravenously to avoid trauma to the heart with intracardiac injection tried as a last resort.

a. True
b. False

20–34. Determine the gestational age of a newborn with the following characteristics:

Sole creases	Occasional creases anterior two-thirds
Breast nodule diameter	4 mm
Scalp hair	Fine and fuzzy
Ear lobe	Some cartilage present
Testes and scrotum	Intermediate

a. 36 weeks or less
b. 37 to 38 weeks
c. 39 weeks or more

20–35. Which of the following statements about the prevention of gonorrheal ophthalmia is correct?

a. Use of a 1 percent silver nitrate solution eliminates the possibility of gonorrheal ophthalmia.
b. In all cases where it is used, silver nitrate causes a transient chemical conjunctivitis.
c. Prophylaxis with penicillin, either as an ointment or by intramuscular injection, reduces the frequency of gonorrheal ophthalmia.
d. Tetracycline ointment instilled into the newborn's eyes affords effective prophylaxis.

20–36. Which of the following statements about proper infant identification procedures is correct?

a. A system should be available at all hours.
b. It is only necessary to retain identification records until the infant leaves the hospital.
c. Fingerprints are superior to footprints because the ridges are more pronounced.
d. Close attention must be paid to technique or the prints will be unsatisfactory.

20–37. Which of the following statements about the temperature of the newborn is correct?

a. The infant's temperature drops rapidly after birth.
b. Chilling increases oxygen requirements.
c. After the 1st hour of life, the infant's temperature stabilizes and becomes less responsive to external stimuli.

20–38. Vitamin K should routinely be administered to the newborn infant.

a. True
b. False

20–39. Which of the following statements about the umbilical cord in the newborn is correct?

a. Loss of water from Wharton's jelly leads to mummification of the cord shortly after birth.
b. Separation of the cord usually occurs in the first 2 weeks of life.
c. A dressing for the cord is recommended.
d. Infection of the umbilical stump may present no physical signs.
e. Hygienic management of the cord serves to minimize the risk of neonatal tetanus.

20–40. Which of the following statements about skin care in the newborn is correct?

a. The infant should be dried promptly to eliminate heat loss due to evaporation.
b. All vernix caseosa must be removed.
c. Immediate bathing should be used to stabilize temperature.
d. The newborn infant should be handled as much as possible.

20–41. The components of meconium include

a. Intestinal tract epithelial cells
b. Epidermal cells
c. Lanugo
d. Bile pigments
e. Blood

20–42. Which of the following statements about stools in the newborn is correct?

a. For a few hours after birth, intestinal contents contain no bacteria.
b. Failure of the infant to pass meconium within the first 12 to 24 hours indicates a congenital defect such as imperforate anus.
c. After ingestion of milk, meconium is replaced by light yellow feces.
d. Stools should not have an odor until the infant is about 1 month of age.

20–43. Which of the following statements about jaundice in the newborn is correct?

a. Typically, there is hyperbilirubinemia at birth in the range of 1.8 to 2.8 mg/dl of serum.
b. About one in ten infants develop physiologic jaundice of the newborn.
c. Physiologic jaundice of the newborn always occurs before the 3rd day of life.
d. Jaundice becomes noticeable when the serum concentration of bilirubin exceeds 5 mg/dl.
e. In premature infants, jaundice is more common and usually more severe than in term infants.
f. In infants who are mature but small-for-gestational age, jaundice is more common and usually more severe than in normal-sized infants.

20–44. Which of the following factors contribute to hyperbilirubinemia in the newborn?

a. Immaturity of hepatic cells
b. Reduced production and excretion of conjugated bilirubin
c. Reabsorption of free bilirubin
d. Increased erythrocyte destruction

20–45. Weight loss in the newborn may be attributed to

a. Lack of nutriment
b. Urine production
c. Sweat production
d. Feces production

20–46. Which of the following statements about weight changes in the infant is correct?

a. Premature infants lose relatively more weight than term infants.
b. Premature infants regain weight more rapidly than term infants.
c. Healthy but small-for-gestational age infants gain weight more rapidly than premature infants.
d. The normal infant regains its birth weight by about the 10th day.
e. The average healthy infant will triple its birth weight by 6 months of age.

20–47. Which of the following statements about feeding the newborn is correct?

a. Nursing should be initiated within the first 12 hours postpartum.
b. All infants thrive best when fed every 6 hours.
c. Only one breast should be used for each feeding.
d. The proper length of each feeding depends on the quantity and availability of breast milk and on the infant's appetite.

20–48. Circumcision should be performed at the time of delivery.

a. True
b. False

20–49. Which of the following are contraindications to circumcision?

a. Prematurity
b. Neonatal illness
c. Family history of penile cancer
d. Presence of coagulation defects

21. OBSTETRIC HEMORRHAGE

21–1. Obstetric hemorrhage is most likely to be fatal for the mother when ______________.

21–2. In pregnancies complicated by bleeding during the second and third trimesters, the rates of premature delivery and perinatal mortality are at least quadrupled.

a. True
b. False

21–3. Which of the following statements about blood loss at the time of delivery is correct?

a. Postpartum hemorrhage is defined as the loss of 500 ml or more of blood.
b. About 1 out of 10 women who are delivered vaginally fulfill the criteria for postpartum hemorrhage.
c. One-half of women who undergo cesarean section fulfill the criteria for postpartum hemorrhage.
d. Blood loss at delivery may approach the amount added during pregnancy without a significant decrease in hematocrit.

21–4. The woman who develops a normal degree of pregnancy induced hypervolemia usually increases her blood volume by ______________ ml.

21–5. Life-threatening obstetric hemorrhage is confined to the third trimester of pregnancy.

a. True
b. False

21–6. List the causes of obstetric hemorrhage related to abnormal placental implantation or development.

21–7. List the causes of obstetric hemorrhage related to trauma during labor or delivery.

21–8. List the causes of obstetric hemorrhage related to uterine atony.

21–9. List the causes of obstetric hemorrhage related to small maternal blood volume.

21–10. List the causes of obstetric hemorrhage related to conditions predisposing to impaired coagulation.

21–11. The term "third trimester bleeding" is useful for distinguishing those patients who are to be managed aggressively from those to be managed conservatively.

a. True
b. False

21–12. Which of the following statements about bleeding from the placental site is correct?

a. The mechanism of hemostasis at the placental implantation site depends on intrinsic vasospasm and formation of local blood clots.
b. Hemostasis after placental separation depends on contraction of the myometrium.
c. Hemostasis at the implantation site may be hindered by large blood clots or placental fragments.
d. Postpartum hemorrhage occurs with a hypotonic uterus in the presence of normal maternal coagulation mechanisms.
e. Postpartum hemorrhage occurs with a well-contracted uterus if the blood coagulation mechanism is impaired.

21–13. Following delivery of an intact placenta, hemorrhage that persists in the presence of a contracted uterus usually indicates bleeding from lacerations of the genital tract.

a. True
b. False

21–14. Oxytocic drugs and uterine massage are ineffective in controlling hemorrhage that does not originate from a hypotonic uterus.

a. True
b. False

21–15. The presence of what three major causes of postpartum hemorrhage must be identified in cases of excessive blood loss?

21–16. Which of the following is needed in the management of obstetric hemorrhage?

a. Intravenous infusion system(s)
b. Available operating room
c. Surgical team
d. Anesthesiologist

21–17. Which techniques provide a precise measurement of the amount of blood loss in cases of obstetric hemorrhage?

a. Visual estimate
b. Vital signs
c. "Tilt test"
d. Urine flow
e. Blood volume measurements

21–18. Which of the following statements about estimating the degree of obstetric hemorrhage is correct?

a. Visual estimates of blood loss are usually low.
b. A normal blood pressure precludes the possibility of dangerous hypovolemia.
c. The "tilt test" is most useful in patients who are hypotensive when recumbent.
d. The rate of urine flow reflects renal perfusion even during the use of potent diuretics.
e. The total absence of urine flow through an indwelling catheter is an indication for diuretic therapy.

21–19. What potential harm can arise from administration of diuretics in cases of obstetric hemorrhage?

21–20. Administration of oxytocin in an isotonic electrolyte solution to a hemorrhaging woman is likely to cause severe oliguria.

a. True
b. False

21–21. Which of the following is a reason that blood volume measurements have not been widely used in cases of obstetric hemorrhage?

a. The ideal blood volume for a given woman is not known.
b. The size of the intravascular compartment changes drastically at delivery.
c. In cases of severe hemorrhage, the blood volume measurement obtained is invalid by the time it has been determined.

21–22. Which of the following statements about fluid replacement in obstetric hemorrhage is correct?

a. Lactated Ringer's is a preferred intravenous replacement solution.
b. Packed cells are more effective therapy than whole blood.
c. Urine flow should be maintained at a minimum of 30 ml per hour.
d. The hematocrit should be maintained at about 30 percent.
e. The best method to monitor central venous pressure is through a catheter in the subclavian vein.

21–23. Fresh whole blood is better for the treatment of hypovolemia than stored blood because ________.

21-24. Which of the following statements about the replacement of blood fractions is correct?

a. An adequate substitute for whole blood is packed red cells plus normal saline.
b. Infusion of large volumes of normal saline results in a drop in the colloid oncotic pressure.
c. Use of reconstituted blood increases the risk of blood-transmitted infection.
d. Infusion of many units of stored blood may result in generalized bleeding due to thrombocytopenia or low levels of Factors V and VIII.

Instructions for Items 21-25 to 21-26: Match the appropriate treatment with the problem arising from blood replacement therapy.

a. Administration of platelets from donors with same blood type as recipient
b. Administration of fresh frozen plasma

21-25. Development of thrombocytopenia after administration of stored whole blood
21-26. Low levels of Factors V and VIII after administration of stored whole blood

21-27. Which of the following coagulation factors is markedly increased in pregnancy?

a. I (fibrinogen)
b. V
c. VII
d. VIII
e. IX
f. X
g. Platelets

Instructions for Items 21-28 to 21-31: Match the clinical circumstance with the proposed mechanism of activation of the blood coagulation system.

a. Activation of extrinsic pathway
b. Activation of intrinsic pathway
c. Direct activation of Factor X
d. Induction of procoagulant activity

21-28. Bacterial toxins
21-29. Collagen exposure due to loss of endothelial integrity
21-30. Thromboplastin released at sites of tissue destruction
21-31. Protease activity in neoplasias

21-32. How do fibrin degradation products contribute to defective hemostasis?

21-33. The laboratory identification of possible stigmas of intravascular coagulation are indications for the prompt use of heparin, fibrinogen, or ϵ-amino caproic acid.

a. True
b. False

21-34. Which of the following statements about consumptive coagulopathy (DIC) is correct?

a. The most important principles for the management of DIC are maintenance of circulation and perfusion of vital organs.
b. Low levels of procoagulants may be the result of impaired synthesis rather than DIC.
c. Low levels of procoagulants may be the result of vigorous treatment with electrolyte solution rather than DIC.
d. The likelihood of hemorrhage in obstetric situations depends only on the extent of the coagulation defect.

21-35. Excessive bleeding from sites of modest trauma is an inaccurate and uninformative sign of defective hemostasis.

a. True
b. False

21-36. Which of the following statements about the identification of defective hemostasis is correct?

a. If severe hypofibrinogenemia is present, whole blood will not clot.
b. Petechiae may be indicative of serious thrombocytopenia.
c. A prolonged prothrombin time may be due to sepsis rather than to DIC.
d. A prolonged partial thromboplastin time is invariably due to consumptive coagulopathy.
e. The thrombin time is prolonged in the presence of low fibrinogen or appreciable amounts of fibrinogen-fibrin products.
f. In some cases of eclampsia, the thrombin time may be prolonged.

21-37. Which statement about uterine bleeding before delivery is correct?

a. Slight bleeding through the vagina is common during labor.
b. Placenta previa and abruptio placentae cause bleeding from a site above the cervix.
c. Vasa previa is a rare cause of uterine bleeding.
d. If uterine bleeding ceases, the pregnancy is not considered at higher risk than if bleeding had not occurred at all.
e. The origin of uterine bleeding from above the cervix is often difficult to identify.

21-38. Which of the following terms are synonomous?

a. Abruptio placentae
b. Ablatio placentae
c. Accidental hemorrhage
d. Premature separation of the normally implanted placenta
e. Placenta previa

Instructions for Items 21-39 to 21-41: Match the type of bleeding from placental abruption with the appropriate statement.

a. External hemorrhage
b. Concealed hemorrhage

21-39. Blood escapes through the cervix.
21-40. Blood is retained between the detached placenta and the uterus.
21-41. It carries a greater risk of intense consumptive coagulopathy.

21-42. Which of the following statements about the frequency and significance of abruptio placentae is correct?

a. The variability of reported frequencies of abruptio placentae is a function of the different diagnostic criteria in use.
b. The reported frequency is between 1 in 75 and 1 in 100 deliveries.
c. The perinatal mortality rate is approximately 5 percent.
d. In recent years, abruptio placentae has become a relatively rare cause of stillbirths as compared to other causes.
e. Maternal mortality from abruptio placentae is common.
f. If the fetus survives, the newborn is at greater risk for morbidity and mortality.

21-43. Suggested causes of abruptio placentae include

a. Trauma
b. Maternal hypertension
c. Sudden uterine decompression
d. Short cord syndrome
e. Uterine anomaly
f. Uterine tumors
g. Hydramnios
h. Multifetal pregnancy
i. Dietary deficiency

21-44. Severe placental abruption is ____________ to be associated with maternal hypertension than are lesser degrees of abruption.

a. More likely
b. Less likely

21-45. In women with a previous placental abruption, the risk of placental abruption in a subsequent pregnancy is higher than is the risk for the general population.

a. True
b. False

21-46. Which of the following are consistently useful in identifying imminent abruptio placentae?

a. Urinary estriol levels
b. Nonstress test
c. Contraction stress test
d. Ultrasonography

21-47. Which of the following statements about the pathology of abruptio placentae is correct?

a. Placental abruption begins with hemorrhage into the decidua basalis, with the resulting decidual hematoma affecting separation of the placenta from its implantation site.
b. All abruptio placentae are symptomatic.
c. Spiral artery rupture is a cause of retroplacental hematoma formation.
d. Decidual spiral artery rupture always results in severe vaginal bleeding.

21-48. In which of the following situations is a concealed hemorrhage likely to occur?

a. Placental margins remain adherent
b. Membranes are attached to uterine wall
c. Blood enters into amnionic cavity
d. Fetal head is closely applied to lower uterine segment

21-49. What is chronic placental abruption?

21-50. Severe hemorrhage from fetus to mother is common with placental abruption.

a. True
b. False

21-51. The intensity of the symptoms of abruptio placentae are ____________ to the severity of the abruption.

a. Directly proportional
b. Inversely proportional
c. Unrelated
d. Variably related

21-52. Which of the following statements about the diagnosis of abruptio placentae is correct?

a. A normal ultrasound excludes life-threatening abruption.
b. Common symptoms include vaginal bleeding and uterine tenderness.
c. Fetal demise is more common than fetal distress.
d. The intensity of shock is out of proportion to the extent of maternal blood loss.
e. Either hypotension or anemia is always associated with placental abruption.

21-53. Signs and symptoms of abruptio placenta which occur in more than 50 percent of cases include

a. Premature labor
b. Vaginal bleeding
c. Fetal demise
d. Fetal distress
e. Uterine hypertonus
f. Uterine tenderness or back pain
g. High frequency contractions

21-54. Painful uterine bleeding is usually associated with abruptio placentae while painless uterine bleeding is usually associated with placenta previa.

a. True
b. False

21-55. The presence of painful uterine bleeding in the third trimester is always indicative of placental abruption.

a. True
b. False

21-56. The most common cause of consumptive coagulopathy in pregnancy is ________.

21-57. Which of the following statements about placental abruption and consumptive coagulopathy is correct?

a. Significant coagulation derangements are relatively uncommon in cases in which the fetus survives.
b. The coagulation defect arises principally from induction of intravascular coagulation.
c. Levels of fibrin degradation products are higher in serum from the uterine cavity than in peripheral blood.
d. At the outset, thrombocytopenia is found as frequently as hypofibrinogenemia.

21-58. Which of the following statements about renal failure and placental abruption is correct?

a. Acute renal failure usually occurs with any degree of placental abruption.
b. The most common renal lesion is acute tubular necrosis.
c. Major etiologic factors probably include impaired renal perfusion and coexistent hypertension.
d. Renal dysfunction may be avoided by the treatment of hemorrhage with blood and fluids.
e. Proteinuria is only rarely seen in placental abruption.

21-59. Describe the characteristics of uteroplacental apoplexy (Couvelaire uterus).

21-60. The Couvelaire uterus must be treated by hysterectomy in order to prevent severe postpartum uterine hemorrhage.

a. True
b. False

Instructions for Items 21-61 to 21-63: Match the clinical circumstance with the indicated management in third trimester bleeding.

a. Administration of whole blood and electrolyte solution
b. Procrastination and close observation
c. Prompt delivery

21-61. Massive external bleeding
21-62. Blood loss at a slow rate with no evidence of fetal distress
21-63. Evidence of fetal distress

21-64. Failure to identify a blood clot in the uterine cavity by sonography excludes the possibility of serious placental abruption.

a. True
b. False

21-65. List the major causes of fetal distress from abruptio placentae.

21-66. Which of the following is recommended in cases of uterine hypertonicity associated with fetal distress and placental abruption?

a. Magnesium sulfate
b. Ritodrine
c. Other β-receptor agonists

21-67. If placental abruption is suspected, facilities for immediate cesarean delivery should be continuously available.

a. True
b. False

21-68. Which of the following statements about placental abruption and vaginal delivery is correct?

a. If fetal death occurs, vaginal delivery is usually preferable.
b. Coagulation defects may be more troublesome in an abdominal delivery than in a vaginal delivery.
c. Postpartum stimulation of the myometrium pharmacologically and with uterine massage can prevent hemorrhage from the implantation site.
d. Postcesarean bleeding may accumulate as troublesome hematomas.

21-69. There is definite evidence that early amniotomy in cases of abruptio placentae decreases bleeding from the implantation site and reduces thromboplastin entry into the maternal circulation.

a. True
b. False

21-70. Which of the following statements about labor in cases of placental abruption is correct?

a. With mild degrees of abruption, labor contractions appear normal.
b. Uterine hypertonus characterizes severe cases of placental abruption.
c. Failure of the cervix to dilate in the presence of definite effacement should be considered as a lack of progress.
d. In severe cases, it is often difficult to determine by palpation if the uterus is contracting and relaxing.

21-71. Delivery of the infant within 6 hours of the diagnosis of placental abruption maximizes fetal and maternal outcome.

a. True
b. False

21-72. In what aspects does the basic management of obstetric hemorrhage differ from the optimal method of treating placental abruption?

a. Use of blood
b. Types of intravenous fluid administered
c. Amount of intravenous fluid administered
d. Hematocrit goal
e. Urine output goal
f. Use of furosemide

21-73. Which of the following statements about the treatment of coagulation defects associated with abruptio placentae is correct?

a. If the clot observation test reveals a small or absent clot, coagulation studies will be grossly abnormal.
b. The platelet count will always fall abruptly and in parallel with the fibrinogen level in severe abruptio placentae.
c. Microangiopathic hemolysis is very common in severe abruptio placentae.
d. Transfusion with packed platelets is indicated in cases of severe thrombocytopenia.
e. Coagulation defects (factors plus low platelets) will usually return to normal levels within a few days of delivery.
f. Intravenous heparin administration to block DIC is not effective and should be avoided.
g. The use of ϵ-aminocaproic acid will aid in controlling fibrinolysis.

21-74. What is the major problem arising from the use of lyophilized fibrinogen in cases of severe hypofibrinogenemia?

21-75. In the presence of coagulation defects due to placental abruption, supracervical hysterectomy is the best prophylactic measure available.

a. True
b. False

21-76. What are causes of consumptive coagulopathy in the newborn?

a. Placental abruption
b. Sepsis
c. Prematurity
d. Trauma
e. Hypoxia

21-77. What is a placenta previa?

Instructions for Items 21-78 to 21-81: Match the type of placenta previa with the correct description.

a. Total placenta previa
b. Partial placenta previa
c. Marginal placenta previa
d. Low-lying placenta previa

21-78. The edge of the placenta is at the margin of the internal os.

21-79. The internal os is partially covered by the placenta.

21-80. The placental edge is in close proximity to the internal os.

21-81. The internal os is completely covered by the placenta.

21-82. The degree of a placenta previa is independent of cervical dilation.

a. True
b. False

21-83. Which of the following statements about placenta previa is correct?

a. As labor progresses, the degree of placenta previa becomes greater.
b. Digital palpation is the most accurate method of monitoring the changing relationship between placental edge and cervical os.
c. As the lower uterine segment forms, some degree of placental separation invariably occurs.

21-84. What are possible outcomes of a zygote implanting very low in the uterine cavity?

a. Abortion
b. Placenta previa
c. Placental migration

21-85. Placenta previa is ______________ placental abruption.

a. More common than
b. About as common as
c. Less common than

21-86. Which of the following factors are associated with placenta previa?

a. Multiparity
b. Previous cesarean delivery
c. Advancing maternal age
d. Erythroblastosis
e. Multiple fetuses
f. Placenta accreta
g. Defective vascularization of the decidua

21-87. The most characteristic event in placenta previa is ______________.

21-88. Which of the following statements about bleeding with placenta previa is correct?

a. The initial bleeding episode is usually fatal to the fetus and often fatal to the mother.
b. Hemorrhage may be better controlled as labor ensues.
c. Excessive bleeding after delivery may be expected.
d. Consumptive coagulopathy is rarely associated with placenta previa.

21-89. Which of the following statements about the diagnosis of placenta previa is correct?

a. The diagnosis of placenta previa can seldom be made without palpation of the placenta through the cervical os.
b. Vaginal examination for placenta previa should only be conducted in the operating room after full preparation for delivery is made.
c. Vaginal examination should be withheld in women with an immature fetus.
d. Ultrasound localization of the placenta is reasonably reliable in the diagnosis of placenta previa.
e. Placentas seen to lie low or over the os in early pregnancy will, in the majority of cases, lie above the lower uterine segment in advanced pregnancy.

21-90. A woman with placenta previa who has no vaginal bleeding and a premature fetus must always be hospitalized.

a. True
b. False

21-91. Aside from fetal lung maturation, what benefits are possible with delayed delivery in cases of placenta previa?

Instructions for Items 21-92 to 21-94: Match the mode of delivery with its advantages in the management of placenta previa.

a. Cesarean
b. Vaginal

21-92. Allows for immediate delivery and consequent uterine contraction to halt hemorrhage
21-93. Tamponade of bleeding vessels
21-94. Avoids cervical lacerations

21-95. Which of the following statements about cesarean delivery for placenta previa is correct?

a. It is the accepted method of delivery in practically all cases.
b. Cesarean delivery may be indicated for a dead fetus if done for the welfare of the mother.
c. With anterior placenta previa, a transverse uterine incision is optimal.
d. With placenta accreta, a vertical uterine incision will avoid the need for hysterectomy.

21-96. The preferred compression (tamponade) method for vaginal delivery in cases of placenta previa is ______________.

21-97. Which of the following statements concerning the outcome of cases of placenta previa is correct?

a. Cesarean section and adequate transfusion have improved maternal outcome.
b. Perinatal outcome has been improved by expectant management for pregnancies remote from term.
c. Labor or hemorrhage may force delivery of a premature fetus.
d. Perinatal mortality is higher in cases of placenta previa for a given fetal weight than for the general population.
e. Serious fetal malformations are more common in cases of placenta previa.

21-98. The primary mode of management of intrauterine fetal demise is "watchful waiting" until spontaneous labor ensues.

a. True
b. False

21-99. What factors have contributed to a more agressive management of the patient whose fetus has died?

a. Psychologic stress on mother
b. Dangers of blood coagulation defects
c. Advent of effective methods of labor induction

21-100. The majority of pregnancies with a fetal demise will deliver within

a. 24 hours
b. 72 hours
c. 1 week
d. 2 weeks

21-101. Which of the following statements about consumptive coagulopathy after fetal demise is correct?

a. Marked disruption of maternal coagulation rarely occurs in less than 1 month after fetal death.
b. If the fetus is retained more than 1 month, approximately 25 percent of cases develop changes in the coagulation mechanism.
c. Thrombocytopenia precedes severe hypofibrinogenemia.
d. Coagulation defects are always irreversible until delivery occurs.

21-102. In women with delayed delivery of a dead fetus, heparin can be used to correct coagulation defects if the maternal circulatory system is intact.

a. True
b. False

21-103. Death of a fetus in a multifetal pregnancy remote from term warrants immediate cesarean delivery to avoid the risks of consumptive coagulopathy.

a. True
b. False

21-104. In the presence of coagulation defects, serious hemorrhage that occurs as the dead products of conception are being expelled should be treated by

a. Heparin
b. ϵ-Aminocaproic acid
c. Fibrinogen
d. Blood
e. Lactated Ringer's solution

21-105. Which of the following is useful in cases of fetal death requiring pregnancy termination?

a. Oxytocin
b. Laminaria
c. Hypertonic saline
d. Prostaglandin E_2 suppositories

Instructions for Items 21-106 to 21-109: Match the means used to terminate pregnancy with its possible complication.

a. Oxytocin
b. Laminaria
c. Prostaglandin E_2
d. Hypertonic saline

21-106. Nausea, vomiting, and diarrhea
21-107. Water intoxication
21-108. Infection
21-109. Coagulation defects

21-110. List the conditions essential to the development of an amnionic fluid embolism.

21-111. Amnionic fluid embolism is characterized by

a. Respiratory distress
b. Circulatory collapse
c. Hemorrhage
d. Coagulation defects

21-112. Which of the following statements about amnionic fluid embolism is correct?

a. The lethality of intravenously infused amnionic fluid appears related to the particulate matter it contains.
b. The clot-accelerating activity of amnionic fluid is greater at term than early in the third trimester.
c. Amnionic fluid embolism can be confirmed by the widespread appearance of amnionic fluid debris in pulmonary vessels.
d. Successful treatment is dependent upon vigorous antibiotic therapy.
e. The benefits of the use of fibrinogen outweigh its risks in cases of amnionic fluid embolism.

21-113. In what circumstances may coagulopathy develop as a consequence of abortion?

a. Prolonged retention of a dead fetus
b. Sepsis
c. Intrauterine instillation of hypertonic saline
d. Medical induction with prostaglandins
e. Use of instrumentation to terminate a pregnancy

21-114. In an abortion induced by hypertonic saline, thromboplastin may be released from the

a. Placenta
b. Fetus
c. Decidua

21-115. In cases of septic abortion, disruption of coagulation is always associated with intravascular hemolysis.

a. True
b. False

21-116. Severe hemorrhage may itself induce coagulation defects.

a. True
b. False

21-117. Which of the following can be associated with consumptive coagulopathy?

a. Eclampsia
b. Diabetes
c. Barlow's syndrome
d. Severe preeclampsia

22. ECTOPIC PREGNANCY

22-1. Ectopic pregnancy is defined as the implantation of the embryo in the fallopian tube.

a. True
b. False

22-2. Which of the following conditions has been implicated as a cause of ectopic pregnancy?

a. Salpingitis
b. Peritubal adhesions
c. Developmental abnormalities of the fallopian tube
d. Tumors that distort the fallopian tube
e. Previous tubal surgery
f. External migration of the ovum
g. Menstrual reflux
h. Ectopic endometrial elements

22-3. Ectopic pregnancy can occur after hysterectomy.

a. True
b. False

22-4. The incidence of ectopic pregnancies in recent years has increased by a factor of

a. 2
b. 3
c. 4
d. 5

22-5. List the causes for the increased incidence of ectopic pregnancy.

22-6. All ectopic pregnancies require surgical intervention.

a. True
b. False

22-7. Order the anatomic portions of the oviduct from the least frequent to the most frequent site for implantation of a tubal pregnancy.

a. Interstitium
b. Fimbria
c. Ampulla
d. Isthmus

22-8. Which of the following statements about implantation in cases of tubal ectopic pregnancy is correct?

a. The fertilized ovum remains on the epithelial surface.
b. The proliferating trophoblast invades the muscularis layer of the tube.
c. Maternal vessels are eroded by the proliferating trophoblast.
d. The fallopian tube does not form an extensive decidua.
e. The embryo is always identifiable.

22-9. Which of the following statements about uterine changes in ectopic pregnancy is correct?

a. The uterus enlarges.
b. The cervix and isthmus soften.
c. External bleeding may be associated with sloughing of the uterine decidua.
d. The absence of decidua excludes the possibility of ectopic pregnancy.

22-10. Which of the following cellular changes are characteristic of the Arias-Stella reaction?

a. Enlarged epithelial cells with hypertrophic nuclei
b. Loss of mitotic capacity
c. Loss of cellular polarity
d. Vacuolated cytoplasm

22-11. The Arias-Stella reaction is not specific for ectopic pregnancy, but is associated with the blighting of the conceptus.

a. True
b. False

22-12. Which type of endometrium has been identified in cases of ectopic pregnancy?

a. Decidua
b. Secretory
c. Proliferative
d. Menstrual

22-13. Tubal abortion is defined as ____________.

22–14. Which of the following statements about tubal abortion is correct?

a. It is more common in ampullary pregnancies than in isthmic pregnancies.
b. Bleeding usually persists as long as the products of conception remain in the oviduct.
c. Immediate laparotomy is required to control hemorrhage.
d. Hematosalpinx may occur if the distal tube is occluded.
e. Incomplete tubal abortion may result in a tubal polyp.

22–15. Which of the following statements about rupture of a tubal pregnancy is correct?

a. Rupture will occur sooner if the pregnancy is located in the isthmus than if it is located in the interstitium.
b. The most usual cause of tubal rupture is coital trauma.
c. If tubal rupture is suspected, the woman should not undergo surgery.
d. Formation of a lithopedion is the most likely outcome following tubal rupture in an early pregnancy.
e. If the placenta is damaged extensively during the process of tubal rupture, consequent abdominal pregnancy is unlikely.

22–16. Rupture of a tubal pregnancy into the broad ligament may result in

a. Abdominal pregnancy
b. Broad ligament hematoma
c. Death of the fetus

22–17. Interstitial pregnancy occurs when the fertilized ovum __________.

22–18. Which of the following statements about interstitial pregnancy is correct?

a. The term is synonomous with cornual pregnancy.
b. Twenty-five percent of all tubal pregnancies are interstitial.
c. No adnexal mass is palpable.
d. Rupture is likely to occur later than in other types of tubal pregnancy.
e. There is the possiblility of severe hemorrhage following rupture.

22–19. Ruptured interstitial pregnancies must commonly be treated by hysterectomy.

a. True
b. False

22–20. A tubal pregnancy in the presence of a coexisting intrauterine pregnancy is referred to as __________.

22–21. Which of the following statements about combined or multifetal ectopic pregnancy is correct?

a. Combined pregnancy is difficult to diagnose clinically.
b. A congested and enlarged uterus observed upon laparotomy confirms the presence of an intrauterine pregnancy.
c. Combined pregnancy is relatively common following clomiphene therapy.
d. Twin tubal pregnancy has been reported.

Instructions for Items 22–22 to 22–24: Match the type of ectopic pregnancy with its definition.

a. Tubouterine pregnancy
b. Tuboabdominal pregnancy
c. Tuboovarian pregnancy

22–22. Fimbrial implantation that extends to the peritoneal cavity

22–23. Interstitial implantation that extends to uterine cavity

22–24. Fetal sac partially attached to both tube and ovary

22–25. Which of the following are "classic" signs or symptoms of a ruptured tubal pregnancy?

a. Sudden onset lower abdominal pain
b. Cul-de-sac bulging
c. Vasomotor symptoms
d. Shoulder or neck pain
e. Cervical motion tenderness
f. Tender, boggy adnexal mass

22–26. The shoulder or neck pain felt on inspiration in cases of ruptured tubal pregnancy occurs because of __________.

22–27. Which of the following statements about pain in a ruptured tubal pregnancy is correct?

a. It is always unilateral.
b. It may be confined to the upper abdomen.
c. Pain is proportional to the amount of intraabdominal blood.
d. Abdominal tenderness occurs with hemorrhage exceeding 1000 ml.

22–28. Which of the following conditions rules out the presence of a ruptured tubal pregnancy?

a. A reported menstrual period
b. Profuse vaginal bleeding
c. A negative pregnancy test
d. A normal blood pressure and pulse rate
e. Leukocytosis

22–29. Which of the following clinical measurements is appropriate to detect significant hypovolemia before hypovolemic shock develops?

a. Blood pressure in supine and upright positions
b. Pulse rate in supine and upright positions
c. Urine output

22–30. What type of anemia may be identified soon after a ruptured tubal pregnancy?

22–31. Which of the following statements about physical signs in a ruptured tubal pregnancy is correct?

a. Both pelvic and abdominal tenderness may be absent.
b. If a pelvic mass is present, it is located anterior to the uterus.
c. The uterus may be the same size and consistency as if a viable intrauterine pregnancy were present.
d. Temperatures greater than 38°C are suggestive of a diagnosis other than ruptured tubal pregnancy.
e. Patients with pelvic hematoceles present with most "textbook" symptoms of a ruptured tubal pregnancy.

22–32. List the conditions most commonly included in the differential diagnosis of a ruptured tubal pregnancy.

22–33. Which of the following suggest salpingitis rather than a ruptured tubal pregnancy?

a. History of abnormal bleeding
b. Bilateral pain and tenderness
c. Unilateral pelvic mass
d. Temperature in excess of 38°C
e. Negative pregnancy test

22–34. Which of the following statements regarding the differentiation of a ruptured tubal pregnancy from abortion of an intrauterine pregnancy is correct?

a. In tubal pregnancy rupture, vaginal bleeding tends to be more profuse.
b. In tubal pregnancy rupture, shock from hypovolemia is usually in proportion to the extent of vaginal hemorrhage.
c. The pain from uterine abortion is less severe.
d. Endometrial biopsy is a reliable diagnostic tool to differentiate the two situations.
e. The shed decidua of a tubal pregnancy can be mistaken for the products from an intrauterine pregnancy.

22–35. The identification of products of conception in the cervical canal or vagina eliminates the possibility of an ectopic pregnancy.

a. True
b. False

Instructions for Items 22–36 to 22–40: Match the statement with the condition with which it is associated.

a. Ruptured tubal pregnancy
b. Appendicitis
c. Twisted ovarian cyst

22–36. Amenorrhea
22–37. Presence of a discrete mass
22–38. Severe pain on cervical motion
22–39. Pain located over McBurney's point
22–40. Surgery required

22–41. It may be extremely difficult to distinguish a ruptured tubal pregnancy from a ruptured follicular cyst or a ruptured corpus luteum.

a. True
b. False

22–42. Which of the following statements about events associated with the occurrence of a tubal pregnancy is correct?

a. The presence of diarrhea, nausea, and vomiting may lead to inappropriate diagnosis and treatment.
b. The use of an IUD prevents extrauterine pregnancy.
c. An IUD may predispose to unilateral adnexal inflammation.
d. Previous tubal sterilization precludes the possibility of tubal pregnancy.

22–43. Which of the following statements about the use of ultrasonography in the identification of a tubal pregnancy is correct?

a. Identification of an intact intrauterine gestational sac eliminates the possibility of a tubal pregnancy.
b. A positive pregnancy test in the absence of sonographic evidence of an intrauterine pregnancy is suggestive of tubal pregnancy.
c. Sonographic findings suggestive of intrauterine pregnancy may lead to the misdiagnosis of a tubal pregnancy.
d. A corpus luteum cyst can be mistaken for a tubal pregnancy.
e. Identification of fetal heart action by real-time ultrasonography outside the uterus suggests ectopic pregnancy.

22–44. Which of the following statements about culdocentesis for the identification of a ruptured tubal pregnancy is correct?

a. It must be performed after admission to the hospital.
b. Failure to aspirate fluid rules out a bleeding tubal pregnancy.
c. Aspiration of blood that subsequently clots indicates a ruptured tubal pregnancy.
d. Previous salpingitis may dispose to an unsatisfactory culdocentesis.
e. When performed correctly, culdocentesis is a definitive test for ruptured ectopic pregnancy.

Instructions for Items 22–45 to 22–47: Match the finding from curettage with the probability of a tubal pregnancy.

a. Tubal pregnancy likely
b. Tubal pregnancy unlikely

22–45. Embryo identified
22–46. No embryo, fetus or placenta identified
22–47. Only decidua identified

22–48. Colpotomy is widely used as the single procedure of choice for the diagnosis and treatment of tubal pregnancy.

a. True
b. False

22–49. Which of the following statements about the use of laparoscopy to diagnose tubal pregnancy is correct?

a. The use of surgical anesthesia is usually required.
b. The presence of blood or inflammation may lead to poor visualization.
c. If the tube is fully visualized, identification of an unruptured tubal pregnancy can be made with certainty.
d. Demonstration of tubal patency does not exclude the presence of tubal pregnancy.

22–50. In the diagnosis of tubal pregnancy, culdoscopy is easier, more convenient, and more accurate than laparoscopy.

a. True
b. False

22–51. If a doubt exists about the presence of a tubal pregnancy, which single procedure should be performed?

a. Culdoscopy
b. Culdocentesis
c. Laparoscopy
d. Laparotomy
e. Colpotomy

22–52. At present, what proportion of women with ectopic pregnancies die?

a. 10 per 1000
b. 5 per 1000
c. 2 per 1000
d. <1 per 1000

22–53. Ectopic pregnancy is responsible for about ________ percent of deaths associated with reproduction.

a. 5
b. 15
c. 25
d. 35
e. 45

22–54. Which of the following statements about the management of tubal pregnancy is correct?

a. Extensive cornual resection should accompany salpingectomy.
b. Fertility is markedly decreased after one tubal pregnancy.
c. After one tubal pregnancy, there is a 10 to 15 percent risk of another occurring in women who are able to conceive.
d. Salpingectomy is the procedure of choice for all tubal pregnancies.
e. The ipsilateral ovary should be removed at the time of salpingectomy.

22–55. Methotrexate administration offers a safe and effective alternative to surgical treatment of an early unruptured ectopic pregnancy.

a. True
b. False

Instructions for Items 22–56 to 22–58: Match the type of autotransfusion with the appropriate description.

a. Transfusion of blood collected from the abdomen
b. Free blood left in abdomen

22–56. Adverse reactions possible
22–57. Too slow to be effective
22–58. Makes the determination of hemostasis difficult

22–59. In which of the following situations should Rh immune globulin be administered to a woman who is Rh negative?

a. After hysterectomy following a tubal pregnancy
b. When Rh positive blood has been administered
c. If platelets were transfused
d. If the woman has not been previously sensitized to Rho (D) antigen

22–60. The most common origin of abdominal pregnancy is primary implantation of the fertilized ovum on the peritoneum.

a. True
b. False

22–61. Which of the following statements about abdominal pregnancy is correct?

a. Perinatal loss is about 20 to 25 percent.
b. There is a significant incidence of congenital malformations.
c. Abscess formation in a dead fetus may eventually rupture into the intestines or the bladder.
d. Lithopedion and adipocere are possible sequelae to abdominal pregnancy.
e. A careful history taken from patients with abdominal pregnancy will often elicit symptoms suggestive of a preceding tubal accident.

22–62. Which of the following symptoms is compatible with the diagnosis of abdominal pregnancy?

a. Nausea
b. Diarrhea
c. Abdominal pain
d. Constipation
e. Flatulence

22–63. Which of the following physical findings is suggestive of abdominal pregnancy?

a. Oblique fetal lie
b. Ease of palpation of fetal parts
c. Displaced cervix
d. Abnormal uterine outline
e. Fetal head felt outside uterus

22–64. In abdominal pregnancy, massage of the abdomen over the pregnancy products ________ the mass to become firmer.

a. Causes
b. Does not cause

22–65. Uterine contractions in response to oxytocin administration rule out the possibility of abdominal pregnancy.

a. True
b. False

22–66. Isotope localization is superior to either radiographic examination or ultrasound for diagnosing an abdominal pregnancy.

a. True
b. False

22–67. Which of the following statements about factors associated with the treatment of abdominal pregnancy is correct?

a. Massive hemorrhage is the major maternal risk in abdominal pregnancy.
b. Immediate operation is indicated given the danger of hemorrhage from the placental site.
c. Once the fetus is removed, the best management is to sever the cord and membranes and leave the placenta attached within the abdomen.
d. Maternal mortality has been recorded at 50 percent and perinatal mortality at 75 percent in cases of abdominal pregnancy.

22–68. What are five common complications of leaving the placenta in place at the time of surgery for abdominal pregnancy?

22–69. The most effective way to prevent abdominal pregnancy is to ________.

22–70. List the criteria formulated by Spiegelberg for the presence of an ovarian pregnancy.

22–71. Which of the following statements about ovarian pregnancy is correct?

a. The usual termination is early rupture.
b. A tumor may originate from an unruptured pregnancy that has undergone degeneration.
c. Ovarian pregnancy can easily be distinguished from tubal pregnancy.
d. Oophorectomy is the procedure of choice for all cases.

22–72. Cervical pregnancy occurs when the ovum implants ________.

22–73. Which of the following statements about cervical pregnancy is correct?

a. Painless bleeding is the most common characteristic.
b. Cervical pregnancy usually proceeds to term.
c. Attempts to remove the placenta can result in heavy bleeding.
d. Hysterectomy is commonly the procedure of choice for treatment of cervical pregnancy.

23. DISEASES AND ABNORMALITIES OF THE PLACENTA AND FETAL MEMBRANES

Instructions for Items 23-1 to 23-3: Match the placental abnormality with the corresponding description.

a. Placenta bipartita
b. Placenta duplex
c. Placenta triplex
d. Placenta succenturiata

23-1. Presence of a small accessory lobe
23-2. Incomplete division into lobes (vessels extend from one lobe to the other)
23-3. Presence of two separate lobes (vessels remain distinct)

23-4. If, on examination of the placenta, defects in the membranes are noted a short distance from the placental margin, retention of a ____________ should be suspected.

23-5. The incidence of a succenturiate lobe is approximately ____________ percent.

a. 1
b. 3
c. 6
d. 12

23-6. Which of the following abnormalities is associated with postpartum hemorrhage?

a. Placenta bipartita
b. Placenta duplex
c. Placenta succenturiata
d. Placenta triplex

23-7. A ring-shaped placenta is associated with

a. Fetal growth retardation
b. Congenital malformations
c. Antepartum bleeding
d. Postpartum bleeding
e. Prematurity

23-8. Which of the following statements about placenta membranacea is correct?

a. All of the fetal membranes are covered by functioning villi.
b. The placenta develops as a thin membranous structure occupying the entire periphery of the chorion.
c. The nutrition of the fetus is compromised.
d. Serious bleeding is rare.
e. During the third stage of labor, the placenta may not separate.

23-9. What is a fenestrated placenta?

23-10. In an extrachorial placenta, the chorionic plate (fetal side) is smaller than the basal plate (maternal side).

a. True
b. False

Instructions for Items 23-11 to 23-15: Match the type of extrachorial placenta with the appropriate description.

a. Circumvallate placenta
b. Marginate placenta

23-11. Fetal surface presents a central depression surrounded by a thickened, grayish white ring
23-12. Ring coincides with the placental margin
23-13. Ring is composed of a double fold of amnion and chorion with degenerated decidua and fibrin in between
23-14. Chorion and amnion are raised at the margin by interposed decidua and fibrin
23-15. Associated with antepartum hemorrhage and fetal malformations

23-16. The normal term placenta weighs about ____________ g.

a. 250
b. 500
c. 750
d. 1000

23-17. Which of the following conditions is associated with an enlarged placenta?

a. Erythroblastosis fetalis
b. Sickle cell disease
c. Epilepsy
d. Syphilis
e. Gonorrhea

23-18. A placental polyp is formed from ____________.

23-19. What etiologic factors do degenerative lesions (e.g., placental infarct) of the placenta have in common?

23-20. Which histopathologic findings are characteristic of placental infarcts?

a. Calcification
b. Ischemic infarction from spiral artery occlusion
c. Fibrinoid degeneration of trophoblasts
d. Marked cellular hyperplasia

23–21. Which of the following statements about placental infarcts is correct?

a. Placental infarcts are the most common lesions of the placenta.
b. The degenerative changes due to trophoblast aging and impairment of the uteroplacental circulation make the term placenta an essentially dying organ.
c. Marginal infarcts occur at the edges of the central cotyledons of the placenta and may be quite extensive.
d. The frequencies of placental infarcts in normal term pregnancies and in pregnancies complicated by hypertension are almost identical.
e. Syncitial degeneration begins during the latter half of pregnancy.

23–22. Which of the following statements about placental calcification is correct?

a. Calcification of the placenta occurs in less than 10 percent of pregnancies.
b. The amount of calcium deposited decreases as the pregnancy progresses.
c. Calcification of the placenta may be detected by sonography.
d. Discovery of placental calcification is an indication for immediate delivery.

23–23. Thrombosis of a fetal villous stem artery produces discrete areas of avascularity.

a. True
b. False

23–24. Enlargement of chorionic villi is associated with

a. Erythroblastosis (hydropic type)
b. Diabetes
c. Sickle cell disease
d. Fetal congestive heart failure
e. Rheumatic fever

23–25. Pyogenic bacteria can invade the fetal surface of the placenta and give rise to generalized fetal infection.

a. True
b. False

23–26. Hydatidiform moles are ________________.

23–27. The villi of an invasive mole may

a. Invade the uterus
b. Metastasize to distant organs

23–28. Choriocarcinoma consists of neoplastic trophoblast __________ stroma.

a. With
b. Without

23–29. Choriocarcinoma occurs when ____________.

Instructions for Items 23–30 to 23–31: Match the type of neoplastic trophoblasts with the correct synonym.

a. Invasive mole
b. Choriocarcinoma

23–30. Chorioadenoma destruens
23–31. Chorionepithelioma

23–32. Hydatidiform moles may occupy the

a. Uterine cavity
b. Oviduct
c. Ovary

23–33. Describe the features of a complete hydatidiform mole.

Instructions for Items 23–34 to 23–40: Match the type of hydatidiform mole with the appropriate description.

a. Complete hydatidiform mole
b. Partial hydatidiform mole

23–34. Chromosomal composition mostly 46, XX
23–35. Karyotype is typically triploid
23–36. Chromosomes are of paternal origin
23–37. Presence of focal trophoblastic hyperplasia
23–38. Absence of fetus and amnion
23–39. Risk of choriocarcinoma is slight
23–40. Associated with ovarian theca lutein cysts

23–41. What is molar degeneration?

23–42. Careful histologic scrutiny of hydatidiform moles can identify those which will eventually give rise to choriocarcinoma.

a. True
b. False

23–43. Which of the following statements about theca lutein cysts is correct?

a. They are exclusively associated with hydatidiform moles.
b. The cysts are lined with lutein cells.
c. Torsion, infarction or hemorrhage may occur in large cysts.
d. Extensive cystectomy or oophorectomy is usually necessary.
e. After molar evacuation, the ovaries may enlarge before they regress.

23–44. The incidence of hydatidiform mole is approximately ______________.

23-45. The demographic groups at greater risk for the development of hydatidiform mole include women

a. Of European origin
b. Less than 20 years old
c. With a history of a previous mole
d. Who have had a previous multifetal pregnancy
e. With a history of ovarian cysts

23-46. Early in its development, hydatidiform mole is difficult to distinguish from a normal pregnancy.

a. True
b. False

23-47. Which of the following aid in the diagnosis of hydatidiform mole?

a. Bleeding
b. Uterine size
c. Fetal activity
d. Hypertension
e. Disturbed thyroid function

23-48. The outstanding clinical sign of hydatidiform mole is ________________.

23-49. Which of the following statements about bleeding with hydatidiform mole is correct?

a. Bleeding always begins just before abortion.
b. Bleeding is always profuse.
c. Iron deficiency anemia is a relatively common finding.
d. Hemorrhage may be concealed as well as external.

23-50. In about one-half the cases of hydatidiform mole, the uterus is __________ than normal for gestational age.

a. Larger
b. Smaller

23-51. In molar pregnancy, the ovaries are often enlarged due to the presence of ______________.

23-52. Which of the following statements about the clinical course of hydatidiform mole is correct?

a. Survival of a fetus in the presence of hydatidiform mole is impossible.
b. Pregnancy-induced hypertension is frequently associated with hydatidiform mole.
c. Hypertension before 24 weeks strongly suggests chronic hypertension rather than a molar pregnancy.
d. Embolization of trophoblastic tissue typically progresses to maternal death.

23-53. In case of hydatidiform mole, the levels of free thyroxine may be elevated due to the effects of

a. Estrogen
b. Human chorionic gonadotropin
c. Thyroid-stimulating hormone

23-54. Spontaneous expulsion of a hydatidiform mole is most likely to occur around which month of pregnancy?

a. Third
b. Fourth
c. Fifth
d. Sixth

23-55. Which of the following must be ruled out in determining the presence of a hydatidiform mole?

a. Myomata
b. Multifetal pregnancy
c. Hydramnios
d. Error in determining gestational age

23-56. The diagnostic technique of choice for determining the presence of hydatidiform mole is

a. An amniogram
b. Ultrasonography
c. Physical examination
d. Urinary chorionic gonadotropin levels
e. Flat plate x-ray of abdomen

23-57. Which of the following statements about the use of hCG in the diagnosis of hydatidiform mole is correct?

a. Serum assays are more reliable than urine assays.
b. Levels far above normal for a certain stage of pregnancy are definitively diagnostic.
c. High values early in pregnancy are particularly characteristic of hydatidiform mole.
d. Rising levels after 100 days of pregnancy are strong evidence for abnormal trophoblastic growth.

23-58. Which of the following is a diagnostic clinical feature of complete hydatidiform mole?

a. Continuous or intermittent bloody vaginal discharge from about 12 weeks' gestation
b. Uterine enlargement out of proportion to the gestational age
c. Absence of fetal parts on palpation and fetal heart sounds on auscultation
d. Characteristic ultrasonographic pattern
e. Very high hCG level in serum 100 days or more after LMP
f. Preeclampsia-eclampsia developing before 24 weeks' gestation

23–59. The maternal mortality from hydatidiform mole is about __________ percent.

23–60. What percent of hydatidiform moles progress to choriocarcinoma?

a. 10
b. 40
c. 70
d. 100

23–61. Which of the following statements about the treatment of hydatidiform mole is correct?

a. If a fetus and a hydatidiform mole coexist, it is necessary to treat the mole to the exclusion of concern for the fetus.
b. Prophylactic chemotherapy reduces the incidence of uterine perforation and hemorrhage at the time of molar evacuation.
c. Molar evacuation should be undertaken with at least 4 units of compatible whole blood available.
d. Intravenous oxytocin should be administered as the uterus is emptied by vacuum aspiration.
e. Uterine relaxation induced by anesthesia reduces intraoperative complications.

23–62. What is the purpose of obtaining a separate sharp curettage specimen at the time molar evacuation is performed?

23–63. The possibility of uterine trauma and/or uncontrollable hemorrhage at the time of molar evacuation necessitates immediate availability of facilities to perform __________.

Instructions for Items 23–64 to 23–65: Match the treatment method for molar pregnancy with its potential negative effect.

a. Incomplete evacuation
b. Hemorrhage

25–64. Oxytocin
25–65. Prostaglandin

23–66. In women over 40 years of age, hysterectomy is a more logical treatment for hydatidiform mole than vacuum aspiration.

a. True
b. False

23–67. What is the prime objective of follow-up after treatment of hydatidiform mole?

23–68. Serial measurement of __________ is the most important component of follow-up after hydatidiform mole.

23–69. Which of the following statements about the evaluation and treatment of persistent trophoblastic disease is correct?

a. Rising hCG titers indicate persistent trophoblastic disease requiring treatment.
b. Estrogen-progestin contraceptives should be given in the 1st year posttreatment to prevent subsequent pregnancy.
c. Chest roentgenograms should be obtained at the first posttreatment visit.
d. Treatment with methotrexate, actinomycin D or other tumoricidal agents is indicated until hCG levels return to normal.
e. Once hCG levels have returned to normal after chemotherapy, no further evaluation is required.

Instructions for Items 23–70 to 23–72: Match the clinical circumstance with the appropriate treatment.

a. Hysterectomy
b. Curettage
c. Chemotherapy

23–70. Rising hCG levels, no disease beyond the uterus, further childbearing desired
23–71. Rising hCH levels, no disease beyond the uterus, no further childbearing desired
23–72. Rising hCG levels, presence of a lung lesion

23–73. Which of the following is a part of the recommended follow-up for persistent trophoblastic disease?

a. Prevent pregnancy
b. Perform urine pregnancy tests weekly
c. Utilize medical therapy for any patient desiring further childbearing
d. Follow for 1 year after hCG levels return to normal
e. Evaluate and treat rising or plateau levels of hCG

23–74. Choriocarcinoma is equally likely to develop from a normal pregnancy as from hydatidiform mole.

a. True
b. False

23–75. Which of the following statements about the pathology of choriocarcinoma is correct?

a. It is classified as a moderately malignant lesion.
b. The main factor involved in the malignant transformation of the trophoblast is the previous use of steroidal contraceptives.
c. The characteristic gross picture of choriocarcinoma is a slowly growing mass spreading through the uterine endometrium.
d. Choriocarcinoma is characterized by the absence of a villous pattern.
e. Only cytotrophoblast is involved in choriocarcinoma.
f. Metastases in choriocarcinoma are generally carried by the lymphatic system.
g. The most common metastatic site for choriocarcinoma is the vagina.

23–76. Theca lutein cysts of the ovary occur in about __________ percent of cases of choriocarcinoma.

a. 10
b. 30
c. 50
d. 70
e. 90

23–77. Which of the following clinical circumstances suggest the possibility of choriocarcinoma?

a. Irregular bleeding after pregnancy termination
b. Bloody cough
c. Uterine subinvolution
d. Vaginal tumor

23–78. The most common cause of death from choriocarcinoma is infection associated with lymphatic system blockage.

a. True
b. False

23–79. Which of the following statements about the diagnosis of choriocarcinoma is correct?

a. All cases of hydatidiform mole should be followed for the appearance of choriocarcinoma.
b. The best method to evaluate unusual bleeding after a term pregnancy or abortion is by curettage.
c. Elevated hCG levels in the absence of pregnancy are indicative of trophoblastic neoplasia.
d. Malignant tissue may be inaccessible to routine surgical diagnostic techniques.

23–80. The overall cure rate for persistent gestational trophoblastic disease is approximately __________ percent.

a. 10
b. 30
c. 50
d. 70
e. 90

23–81. Which of the following statements about the treatment of choriocarcinoma is correct?

a. Methotrexate and actinomycin D are effective in the treatment of choriocarcinoma.
b. Hysterectomy is usually not necessary for successful treatment.
c. Patients in the low-risk category have an overall cure rate approaching 100 percent.
d. Cerebral metastases may respond to high-voltage radiation and combination chemotherapy.

23–82. List the criteria for low-risk (good prognosis) cases of choriocarcinoma.

23–83. What treatment modality should be used for low-risk choriocarcinoma patients?

a. Combination chemotherapy
b. Single agent chemotherapy
c. Radiation

23–84. Which of the following statements about invasive mole (chorioadenoma destruens) is correct?

a. The incidence is markedly greater than that of choriocarcinoma.
b. It is locally invasive.
c. Trophoblastic elements penetrate the myometrium.
d. Methotrexate may be curative when used alone.

23–85. Which of the following statements about chorioangioma (hemangioma) of the placenta is correct?

a. They are most likely hamartomas of primitive chorionic mesenchyme.
b. Large tumors may be associated with antepartum hemorrhage or hydramnios.
c. Fetal malformations are common complications.
d. Infants tend to be large for gestational age.
e. Fetal to maternal hemorrhage may occur.

23–86. What is the most common tumor metastatic to the placenta?

Instructions for Items 23–87 to 23–90: Match the abnormality of umbilical cord length with the problem with which it has been associated.

a. Short cord
b. Long cord

23–87. True knots
23–88. Umbilical cord prolapse
23–89. Abruptio placentae
23–90. Rupture with intrafunicular hemorrhage

23-91. Which of the following statements about abnormalities of the umbilical cord (funis) is correct?

a. A single umbilical artery is associated with an increased incidence of fetal malformations.
b. A battledore placenta occurs when the umbilical cord inserts at the placental margin.
c. Velamentous insertion occurs in almost all cases of triplets and in about 1 percent of singleton pregnancies.
d. Vasa previa occurs when a velamentous insertion crosses the internal os.
e. Vasa previa is associated with an increased risk of maternal exsanguination.
f. Vasa previa may be identified by the demonstration of nucleated red blood cells in a patient with antepartum hemorrhage.

23-92. Which of the following statements about impeded blood flow in the umbilical cord is correct?

a. Nuchal cord is a common cause of fetal death.
b. Extreme degrees of torsion in the cord commonly cause fetal demise.
c. Cord stricture is associated with a focal deficiency of Wharton jelly.
d. True cysts of the cord are derived from remnants of the umbilical vesicle or the allantois.

23-93. Which of the following statements about diseases of the amnion is correct?

a. Meconium staining of the amnion is always associated with significant fetal distress.
b. Chorioamnionitis is characterized by mononuclear and polymorphonuclear infiltration of the chorion.
c. Amnion nodosum is associated with multiple congenital abnormalities.
d. Amnionic bands are associated with intrauterine amputations.

23-94. What is hydramnios?

23-95. Which of the following statements about hydramnios is correct?

a. Most hydramnios is of gradual onset.
b. Moderate hydramnios (2 to 3 liters) is rather common.
c. The diagnosis of hydramnios rests primarily on clinical evaluation and ultrasonographic estimation of the amount of amnionic fluid.
d. Hydramnios severe enough to be symptomatic occurs in about 0.1 percent of singleton pregnancies.

23-96. Which of the following conditions is highly associated with hydramnios?

a. Multifetal pregnancy
b. Esophageal atresia
c. Maternal diabetes
d. Anencephaly
e. Erythroblastosis fetalis, hydropic variety
f. Cleft lip and palate
g. Intrauterine growth retardation
h. Maternal hypertension
i. Spina bifida

23-97. Hydramnios may be associated with

a. Maternal dyspnea
b. Edema of the lower extremities
c. Oliguria
d. Pain
e. Premature labor

23-98. List the signs and symptoms that are helpful in diagnosing hydramnios.

23-99. Which of the following complications are commonly associated with hydramnios?

a. Placental abruption
b. Uterine dysfunction
c. Postpartum hemorrhage
d. Abnormal presentation

23-100. Which of the following is an effective treatment method for hydramnios?

a. Diuretics
b. Salt restriction
c. Water restriction
d. Removal of excess fluid

Instructions for Items 23-101 to 23-104: Match the complication with the method of extracting excess amnionic fluid.

a. Transcervical
b. Transabdominal

23-101. Infection
23-102. Prolapsed cord
23-103. Placental abruption
23-104. Fetal vessel injury

23–105. Which of the following statements about oligohydramnios is correct?

a. Oligohydramnios is most often associated with postmature or prolonged pregnancy.
b. Oligohydramnios is associated with fetal renal agenesis or obstruction of the fetal urinary tract.
c. Fetal distress is no more common with oligohydramnios than in a pregnancy with a normal amount of amnionic fluid.
d. There is increased risk of fetal amnionic band amputation with oligohydramnios.
e. Pulmonary hypoplasia is associated with oligohydramnios.
f. Esophageal atresia is associated with oligohydramnios.

23–106. Oligohydramnios may be the cause of serious fetal musculoskeletal deformities.

a. True
b. False

24. ABORTION

24–1. An abortion is defined as the elective termination of pregnancy by artificial means.

a. True
b. False

Instructions for Items 24–2 to 24–3: Match the category of abortion with the appropriate definition.

a. Elective (voluntary)
b. Therapeutic
c. Criminal

24–2. The interruption of pregnancy before viability at the request of the woman but not for reasons of impaired maternal health or fetal disease

24–3. The interruption of pregnancy before the time of fetal viability for the purpose of safeguarding the health of the mother

24–4. Which of the following is now the most common category of abortion?

a. Therapeutic
b. Criminal
c. Elective (voluntary)

24–5. According to a United States Supreme Court decision, during what period of gestation is the decision to perform an abortion left solely to the judgment of the woman's physician?

a. During the first trimester
b. After the first trimester but before the fetus is viable
c. After the fetus is viable

24–6. Define viability as it is commonly used with respect to abortion.

24–7. Describe what is meant by the preterm delivery of a premature infant.

24–8. In many states, abortion is defined as occurring at less than ________ (1) weeks of completed gestation or less than ________ (2) grams of fetal weight.

24–9. The determination of the degree of prematurity or immaturity should be based on

a. Fetal length
b. Fetal weight
c. Fetal gestational age
d. Reported date of the LMP

24–10. Why is the commonly quoted incidence of spontaneous abortion (10 percent of all pregnancies) believed to be unreliable?

24–11. Which of the following is a possible cause of embryonic or fetal death?

a. Abnormalities of the ovum
b. Abnormalities of the generative tract
c. Maternal systemic disease
d. Paternal disease

24-12. Which of the following statements about abnormalities of embryonic development associated with spontaneous abortion is correct?

a. In the very early months of pregnancy, spontaneous abortion is most often preceded by the death of the embryo or fetus.
b. The most common morphologic findings in early spontaneous abortions are developmental abnormalities of the embryo (fetus) or the placenta.
c. Chromosomal abnormalities are associated with about 25 percent of early spontaneous abortions.
d. Most chromosomal abnormalities involve some abnormality of chromosome structure.
e. Monosomies, trisomies, and polyploidies are the most frequent abnormalities of chromosome number.
f. Cases of abnormal chromosome number in the fetus usually reflect an abnormal chromosome number in one or both parents.

24-13. The missing chromosome in monosomic zygotes is usually a(n) ________ (1), and in trisomic zygotes the extra chromosome is usually a(n) ________ (2).

a. Autosome
b. Sex chromosome

24-14. The longer both male and female gametes spend within the female reproductive tract, the higher the rate of spontaneous abortion.

a. True
b. False

24-15. Which of the following factors may affect the normal intrauterine environment and, consequently, lead to a defective conceptus?

a. Hormonal control of tubal and uterine peristalsis
b. Endocrine control of the maturation of the endometrium
c. Blastocyst response to implantation
d. Trophoblast ability to obtain nutrition

24-16. Which of the following maternal infections has been clearly implicated as a cause of spontaneous abortion?

a. *Brucella abortus*
b. *Toxoplasma*
c. *Listeria monocytogenes*
d. Syphilis
e. Mycoplasma infection

24-17. Severe hypertension is a common cause of spontaneous abortion.

a. True
b. False

24-18. Measurement of the levels of which of the following hormones is of benefit in predicting the outcome of a pregnancy?

a. Progesterone
b. Human placental lactogen
c. Estrogen
d. Thyroid hormone

24-19. Which of the following situations predisposes to a greater frequency of spontaneous abortion?

a. Moderate to heavy alcohol consumption
b. Smoking
c. Severe general malnutrition
d. Micronutrient deficiency
e. Maternal-fetal Rh incompatibility

24-20. Women who share a large number of major antigens of the histocompatibility complex with their sex partners abort more often than the general population.

a. True
b. False

24-21. Which of the following statements about spontaneous abortion after laparotomy is correct?

a. Use of postoperative progesterone minimizes the risk of spontaneous abortion.
b. Abortion is more likely if surgery involves the pelvic organs.
c. Ovarian cystectomy may be performed without usually compromising pregnancy.
d. Pedunculated myomas may be removed without usually compromising pregnancy.
e. Postoperative peritonitis appears to have no adverse effect on pregnancy outcome.

24-22. Which of the following statements about spontaneous abortion resulting from abnormalities of the reproductive tract is correct?

a. Chronic adnexal inflammation is a frequent cause of abortion.
b. Large, multiple subserous or intramural myomas are more likely to result in abortion than smaller ones.
c. Submucous myomas are more likely to result in abortion than subserous myomas.
d. It is best to remove any myoma prior to pregnancy.
e. Uncomplicated uterine displacement does not usually cause abortion.
f. Faulty Müllerian duct development may result in an increased frequency of abortion.

24-23. Uterine incarceration may cause late spontaneous abortion.

a. True
b. False

24–24. How can abnormal development of spermatozoa cause abortion?

Instructions for Items 24–25 to 24–29: Match the type of spontaneous abortion with the correct description.

a. Blighted ovum
b. Carneous mole
c. Tuberous mole
d. Macerated fetus
e. Fetus papyraceus

24–25. The ovum is surrounded by a capsule of clotted blood
24–26. There is no visible fetus in the gestational sac
24–27. The fetus resembles parchment
24–28. There is a nodular amnion
24–29. The skin peels off in utero, the skull bones are collapsed, and the abdomen distended

24–30. Which of the following statements about the pathology of abortion is correct?

a. Hemorrhage into the decidua basalis and necrotic changes in adjacent tissues usually occur.
b. After fetal death, the ovum or gestational sac acts as a foreign body, usually resulting in uterine contractions and expulsion of the products of conception.
c. Fetus compressus and fetus papyraceus are progressive stages in the decomposition of a retained dead fetus.
d. Fetus papyraceus is relatively common in twin pregnancies when one of the fetuses has died and the pregnancy continues to viability.

Instructions for Items 24–31 to 24–35: Match the type of abortion with the appropriate description.

a. Threatened
b. Inevitable
c. Incomplete
d. Missed
e. Habitual

24–31. Vaginal bleeding with or without cramping in the first half of pregnancy
24–32. Partial expulsion of the placenta or fetus
24–33. Rupture of the membranes and cervical dilation
24–34. Repeated spontaneous abortion
24–35. Prolonged retention (>8 weeks) of a fetus who died during the first half of pregnancy

24–36 Which of the following statements about threatened abortion is correct?

a. Signs of threatened abortion occur in about 25 percent of pregnancies.
b. About 75 percent of women with threatened abortion will eventually abort.
c. Bleeding at the time of the first expected menses may be physiologic.
d. Bleeding early in pregnancy may result from cervical lesions or polyps rather than from the endometrium.

24–37. What outcomes are associated with threatened abortion?

a. Congenital malformations
b. Prematurity
c. Low birth weight
d. Perinatal death

24–38. A gush of fluid from the uterus during the first half of pregnancy always signals an inevitable abortion.

a. True
b. False

24–39. Which of the following statements about incomplete abortion is correct?

a. The fetus and placenta are more likely to be expelled together before the tenth week of gestation.
b. The main sign of incomplete abortion is bleeding.
c. Whatever the duration of gestation, serious hemorrhage is very rare.

24–40. Which of the following statements about missed abortion is correct?

a. Signs of a threatened abortion always occur at the time of fetal death.
b. The uterus begins to regress in size at the time of fetal death.
c. Most missed abortions terminate spontaneously.
d. Maternal coagulopathy secondary to missed abortion usually occurs when the fetus has died early in gestation.

24–41. A woman should be instructed to notify her physician whenever vaginal bleeding, however slight, occurs during pregnancy.

a. True
b. False

24–42. In threatened abortion, usually ______ (1) begins first, followed a few hours later by ______ (2).

a. Bleeding
b. Cramping

24–43. Which of the following types of pain are commonly associated with threatened abortion?

a. Anterior pelvic pain that is clearly rhythmic
b. Persistent low back pain associated with a feeling of pelvic pressure
c. Dull, midline, suprasymphyseal discomfort, with tenderness over the uterus
d. Sharp, intermittent pain in the epigastric region

24–44. Which of the following statements about the management of threatened abortion is correct?

a. If pain and/or bleeding is minimal, physical examination is not necessary.
b. If bleeding continues after an interval of bed rest, the patient should be examined and her hematocrit determined.
c. Termination of the pregnancy is generally indicated when bleeding is sufficient to cause anemia or hypovolemic symptoms.
d. Progesterone given in regular oral doses is effective in reducing the risk of pregnancy loss.
e. Daily quantitative measurements of hCG that do not show an increase in concentration are usually indicative of eventual pregnancy loss.
f. If the uterus does not increase in size or becomes smaller over time, the fetus is almost certainly dead.

24–45. Which of the following statements about the use of ultrasonography in threatened abortion is correct?

a. A distinct, well-formed gestational ring with central echoes implies that the embryo/fetus is reasonably healthy.
b. A gestational sac with no central echoes proves the conceptus is dead.
c. Heart action in a living fetus is observable at 5 to 6 weeks of gestation.
d. A single examination is usually sufficient to determine the likelihood of abortion.

24–46. If bleeding and pain persist unabated for at least __________, an abortion is probably inevitable.

a. 1 hour
b. 6 hours
c. 1 day
d. 3 days

24–47. Which finding accompanying or following a gush of amnionic fluid warrants uterine evacuation?

a. Fever
b. Severe pain
c. Foamy vaginal discharge
d. Bleeding

24–48. Which of the following statements about incomplete abortion is correct?

a. Dilation is often unnecessary prior to curettage.
b. Suction curettage should only be used for intact pregnancies.
c. Curettage should not be performed if the patient is febrile.
d. Hemorrhage from incomplete abortion is rarely fatal.

24–49. Optimal therapy for a missed abortion is to await the spontaneous expulsion of the uterine contents.

a. True
b. False

24–50. What is the most generally accepted definition of habitual spontaneous abortion?

Instructions for Items 24–51 to 24–52: Match the time during gestation when spontaneous abortion occurs with the most probable cause.

a. Cytogenetic abnormalities in the conceptus
b. Maternal abnormalities

24–51. Early abortions
24–52. Late abortions

24–53. Which of the following statements about habitual spontaneous abortion is correct?

a. Following the first spontaneous abortion, the likelihood of future spontaneous abortions rises by about 25 percent for each subsequent pregnancy.
b. After the first spontaneous abortion, the parents should be karyotyped.
c. Chromosomal banding techniques should be used when karyotyping is done.
d. After two or more spontaneous abortions, a pregnancy carried to term is at greatly increased risk of congenital anomalies.

24–54. Which of the following is characteristic of an incompetent cervix?

a. Painless cervical dilation in the second or early third trimester
b. Rupture of the membranes
c. Expulsion of the immature fetus
d. Severe hemorrhage

24–55. Unless treated, the events characteristic of an incompetent cervix will tend to repeat in subsequent pregnancies.

a. True
b. False

24–56. Which of the following is a potential cause of an incompetent cervix?

a. In utero exposure to stilbesterol
b. Previous trauma to the cervix
c. Early menarche
d. Heavy, irregular menstrual flows

24–57. Cervical dilation with an incompetent cervix seldom occurs prior to ________ weeks of gestation.

a. 12
b. 16
c. 20
d. 24

24–58. What are the contraindications to surgical treatment of an incompetent cervix?

24–59. Which of the following statements about the management of incompetent cervix is correct?

a. A surgical "purse-string" suture (cerclage) is the best treatment for incompetent cervix.
b. Cerclage is best performed in the second trimester, before the cervix has dilated 4 cm.
c. Both the McDonald and the Shirodkar cerclage techniques have an overall success rate of 85 to 90 percent.
d. The McDonald cerclage procedure is usually accompanied by greater blood loss and longer operative time than the Shirodkar procedure.
e. With the development of clinical infection, the cerclage suture should be cut and the uterus emptied.
f. Beta mimetic tocolytics and prophylactic antibiotics will decrease the risks of premature labor and infection.

24–60. What grave consequence can occur if vigorous uterine contractions begin while the ligature used to repair an incompetent cervix is still in place?

24–61. Following the ________ procedure, the suture can be left in place for future pregnancies.

a. McDonald
b. Shirodkar

24–62. List the medical indications for therapeutic abortion proposed by the American College of Obstetricians and Gynecologists.

24–63. Elective abortion is strictly a medical issue.

a. True
b. False

24–64. Which of the following is a potential complication of transvaginal abortion?

a. Infection
b. Uterine perforation
c. Cervical laceration
d. Incomplete removal of the fetus or placenta
e. Hemorrhage

24–65. The likelihood of complication is increased if suction curettage or dilation and curettage are performed after ________ weeks of gestation.

a. 16
b. 17
c. 18
d. 19
e. 20

24–66. Dilation and curettage or suction curettage should be performed on an inpatient basis.

a. True
b. False

24–67. Which of the following statements about transvaginal abortion is correct?

a. Trauma can be minimized by using laminaria tents to slowly dilate the cervix.
b. The laminaria may cause cramping pain.
c. Prostaglandins have been shown to be effective in softening the cervix.
d. Paracervical or local block anesthesia is mandatory prior to uterine evacuation.
e. Suction aspiration is used to remove any tissue remaining after initial vigorous curettage with a dull curet.

24–68. Which instrument, when used in the uterine cavity, is not associated with the possibility of uterine wall perforation?

24–69. What procedural elements can minimize short- and long-term morbidity from vaginal abortion?

24–70. Perforation of the uterus is associated with which step in abortion?

a. Dilation
b. Curettage
c. Sounding of the uterus

24–71. Which of the following statements about uterine perforation during abortion is correct?

a. Perforation is more likely if the operator is inexperienced.
b. Uterine position does not affect the frequency of perforation.
c. All perforations require laparotomy to evaluate the potential intraabdominal damage.
d. Vacuum aspiration has a lower perforation rate than mechanical curettage.

24–72. Which of the following is a rare complication of transvaginal abortion?

a. Uterine synechiae
b. Cervical incompetence
c. Consumptive coagulopathy

24–73. Which of the following terms refers to the aspiration of the endometrial cavity using a flexible 5- or 6-millimeter Karman cannula and syringe?

a. Menstrual extraction
b. Menstrual induction
c. Instant period
d. Atraumatic abortion
e. Miniabortion

24–74. List the problems that may be associated with the technique of menstrual aspiration.

24–75. Postabortion treatment of Rh negative women with anti-Rho (anti-D) immunoglobulin is recommended.

a. True
b. False

24–76. In an abortion by menstrual aspiration, the identification of placenta can only be made using standard fixation and staining techniques.

a. True
b. False

24–77. Which of the following statements about surgical methods of abortion is correct?

a. Hysterotomy or hysterectomy may be indicated after failed medical induction of abortion in the second trimester.
b. Hysterectomy is the best treatment if significant uterine disease is also present.
c. Uterine rupture in subsequent pregnancies is more likely following hysterotomy.
d. Hysterotomy is now outdated as a routine method for pregnancy termination.

24–78. Which of the following statements about the use of oxytocin in pregnancy termination is correct?

a. Intravenous oxytocin is an effective drug for terminating an intact second trimester pregnancy in a healthy woman.
b. Oxytocin is more effective after the cervix has already undergone some dilation and effacement.
c. Water intoxication may develop if a large volume of electrolyte-free solution is administered along with the oxytocin.
d. Oxytocin has no cardiovascular effects.
e. Uterine rupture is unlikely in women who are not of high parity.

24–79. Which of the following statements about the use of prostaglandins in abortion is correct?

a. Prostaglandin $F_2\alpha$ is the only safe prostaglandin for pregnancy termination.
b. Vaginal, transcervical, and intraamnionic administration of prostaglandins have proven effective in the induction of abortion.
c. Vaginal or intraamnionic modes of delivery eliminate any gastrointestinal side effects.
d. A fetus with signs of life may be the result of a prostaglandin-induced abortion.
e. Consumptive coagulopathy is a rare complication of the use of prostaglandins.

24–80. Which of the following statements about the use of hyperosmotic solutions to induce abortion is correct?

a. Hyperosmotic dextrose is more effective than either urea or saline.
b. The fetus is most often killed after the administration of hyperosmotic solutions.
c. The mechanism of action may be related to decidual damage and consequent prostaglandin formation.
d. Hyperosmotic solutions may be used in conjunction with other abortifacients.

24–81. Which of the following complications has been associated with the use of hyperosmotic saline for pregnancy termination?

a. Hyperosmolar crisis
b. Septic shock
c. Cardiac failure
d. Peritonitis
e. Hemorrhage
f. Consumptive coagulopathy
g. Water intoxication
h. Myometrial necrosis
i. Uterine rupture
j. Fistula formation
k. Lacerations

24–82. Which of the following statements about the consequences of abortion is correct?

a. The risk of death from legal abortion is about one-fourth the risk from childbirth.
b. Abortion has not been shown to be associated with adverse late outcomes in subsequent pregnancies.
c. Foreceful dilation of the cervix may predispose to cervical incompetence.
d. Asherman's syndrome predisposes to both infertility and obstetric complications.

24–83. Ovulation may occur as early as ________ weeks after an abortion.

a. 2
b. 4
c. 6
d. 8
e. 12

24–84. What are the main therapeutic steps in managing a patient with septic abortion?

24–85. What pathophysiologic changes are associated with septic shock?

a. Damage to the vascular endothelium
b. Inappropriate vasomotor tone
c. Impaired myocardial function
d. Decreased cardiac output
e. Decreased effective blood volume

24–86. Which of the following statements about the diagnosis and treatment of septic shock is correct?

a. Hypotension or oliguria in an infected patient should arouse suspicion of septic shock.
b. In the absence of hemorrhage, hypotension and oliguria that are unresponsive to fluid therapy are likely due to sepsis.
c. Antibiotics should be initiated after culture results are obtained.
d. Hysterectomy is seldom indicated.

24–87. The primary goal in treatment of septic shock is to reestablish effective ________.

24–88. Which of the following statements about fluid therapy in septic shock is correct?

a. Blood should be given to maintain the hematocrit at or above 30.
b. Urinary flow should be at least 30 ml/hr.
c. Pulmonary edema and adult respiratory distress syndrome may occur.
d. Frequent measurement of pulmonary arterial wedge pressure, central venous pressure, and systemic blood pressure can be of help in monitoring fluid replacement therapy.

24–89. Which of the following is recommended in certain cases of septic shock?

a. Adrenocorticosteroids
b. Pressor agents
c. Vasodilator agents
d. Oxygenation
e. Heparin

24–90. Which of the following statements about renal failure in septic shock is correct?

a. Renal failure usually arises solely as a result of the infection.
b. Mild bacterial shock rarely leads to renal failure.
c. Renal failure may be especially intense when sepsis is due to the exotoxin from *Clostridium perfringens*.
d. Intense hemoglobinemia associated with clostridial infection should be aggressively managed by dialysis.

25. ABNORMALITIES OF THE REPRODUCTIVE TRACT

25–1. Which of the following statements about inflammation of the Bartholin glands is correct?

a. An abscess may result in a puerperal infection.
b. Drainage should be accomplished at the time of delivery.
c. The principal organism found in Bartholin gland abscesses is *Neisseria gonorrhoeae*.
d. Oral antibiotics may be as effective as drainage of an abscess.

25–2. A Bartholin duct cyst is best excised under the anesthetic used for delivery.

a. True
b. False

25–3. Which of the following should be surgically excised during pregnancy?

a. Periurethral abscess
b. Periurethral cyst
c. Urethral diverticula

25–4. Which of the following statements about condylomas is correct?

a. The causative agent is unknown.
b. Condylomas tend to enlarge during pregnancy.
c. Use of podophyllin in pregnancy may be toxic to the mother or the fetus.
d. Condyloma acuminatum may occasionally necessitate cesarean delivery.
e. Condyloma latum is a synonomous term for condyloma acuminatum.

25–5. Large vulvar varicosities usually decrease in size and become asymptomatic after delivery.

a. True
b. False

25–6. What events during delivery predispose to the development of cystocele or rectocele?

25–7. Which of the following statements about cystocele and rectocele is correct?

a. Rectocele and cystocele always coexist in the same patient.
b. Large symptomatic cystoceles and rectoceles are now relatively uncommon.
c. Surgical repair should not be carried out in the antepartum or intrapartum periods.
d. Use of cesarean delivery and episiotomy have contributed to the increased incidence of cystoceles and rectoceles.

25–8. The development of stress incontinence during pregnancy is due to the progressive lengthening of the urethra.

a. True
b. False

25–9. Most vaginal cysts are derived from __________.

25–10. Due to their malignant potential, all vaginal cysts should be excised soon after diagnosis.

a. True
b. False

25–11. Which of the following statements about cervical neoplasia during pregnancy is correct?

a. Pregnancy has a small but measurable tendency to increase the rate of progression of cervical dysplasia.
b. Fungating or ulcerating lesions should be evaluated by biopsy or colposcopy.
c. All degrees of dysplasia identified by pap smear must be biopsied as soon as possible.
d. Directed focal biopsy of the cervix is safe to perform in pregnancy.
e. Staining with Lugol solution is more specific than colposcopy in locating dysplastic epithelium.

25–12. Possible problems associated with conization in pregnancy include

a. Risk of membrane rupture
b. Inability to obtain an adequate tissue sample
c. Appreciable blood loss
d. Risk of abortion or premature delivery

25–13. If care is taken, endocervical curettage should be performed in all pregnant patients with cervical dysplasia.

a. True
b. False

25–14. Patients previously treated for cervical dysplasia should

a. Avoid pregnancy
b. Be encouraged to conceive as quickly as possible
c. Be followed for recurrence of the dysplasia

25–15. Staging errors in pregnant women with invasive cervical carcinoma tend to __________ the extent of the tumor.

a. Underestimate
b. Overestimate

25–16. Which of the following statements about invasive cervical carcinoma in pregnancy is correct?

a. Staging is more difficult.
b. The type of delivery (vaginal or abdominal) does not significantly affect maternal survival.
c. Survival rates are relatively similar for pregnant and nonpregnant women with a given disease stage.
d. During the first half of pregnancy, treatment for invasive carcinoma should be initiated immediately.

Instructions for Items 25–17 to 25–20: Match the degree of cervical neoplasia with the appropriate treatment.

a. Vaginal delivery and follow-up with colposcopy and biopsy
b. Cesarean hysterectomy
c. Radiation therapy
d. (Cesarean) radical hysterectomy and pelvic lymphadenectomy

25–17. Severe cervical dysplasia
25–18. Carcinoma in situ
25–19. Cervical carcinoma—stage 1
25–20. Extensive cervical carcinoma

25–21. Which of the following is common in pregnancy?

a. Endometrial carcinoma
b. Uterine myoma
c. Tubal carcinoma
d. Ovarian cancer

25–22. List the groups of developmental abnormalities of the female reproductive tract.

Instructions for Items 25-23 to 25-26: Match the type of uterus with the appropriate description.

a. Single
b. Septate
c. Bicornuate
d. Double
e. Single hemiuterus

25-23. Two hemiuteri, each with a distinct cervix
25-24. Y-shaped, forked uterus; single cervix
25-25. Externally the uterus appears normal; internally the uterine cavity is divided into two or more compartments
25-26. Normal, symmetrical uterus

25-27. List and describe the four types of cervix.

25-28. A longitudinally septate vagina occurs when ________ (1) and a transversely septate vagina results from ________ (2).

25-29. Most major obstetric difficulties related to abnormalities of the reproductive tract are associated with anomalies of the

a. Vagina
b. Cervix
c. Uterus

25-30. A hemiuterus that fails to dilate and hypertrophy during pregnancy can lead to

a. Abortion
b. Premature birth
c. Abnormal presentation
d. Uterine dysfunction
e. Uterine rupture

25-31. Women with minor uterine abnormalities may be expected to have relatively normal deliveries.

a. True
b. False

25-32. All anatomic abnormalities of the female reproductive tract must be confirmed using some form of radiologic imaging technique.

a. True
b. False

25-33. Anomalies of the reproductive tract are frequently associated with anomalies of the ________ tract.

25-34. What obstetric outcomes are more common in women with major anatomic abnormalities of the uterus?

a. Cesarean delivery
b. Low birth weight infants
c. Perinatal loss
d. Abortion

25-35. Which of the following therapies have been found to be beneficial in improving pregnancy outcomes in patients with major anatomic abnormalities of the reproductive tract?

a. Progestational agents
b. β-Mimetic drugs
c. Metroplasty
d. External podalic version
e. Cerclage

25-36. What type of chemical compound is stilbesterol (diethyl stilbesterol)?

25-37. Which of the following statements about stilbesterol use during pregnancy is correct?

a. It prevents most forms of pregnancy wastage.
b. In utero exposure increases the risk of clear cell adenocarcinoma of the vagina.
c. Lower conception rates have been reported in women who were exposed to stilbesterol in utero.
d. One in ten women exposed in utero exhibit structural anomalies of the reproductive tract.
e. Structural abnormalities in exposed women are confined to the cervix and vagina.

25-38. Which of the following statements about uterine malposition is correct?

a. Extreme anteflexion of the uterus in early pregnancy is uncommon but associated with an increased incidence of spontaneous abortion.
b. Retroversion of the uterus probably has no adverse effects on early pregnancy.
c. Incarceration of a retroverted uterus first manifests in abdominal discomfort and paradoxic incontinence.
d. Sacculation will often occur if the uterus remains incarcerated.
e. Pregnancy associated with a partially prolapsed uterus usually proceeds without problems, with the uterus "rising" as the pregnancy advances.

25-39. Sacculation of the uterus is characterized by ________.

25-40. What therapies are appropriate for treatment of uterine prolapse during pregnancy?

a. Expectant management
b. Use of a pessary
c. Bed rest
d. Attention to careful hygiene

25-41. Cystocele and rectocele may prolapse even though the uterus is in normal position.

a. True
b. False

25–42. Why is primary acute inflammation of the tubes and ovaries rarely, if ever, seen in pregnancy?

25–43. The rare situation where there is a continuous loss of clear fluid, often believed to represent a persistent amniorrhea following rupture of the membranes, is termed ________.

25–44. Endometriosis is a frequent cause of

a. Premature labor
b. Uterine dysfunction
c. Third trimester bleeding
d. Preeclampsia

26. MULTIFETAL PREGNANCY

26–1. List the complications common to multifetal pregnancy.

26–2. Two infants who resulted from the division of one fertilized zygote are referred to as ________ twins.

a. Monozygotic
b. Dizygotic

26–3. Monozygotic twins are always "identical."

a. True
b. False

Instructions for Items 26–4 to 26–10: Match the type of monozygotic twin pregnancy with the appropriate statement.

a. Diamnionic, dichorionic
b. Diamnionic, monochorionic
c. Monoamnionic, monochorionic
d. Conjoined

26–4. Division after the amnion has become established
26–5. Division of the fertilized ovum before the inner cell mass is formed
26–6. Division after cells destined to become chorion have differentiated
26–7. Division after the embryonic disc has formed
26–8. Two embryos within a common amnionic sac
26–9. Two embryos, two amnions, and two chorions
26–10. Two amnionic sacs covered by a single chorion

26–11. In which type of monozygotic twinning do two distinct placentas or a single fused placenta develop?

a. Diamnionic, dichorionic
b. Diamnionic, monochorionic
c. Monoamnionic, monochorionic
d. Conjoined

26–12. The frequency of monozygotic twins is approximately ________.

26–13. Which of the following factors strongly influences the incidence of monozygotic twins?

a. Race
b. Heredity
c. Maternal age
d. Parity
e. Therapy for infertility

26–14. Which of the following factors strongly influences the incidence of dizygotic twins?

a. Race
b. Heredity
c. Maternal age
d. Parity
e. Therapy for infertility

26–15. Which of the following statements about factors influencing the frequency of twins is correct?

a. Once twinning occurs, delivery of viable twins is the most likely outcome.
b. Paternal and maternal genotypes are equally important in determining the probability of twinning.
c. Twinning is inversely proportional to maternal age and parity.
d. There is a higher rate of dizygous twinning in women who conceive within 1 month after discontinuing oral contraceptives.
e. The induction of ovulation is associated with the release of multiple ova.
f. In humans, the percentage of male conceptuses increases as the number of fetuses per pregnancy increases.

26–16. If one amnionic sac is found on examination of a delivered placenta, the two infants are always classified as monozygotic twins.

a. True
b. False

26–17. If adjacent amnions are separated by chorion, the two infants are always classified as dizygotic twins.

a. True
b. False

26–18. Which of the following statements about the determination of zygosity is correct?

a. Careful examination of the placenta will establish zygosity in virtually all cases.
b. A difference in major blood group between twins is indicative of dizygosity.
c. Monozygotic twins may be of different phenotypic sex.
d. The determination of zygosity is of little practical importance.

Instructions for Items 26–19 to 26–22: Match the type of conjoined twins with the appropriate description.

a. Thoracopagus
b. Pyopagus
c. Craniopagus
d. Ischiopagus

26–19. Joining is anterior
26–20. Joining is caudal
26–21. Joining is cephalic
26–22. Joining is posterior

26–23. The most common type of conjoined twins are ________________.

26–24. Vaginal delivery of conjoined twins may be possible.

a. True
b. False

Instructions for Items 26–25 to 26–31: Match the characteristics of monozygous twins in which there is an arteriovenous anastomosis with the appropriate potential problem.

a. "Donor" twin
b. "Hypertransfused" twin

26–25. Hypotension
26–26. Hypertension
26–27. Cardiac hypertrophy
26–28. Microcardia
26–29. Hydramnios
26–30. Polycythemia
26–31. Anemia

26–32. Which of the following problems may occur in the neonatal period in a hypertransfused twin?

a. Circulatory overload with heart failure
b. Occlusive thrombosis
c. Hyperbilirubinemia
d. Kernicterus

26–33. In ______1______, cell lines are derived from different zygotes, whereas in ______2______, two or more cell lines of different chromosomal composition arise from the same zygote.

a. Mosaicism
b. Chimerism

26–34. Blood chimerism as a result of twin to twin transfusion occurs in

a. Monozygotic twins
b. Dizygotic twins

26–35. List the items in the differential diagnosis of a uterus larger than expected for the calculated gestational age.

26–36. Which of the following statements about the diagnosis of multifetal pregnancy is correct?

a. Twin pregnancy is undiagnosed until labor in 5 to 50 percent of cases.
b. In late pregnancy, it is sometimes possible to distinguish separate fetal parts by palpation.
c. Ultrasonography may be used to detect multifetal pregnancy early in the gestation.
d. The number of fetuses does not affect the ease and accuracy of sonographic diagnosis.
e. Discordant fetal growth in multifetal pregnancy may be evaluated by sonographic measurements of biparietal diameters of all fetuses.
f. X-ray examination should generally be avoided for the diagnosis of multifetal pregnancy.

26–37. Which of the following clearly differentiates between the presence of one or multiple fetuses?

a. hCG levels
b. Placental lactogen levels
c. α-Fetoprotein levels
d. Urinary estriol levels
e. Plasma estrogen levels

26–38. Which of the following statements about pregnancy outcome in multifetal pregnancy is correct?

a. Spontaneous abortion and premature delivery are more common in multifetal than singleton pregnancy.
b. Intrauterine fetal demise of one member of a multifetal pregnancy will always lead to loss of the entire pregnancy.
c. Intrauterine fetal demise of one member of a multifetal pregnancy always leads to significant maternal coagulopathy.
d. The perinatal mortality rate for pregnancies with twin fetuses is higher than for singleton pregnancies.
e. The perinatal death rate for monozygotic and dizygotic twins is approximately equal.

26–39. Complete the following table comparing the average length of gestation with the number of fetuses in a multifetal pregnancy.

No. of Fetuses	Weeks Completed
1	(1)
2	(2)
3	(3)
4	(4)

26–40. In general, the larger the number of fetuses the greater the degree of growth retardation.

a. True
b. False

26–41. When two or more fetuses are derived from a single ovum, the degree of growth retardation is likely to be ________ when each fetus in a multifetal pregnancy is derived from a different ovum.

a. Greater than
b. The same as
c. Less than

26–42. Most growth-retarded infants from multifetal pregnancies "catch up" to their normal twins in height and weight within a few years.

a. True
b. False

Instructions for Items 26–43 to 26–44: Match the term with the appropriate definition.

a. Superfetation
b. Superfecundation

26–43. Fertilization with an intervening time as long or longer than an ovulatory cycle
26–44. Fertilization of two ova within a short period of time, but not at the same coitus

26–45. Which of the following statements about maternal adaptation in multifetal pregnancy is correct?

a. The average increase in maternal blood volume is significantly higher in multifetal pregnancy than in singleton pregnancy.
b. The average blood loss in vaginal delivery of twins is nearly twice that in vaginal delivery of a single fetus.
c. Maternal anemia is more common in multifetal pregnancy than in singleton pregnancy.
d. Acute hydramnios may develop, especially with monozygotic twins.
e. Maternal renal function may be impaired in multifetal pregnancy complicated by hydramnios.

26–46. Perinatal mortality and morbidity may be markedly reduced by attention to what management precepts?

26–47. Which of the following statements about the management of multifetal pregnancy is correct?

a. An additional 300 kcal per day should be consumed by a woman carrying twins beyond the caloric increases recommended for normal singleton pregnancy.
b. Iron supplementation of 60 to 100 mg per day is recommended in multifetal pregnancy.
c. Pregnancy-induced hypertension tends to develop earlier and be more severe than in singleton pregnancy.
d. Bed rest may be beneficial in twin pregnancy by enhancing uterine perfusion.
e. The routine use of β-mimetics will decrease the probability of premature labor in twin pregnancy.
f. Progestin administration has not been shown to prevent premature delivery in twins.

26–48. The L/S ratio obtained for one fetus in a multifetal pregnancy is an accurate reflection of fetal lung maturity for all fetuses.

a. True
b. False

26–49. List the major complications of labor and delivery more commonly encountered in multifetal pregnancy.

26–50. Which of the following factors may complicate the use of analgesia and anesthesia during labor and delivery in a multifetal pregnancy?

a. Prematurity
b. Maternal hypertension
c. Desultory labor
d. Need for intrauterine manipulation
e. Uterine atony and hemorrhage after delivery

26–51. Which of the following statements about the delivery of multiple fetuses is correct?

a. Determination of fetal presentations may be made by ultrasonography during labor, or, if necessary, confirmed by x-ray.
b. The use of oxytocin for induction or stimulation of labor in multifetal pregnancy is of uncertain value and safety.
c. Vaginal delivery of the first of twins when the fetus is in cephalic presentation is usually quite normal.
d. Delivery of the second twin if breech may be accomplished by vaginal breech delivery or cesarean section depending on the status of the second twin.
e. In a pregnancy with three or more fetuses, delivery is best accomplished by cesarean section.

27. HYPERTENSIVE DISORDERS IN PREGNANCY

27–1. Which of the following statements about hypertension in pregnancy is correct?

a. Pregnancy usually alleviates chronic hypertension.
b. Normotensive women may become hypertensive in pregnancy.
c. Convulsions may develop in association with hypertension.
d. Proteinuria and/or edema may accompany hypertension.
e. Prenatal care with appropriate therapy can ameliorate the outcome of pregnancies complicated by hypertension.

27–2. The definition of hypertension in pregnancy is ________.

Instructions for Items 27–3 to 27–5: Match the term with its definition according to the Committee on Terminology of the American College of Obstetricians and Gynecologists.

a. Preeclampsia
b. Eclampsia
c. Superimposed preeclampsia
d. Chronic hypertensive disease

27–3. The presence of persistent hypertension in the absence of hydatidiform mole before the 20th week of gestation or beyond 6 weeks postpartum
27–4. Hypertension with proteinuria or edema induced by pregnancy after the 20th week of gestation
27–5. The development of preeclampsia in a woman with chronic hypertensive vascular disease

27–6. The definition of eclampsia is ________.

27–7. Gestational hypertension is a synonym for preeclampsia.

a. True
b. False

27–8. Which of the following is associated with the development of preeclampsia?

a. Nulliparity
b. Pregnancy at extremes of reproductive age
c. Multifetal pregnancy
d. Fetal hydrops
e. Chronic hypertension
f. Diabetes mellitus
g. Renal disease
h. Family history of preeclampsia–eclampsia

27–9. The definition of proteinuria in pregnancy is ________.

27–10. Which of the following statements about pregnancy-induced hypertension (PIH) is correct?

a. For a diagnosis of preeclampsia to be made, there must be evidence of edema.
b. The edema of preeclampsia most usually involves the ankles and legs.
c. Perinatal mortality is markedly increased in the fetuses of women with edema alone.
d. Proteinuria usually develops early in the course of pregnancy-induced hypertension.
e. Proteinuria without associated hypertension has little overall influence on the frequency of fetal death.

27–11. List the most common causes of perinatal mortality associated with pregnancy-induced hypertension.

27–12. Eclampsia is always preceded by some measurable proteinuria.

a. True
b. False

27–13. The factor most associated with decreased perinatal survival in pregnancy-induced hypertension is the presence of maternal

a. Hypertension
b. Proteinuria
c. Edema

27–14. Complete the following table that distinguishes mild from severe pregnancy-induced hypertension by indicating whether the abnormality is typically present or absent.

Abnormality	Mild	Severe
Headache	(1)	(2)
Visual disturbance	(3)	(4)
Upper abdominal pain	(5)	(6)
Oliguria	(7)	(8)
Convulsions	(9)	(10)
Thrombocytopenia	(11)	(12)
Hyperbilirubinemia	(13)	(14)

27–15. Intrauterine growth retardation is as common with pregnancy-induced hypertension as with pregnancy-aggravated hypertension (superimposed preeclampsia).

a. True
b. False

27–16. Which of the following statements about eclampsia is correct?

a. Convulsions will develop in any case of untreated pregnancy-induced hypertension.
b. Seizures are of the grand mal type.
c. Seizures only occur during the intrapartum period.
d. Seizures occurring more than 48 hours postpartum cannot be due to eclampsia.

27–17. The diagnosis of chronic (coincidental) hypertension should be supported by what findings?

27–18. Which of the following statements about chronic hypertension in pregnancy is correct?

a. All chronic hypertensive disorders predispose to the development of superimposed preeclampsia.
b. A woman who is normotensive at 20 weeks of gestation and hypertensive during the third trimester cannot have chronic hypertension.
c. Essential hypertension is the most common cause of hypertension in women.
d. The fetus of a woman with chronic hypertension is at greater risk of growth retardation and intrauterine death.

27–19. Which of the following maternal complications may result from chronic hypertension in pregnancy?

a. Cardiac decompensation
b. Cerebrovascular accidents
c. Renal damage
d. Placental abruption

27–20. What two criteria must be met to establish the diagnosis of pregnancy-aggravated hypertension (superimposed preeclampsia)?

27–21. Which of the following statements about vasospasm in preeclampsia or eclampsia is correct?

a. Segmental vascular spasm with alternate regions of contraction and dilation is characteristic of preeclampsia and eclampsia.
b. Vascular constriction accounts for the development of arterial hypertension.
c. Depressed circulation in the vasa vasorum is the sole factor contributing to blood vessel damage arising from vasospasm.
d. Vascular changes and local hypoxia of the surrounding tissues lead to the hemorrhage and necrosis observed in severe pregnancy-induced hypertension.

27–22. Which of the following statements about the pathophysiology of preeclampsia and eclampsia is correct?

a. Normally, pregnant women develop refractoriness to the pressor effects of angiotensin II.
b. Normotensive primigravid women who will develop pregnancy-induced hypertension (PIH) can demonstrate a loss of refractoriness to angiotensin II before the onset of hypertension.
c. Women with chronic hypertension who will develop PIH do not demonstrate a loss of refractoriness to angiotensin II.
d. Refractoriness to angiotensin II during normal pregnancy is a generalized phenomenon affecting all tissues.
e. Refractoriness to angiotensin II can be abolished by prostaglandin synthetase inhibitors.

27–23. Nulliparous women who exhibit an increase in blood pressure when turned from the lateral recumbent to the supine position are at considerable risk for pregnancy-induced hypertension.

a. True
b. False

Instructions for Items 27-24 to 27-25: Match the cardiovascular changes in pregnancy with the clinical situation.

a. Cardiac output increased
b. Cardiac output decreased
c. Peripheral resistence increased
d. Peripheral resistance decreased

27-24. Normal pregnant woman
27-25. Pregnant woman with pregnancy-induced hypertension

27-26. In assessing cardiac function, which of the following areas must be considered?

a. Preload (end diastolic pressure and chamber volume)
b. Afterload (intramyocardial systolic tension)
c. Inotropic state of the myocardium
d. Heart rate

Instructions for Items 27-27 to 27-28: Match the effect on cardiac function with the appropriate cause.

a. Increases the preload
b. Decreases the preload
c. Increases the afterload
d. Decreases the afterload

27-27. Modulation of the α-adrenergic system
27-28. Administration of crystalloid, colloid or blood

27-29. Which antihypertensive agent is most commonly used in the treatment of severe preeclampsia and eclampsia?

27-30. In pregnancy-induced hypertension, the afterload is __________.

a. Increased
b. Decreased

27-31. In cases of pregnancy-induced hypertension, volume expansion causes cardiac output and peripheral resistance to return to normal.

a. True
b. False

27-32. Which of the following hematologic changes are identified in many women with preeclampsia and eclampsia?

a. Decreased or absent pregnancy-induced hypervolemia
b. A hematocrit below that in normal pregnancy
c. Alterations of the coagulation mechanism
d. Increased destruction of erythrocytes

27-33. What two causes may play a role in the accumulation of extracellular fluid that occurs in preeclampsia?

27-34. Even in the absence of hemorrhage, the intravascular compartment in preeclampsia-eclampsia is usually underfilled.

a. True
b. False

27-35. The woman with eclampsia is __________ sensitive to vigorous fluid therapy or to blood loss at delivery than the average pregnant woman.

a. More
b. Less

27-36. Which of the following may frequently be significantly abnormal in preeclampsia–eclampsia relative to normal pregnancy?

a. Number of platelets in cord blood
b. Maternal platelet count
c. Fibrinogen level in maternal plasma
d. Thrombin time
e. Concentration of fibrin split products

27-37. In cases of preeclampsia and eclampsia, the coagulation changes observed are most likely the sequelae of the disease process rather than the cause.

a. True
b. False

Instructions for Items 27-38 to 27-41: Indicate whether the level of each hormone is raised, lowered, or unchanged in patients with pregnancy-induced hypertension relative to the normal pregnant state.

a. Raised
b. Lowered
c. Unchanged

27-38. Plasma renin
27-39. Angiotensin II
27-40. Aldosterone
27-41. Deoxycorticosterone

27-42. Which of the following statements about endocrine and metabolic changes in patients with pregnancy-induced hypertension (PIH) is correct?

a. Compromised adrenal and pituitary function is common in PIH.
b. Extra-adrenal formation of deoxycorticosterone may play an important role in the pathogenesis of PIH.
c. The oliguria common in PIH can be accounted for by increased levels of aldosterone.
d. Moderate hyponatremia is common in preeclampsia.
e. Severe edema in PIH is indicative of a poor prognosis.

27–43. Which of the following statements about renal changes in pregnancy-induced hypertension (PIH) is correct?

a. In severe cases, renal perfusion and glomerular filtration may be below nonpregnant levels.
b. Plasma uric acid concentration is typically elevated in women with PIH.
c. Plasma uric acid levels are of great prognostic value in PIH.
d. The renal changes identified using electron microscopy are pathognomonic for preeclampsia.

27–44. What microscopic renal changes are characteristic of preeclampsia–eclampsia?

27–45. What lesions associated with pregnancy-induced hypertension may give rise to acute renal failure?

27–46. Which of the following statements about hepatic changes in pregnancy-induced hypertension is correct?

a. Severe hyperbilirubinemia is the most common initial abnormality.
b. Much of the elevation in serum alkaline phosphatase is due to placental synthesis.
c. Periportal necrosis of the liver can be the result but not the cause of eclampsia.
d. The most characteristic feature of the hepatic lesion in eclampsia is its variability in extent and severity.

27–47. Subcapsular hemorrhage in the liver in pregnancy-induced hypertension may be life threatening.

a. True
b. False

27–48. Which of the following is abnormal in the brains of women with pregnancy-induced hypertension?

a. Cerebral blood flow
b. Oxygen consumption
c. Vascular resistance

27–49. Certain women may be genetically predisposed to develop convulsions as a consequence of pregnancy-induced hypertension.

a. True
b. False

27–50. Which of the following has been identified in the brains of women who died with eclampsia?

a. Edema
b. Hyperemia
c. Focal anemia
d. Thrombosis
e. Hemorrhage

27–51. Various studies have shown that uterine blood flow in the normal term pregnancy is

a. 100 to 200 ml/min
b. 300 to 400 ml/min
c. 500 to 700 ml/min
d. 1000 to 1200 ml/min

27–52. There is a ________-fold decrease in uteroplacental perfusion in hypertensive women relative to normotensive gravidas.

a. 0.5 to 1
b. 2 to 3
c. 4 to 5
d. 6 to 7

27–53. Which of the following statements about uteroplacental perfusion in pregnancy-induced hypertension is correct?

a. The mean diameter of myometrial spiral arterioles in normal primigravid women is greater than in women with preeclampsia.
b. The placental clearance rate of dehydroisoandrosterone sulfate may be decreased in PIH.
c. Uteroplacental perfusion is decreased by the administration of thiazide diuretics.
d. The use of intravenous hydralazine to lower diastolic blood pressure does not decrease uteroplacental perfusion.
e. The fetus in cases of PIH may not be as able to tolerate decreased uteroplacental perfusion as the fetus in a normal pregnancy.

27–54. The incidence of preeclampsia is commonly reported to be about ________ (1) and the incidence of eclampsia about ________ (2).

27–55. Which of the following has been clearly shown to be linked to the development of pregnancy-induced hypertension?

a. Social class
b. Diet
c. Infection with *Hydatoxi lualba*
d. Immunologic mechanisms
e. Number of sexual partners

27–56. The tendency to develop pregnancy-induced hypertension may in part be genetically determined.

a. True
b. False

27–57. In preeclampsia, symptoms such as headache or visual disturbance tend to occur ________ the development of hypertension or proteinuria.

a. Before
b. After

27–58. Which of the following statements about blood pressure measurements in preeclampsia is correct?

a. A rise in blood pressure is the most dependable warning sign of preeclampsia.
b. The systolic pressure is a more reliable prognostic sign than the diastolic pressure.
c. A persistent diastolic pressure of 90 or above is generally considered abnormal.
d. Diastolic blood pressures between 90 and 100 are not considered abnormal in edematous or obese patients.

27–59. Which of the following statements about the clinical presentation of preeclampsia is correct?

a. Incipient preeclampsia should be suspected if a patient gains 2 pounds or more in a given week or 6 pounds or more in a given month.
b. In both mild and severe preeclampsia, proteinuria manifests simultaneously with weight gain and hypertension.
c. Frontal headache is common in all preeclamptic patients.
d. Epigastric or right upper quadrant pain is often indicative of imminent convulsions.
e. Visual disturbances such as blurring or blindness usually carry a poor prognosis for return to normal vision.

27–60. The prognosis for the fetus in a pregnancy complicated by pregnancy-induced hypertension is solely dependent on its gestational age.

a. True
b. False

27–61. List the factors predisposing to preeclampsia which warrant careful attention in the antepartum period.

27–62. Which of the following steps should be taken by the health care provider to detect early evidence of pregnancy-induced hypertension?

a. Weigh patient at each visit.
b. Monitor blood pressure at each visit.
c. Instruct patient to immediately report symptoms of PIH.
d. Immediately evaluate patients reporting symptoms of PIH.

27–63. The development of pregnancy-induced hypertension can be controlled by limiting weight gain during pregnancy to 20 pounds or less.

a. True
b. False

27–64. What are possible effects of the routine use of diuretics during pregnancy?

a. Reduced incidence of pregnancy-induced hypertension
b. Decreased renal perfusion
c. Reduced uteroplacental perfusion
d. Increased incidence of fetal thrombocytopenia

27–65. There is little evidence that rigid dietary restriction of sodium is helpful in preventing preeclampsia.

a. True
b. False

27–66. Which of the following statements about the treatment of pregnancy-induced hypertension is correct?

a. The sole objective in the treatment of PIH is the survival of the fetus.
b. Most women with PIH can be successfully managed as outpatients.
c. Hospitalized patients should have oral fluids limited.
d. Hospitalized patients should be sedated with phenobarbital.

27–67. The systematic hospital management of mild preeclampsia includes

a. Daily clinical evaluation for the development of symptoms
b. Weight measurement every other day
c. Urine test for proteinuria at least every 2 days
d. Blood pressure measurements every 4 hours around the clock
e. Measurement of plasma creatinine
f. Measurement of hematocrit, platelets, and SGOT
g. Frequent evaluation of fetal size clinically or by serial ultrasonography
h. Bed rest throughout much of the day

27–68. The correct management of a pregnancy complicated by preeclampsia depends on what factors?

27–69. Which cases of pregnancy-induced hypertension can await spontaneous onset of labor?

27–70. Which of the following statements about the management of worsening or severe preeclampsia is correct?

a. Blood pressure in excess of 160/110, edema, and proteinuria are signs of imminent eclampsia.
b. Oliguria is a sign of impending eclampsia.
c. All women in labor who have severe preeclampsia or eclampsia should be treated with magnesium sulfate.
d. Hydralazine (apresoline) in small intermittent doses can be safely used for the control of blood pressure.
e. In severe cases of preeclampsia, the risk to the fetus even if remote from term may be less if delivery is accomplished than if the pregnancy is allowed to continue.

27–71. Which of the following is an argument against using glucocorticoids to enhance fetal lung maturation in severe preeclampsia or eclampsia?

a. Risk to the mother
b. Risk to the fetus
c. Rarity of severe respiratory distress in infants from pregnancies complicated with severe PIH

27–72. Which of the following assessments of fetal well-being and placental function provide unique information for the management of a pregnancy complicated by pregnancy-induced hypertension?

a. Serial plasma estriol
b. Serial urinary estriol
c. Placental lactogen
d. Fetal biophysical profile
e. Contraction stress test

27–73. In cases of pregnancy-induced hypertension, failure of the fetus to grow is an ominous sign of fetal jeopardy.

a. True
b. False

27–74. Which of the following statements about the postpartum period in cases of severe preeclampsia or eclampsia is correct?

a. The mother's condition usually improves rapidly after delivery.
b. Anticonvulsant medication should be continued for at least 24 hours postpartum.
c. Patients should remain hospitalized until they are normotensive.
d. Patients should be discharged on oral antihypertensive medication.
e. Pregnancy-induced hypertension is a contraindication to later use of oral contraceptives.

27–75. Eclampsia is most common in the last third of pregnancy, although it can occur anytime in the antepartum period.

a. True
b. False

27–76. Which of the following statements about eclampsia is correct?

a. Eclampsia is most serious when it occurs postpartum.
b. Eclampsia is almost always preceded by preeclampsia.
c. Convulsions begin in the lower extremities and ascend throughout the body.
d. During the eclamptic convulsion, the diaphragm is fixed.
e. The patient has no memory of the convulsion.
f. There is a "refractory period" of about 6 minutes after a convulsion when another seizure cannot occur.

27–77. Which of the following are grave signs in association with eclampsia?

a. Pulmonary edema
b. Coma
c. Fever of >39.5°C
d. Increased urinary output
e. Blindness

27–78. Define and describe intercurrent eclampsia.

27–79. What is the significance of sustained hypertension after delivery in a patient with severe preeclampsia or eclampsia?

27–80. The differential diagnosis of eclampsia includes

a. Epilepsy
b. Ruptured cerebral aneurysm
c. Hysteria
d. Acute porphyria
e. Encephalitis
f. Meningitis
g. Cerebral tumor

27–81. All pregnant women with convulsions should be considered to be eclamptic until proven otherwise.

a. True
b. False

27–82. List the essential components in the treatment of eclampsia.

27–83. Which changes arising from eclampsia generally tend to be permanent?

a. Central nervous system
b. Kidney
c. Liver
d. Thrombocytopenia
e. Hemolysis

27-84. Summarize the Parkland Memorial Hospital regimen for treatment of eclampsia.

27-85. Magnesium sulfate

a. Arrests and prevents convulsions in eclampsia
b. Is not effective as an antihypertensive agent
c. Is initially administered intravenously and intramuscularly
d. Is administered in subsequent doses when patellar reflexes are present, respirations are not decreased, and urine output is 100 cc/4 hours
e. Intoxication is avoided by rapid renal clearance

Instructions for Items 27-86 to 27-88: Match the level of magnesium sulfate with the appropriate effect.

a. 12 mEq/L
b. 8 to 10 mEq/L
c. 4 to 7 mEq/L

27-86. Convulsions prevented
27-87. Loss of patellar reflex
27-88. Respiratory depression and arrest

27-89. What is the drug of choice to treat respiratory depression due to magnesium sulfate toxicity?

27-90. The goal of intermittent intravenous hydralazine therapy in preeclampsia and eclampsia is to maintain diastolic blood pressure at about 90, thus decreasing the risk of intracranial hemorrhage while not compromising uteroplacental perfusion.

a. True
b. False

Instructions for Items 27-91 to 27-94: Match the antihypertensive drug with its possible side effects.

a. Diazoxide
b. Sodium nitroprusside

27-91. Cyanide poisoning in the fetus
27-92. Arrest of labor
27-93. Maternal and neonatal hyperglycemia
27-94. Increased intracranial pressure

27-95. Why should diuretics and hyperosmotic agents not be used to treat eclampsia?

a. They constrict maternal blood volume.
b. They compromise uteroplacental perfusion.
c. They are not needed since postpartum diuresis occurs naturally.
d. Hyperosmotic agents cause edema in vital organs.
e. There is a lack of documented efficacy with their use.

27-96. Which of the following statements about fluid therapy in eclampsia is correct?

a. Five percent dextrose in water is the intravenous solution of choice.
b. Administration of large volumes of fluid may enhance the maldistribution of extracellular and intracellular fluids.
c. A significant postpartum fall in hematocrit after delivery is usually due to the relief of vasospasm.
d. A significant decrease in blood pressure just after delivery most often is related to excessive blood loss.
e. On a regimen of limited fluid therapy, postpartum dialysis for renal failure is usually not required.

27-97. The use of magnesium sulfate in the treatment of pregnancy-induced hypertension has made induction of labor extremely difficult.

a. True
b. False

27-98. At Parkland Memorial Hospital, which of the following is the anesthesia of choice for vaginal delivery of eclamptic patients?

a. General anesthesia
b. Demerol with promethazine
c. Epidural
d. Spinal
e. Pudendal or local

27-99. What are potential risks from the use of conduction anesthesia for delivery of eclamptic patients?

a. Splanchnic blockade (hypotension)
b. Danger from pressor agents
c. Danger from the large volumes of fluid needed to correct hypotension
d. Edema formation (cerebral, pulmonary, laryngeal)

27-100. Which of the following statements about magnesium sulfate use in the treatment of preeclampsia and eclampsia is correct?

a. Magnesium sulfate is associated with depressed myometrial contractility.
b. Magnesium sulfate is not transferred across the placenta.
c. In high doses, magnesium sulfate may be associated with neonatal depression.
d. Magnesium sulfate acts both centrally and peripherally in the nervous system.

27–101. Which of the following statements about treatment of eclampsia is correct?

a. Diazepam is a well-documented substitute for magnesium sulfate.
b. Most sedatives including morphine can be used to manage eclampsia with minimal risk.
c. Heparin has not been shown to be effective in the treatment of eclampsia.
d. Eclampsia should be considered one of the hypertensive encephalopathies in planning appropriate treatment mechanisms.

27–102. What percent of eclamptic patients will be eclamptic in a subsequent pregnancy?

a. <5
b. 15 to 20
c. 40 to 50
d. 75 to 80

27–103. Women who had eclampsia associated with a multifetal pregnancy are at no greater risk for future health problems than nulliparous eclamptics.

a. True
b. False

27–104. Preeclampsia probably neither causes residual hypertension nor aggravates preexisting hypertension.

a. True
b. False

27–105. Which of the following statements about the diagnosis of chronic hypertension in pregnancy is correct?

a. Hypertension appearing late in repeated pregnancies may signal latent hypertensive vascular disease.
b. In most women with chronic hypertension, elevated blood pressure is the only abnormal finding.
c. Heredity, obesity, and age play a role in chronic hypertension.
d. The incidence of placental abruption is increased in women with chronic hypertension.
e. Babies of hypertensive mothers tend to be large for gestational age.

27–106. Which of the following statements about the treatment of chronic hypertension in pregnancy is correct?

a. Treatment with antihypertensive drugs reduces the incidence of superimposed preeclampsia.
b. The administration of antihypertensive medications significantly reduces the perinatal mortality rate.
c. The use of α-methyldopa is associated with significant fetal abnormalities.
d. Perinatal mortality is unacceptably high unless antihypertensive medications are begun in the first trimester.
e. Captopril should not be used in pregnancy.

27–107. Describe the typical manifestations of pregnancy-aggravated hypertension.

28. MEDICAL AND SURGICAL ILLNESSES DURING PREGNANCY AND THE PUERPERIUM

28–1. Which of the following statements about the presence of medical disease during pregnancy is correct?

a. Essentially all diseases that affect the nonpregnant woman may be contracted during pregnancy.
b. The presence of most diseases does not prevent conception.
c. Normal pregnancy affects the signs, symptoms, and laboratory values in most diseases.
d. A disease may be misdiagnosed if the possibility of pregnancy is not considered.

28–2. The definition of anemia may be complicated by which of the following factors?

a. Altitude
b. Sex
c. Race
d. Pregnancy

28–3. At low altitudes, which of the following hemoglobin levels may be considered to constitute anemia?

a. <12 g/dl in a nonpregnant woman
b. <10 g/dl in a pregnant woman
c. <10 g/dl immediately postpartum

28–4. During pregnancy, the volume of plasma expansion is ______________ than the increase in hemoglobin mass and erythrocyte volume.

a. Greater
b. Less

28–5. Which of the following statements about anemia in pregnancy is correct?

a. Anemia is more common among indigent patients.
b. Laboratory error may contribute to the misdiagnosis of anemia.
c. A decreased hemoglobin mass is normal in pregnancy.
d. Women who take iron supplements are likely to have higher hemoglobin levels than women who do not receive supplements.

28–6. What are the two most common causes of anemia during pregnancy and the puerperium?

Instructions for Items 28–7 to 28–10: Match the quantity of iron with its utilization in pregnancy.

a. 200 mg
b. 300 mg
c. 500 mg
d. 800 mg
e. 1200 mg

28–7. Total maternal need for iron in pregnancy
28–8. Amount of iron needed for fetus and placenta
28–9. Amount of iron needed to expand maternal hemoglobin mass
28–10. Amount of iron shed through the gut, urine, and skin

28–11. The newborn infant of a severely anemic mother does not usually suffer from iron deficiency anemia.

a. True
b. False

28–12. Which of the following statements about the identification of iron deficiency anemia is correct?

a. The serum iron binding capacity is the best single diagnostic indicator.
b. Examination of the bone marrow is usually necessary to diagnose iron deficiency.
c. Hematologic response to iron may be first detected in a peripheral blood smear.
d. Pregnancy is known to depress erythropoiesis and hemoglobin formation.
e. Evidence of Plummer-Vinson's syndrome is rarely seen in pregnancy.
f. In severe iron deficiency anemia during pregnancy, erythrocytes demonstrate hypochromia and microcytosis.

28–13. Which of the following may be appropriate for the evaluation of moderate anemia in a pregnant woman?

a. Hemoglobin concentration
b. Hematocrit
c. Red cell indices
d. Peripheral blood smear
e. Sickle cell preparation
f. Serum ferritin level

28–14. What is the preferred therapy for simple iron deficiency anemia in pregnancy?

a. Parenteral iron
b. Blood transfusion
c. Oral iron

28–15. Which of the following statements about oral iron therapy is correct?

a. Therapy should provide 200 mg of iron daily.
b. Oral therapy should be discontinued as soon as the anemia has been corrected.
c. Patients receiving iron and folic acid do considerably better than those receiving only iron.
d. Ferrous sulfate is a better iron source than ferrous fumarate or ferrous gluconate.
e. Iron preparations totally free of adverse effects are likely to be poorly absorbed.

28–16. What type of transfusion is an effective way of raising the hemoglobin concentration of severely anemic women without inducing circulatory overload?

28–17. Which of the following statements about acute blood loss anemia is correct?

a. It is more likely in the puerperium than during pregnancy.
b. Acute hemorrhage may have little immediate effect on hemoglobin concentration.
c. Immediate blood replacement with whole blood is indicated.
d. Once stable, the patient can be satisfactorily treated with oral iron.

28–18. Which of the following statements about anemia with chronic disease in pregnancy is correct?

a. Erythrocytes are usually normocytic or slightly microcytic.
b. Bone marrow cytology is typically bizarre.
c. There is decreased erythropoiesis and slightly increased destruction of erythrocytes.
d. The anemia of infection, renal disease, and malignancy is not corrected with iron, folic acid, or vitamin B_{12}.
e. Iron and folate therapy is not worthwhile in pregnancy when anemia with chronic disease is present.

28–19. Which of the following statements about megaloblastic anemia in pregnancy is correct?

a. It is a common complication of pregnancy in the United States.
b. It is usually found in pregnant women who consume neither fresh vegetables nor animal protein.
c. It is most commonly due to vitamin B_{12} deficiency.
d. The earliest morphologic finding in cases of folate deficiency is hypersegmentation of neutrophils.
e. Severe cases of folate deficiency may be accompanied by thrombocytopenia and leukopenia.
f. The fetus of a mother who is anemic due to severe folate deficiency will also be severely anemic.
g. Megaloblastic anemia tends to recur in subsequent pregnancies.

28–20. Which of the following statements about the treatment of folic acid deficiency in pregnancy is correct?

a. One mg of oral folic acid per day produces a significant response.
b. The rate of hemoglobin increase is tempered by the expanding blood volume of pregnancy.
c. Iron as well as folic acid should usually be supplemented.

28–21. Pernicious anemia

a. Caused by the failure to absorb vitamin B_{12} is rare in women of reproductive age
b. If left untreated, may result in infertility
c. Should not be treated during pregnancy

28–22. Breast fed infants of mothers who suffer vitamin B_{12} deficiency may develop megaloblastic anemia during infancy.

a. True
b. False

28–23. Which of the following statements about acquired hemolytic anemia in pregnancy is correct?

a. Pregnancy may accelerate hemolysis in women with autoimmune acquired hemolytic anemia.
b. In autoimmune hemolytic anemia, both the indirect and direct Coombs tests are positive.
c. Pregnancy-induced hemolytic anemia is a rare but treatable disease.
d. The most fulminant acquired hemolytic anemia during pregnancy is caused by the exotoxin of *Clostridium perfringens.*
e. Hemolysis may rarely be due to pregnancy-induced hypertension.
f. Pregnancy is a contraindication to the use of steroids for treatment of acquired hemolytic anemia.

28–24. Which of the following is a clinical aspect of paroxysmal nocturnal hemoglobinuria?

a. The hemoglobinuria only occurs at night.
b. There is a defect in the membranes of red cells, platelets, and granulocytes that makes then susceptible to lysis.
c. Heparin therapy has proven to be of considerable value.
d. The disease is familial, inherited as a sex-linked recessive trait.

28–25. Deficiency of glucose-6-phosphate dehydrogenase is an inherited enzymatic defect that accounts for drug-induced hemolysis in many black women.

a. True
b. False

28–26. Which of the following is characteristic of aplastic anemia in pregnancy?

a. It is relatively rare.
b. Anemia is coupled with thrombocytopenia and leukopenia.
c. Bone marrow is markedly hypocellular.
d. It is always congenital.
e. It is never pregnancy related.
f. Bone marrow transplantation is the most effective therapy.
g. Antithymocyte globulin is the appropriate therapy for patients without a suitable bone marrow donor.

28–27. What are the two greatest risks to women with aplastic anemia during pregnancy?

28–28. List the most common sickle cell hemoglobinopathies.

28–29. Which of the following statements about sickle cell anemia is correct?

a. Sickle cell crises are more common in pregnancy.
b. Maternal and neonatal mortality rates are elevated in the presence of sickle cell anemia.
c. Supplemental folic acid is indicated.
d. Bone pain is best treated with heparin.
e. Red cell transfusion after the onset of a painful crisis alleviates the pain dramatically.

28–30. Which of the following contraceptive techniques is probably contraindicated for women with sickle cell disease?

a. Oral contraceptive
b. Intrauterine device
c. Diaphragm
d. Condom
e. Spermicidal jelly

28–31. Which of the following statements about sickle cell-hemoglobin C disease (SC) is correct?

a. The gene for hemoglobin C is more common than the gene for hemoglobin S.
b. In the nonpregnant woman, SC morbidity is lower and life span is longer than in the woman with sickle cell anemia.
c. Attacks of bone pain and episodes of pulmonary dysfunction are increased during pregnancy and the puerperium.
d. Perinatal mortality rates are as high for SC as for sickle cell anemia.
e. Iron and folic acid supplementation is necessary.
f. Prophylactic exchange transfusion may reduce maternal morbidity.

28–32. Perinatal morbidity and mortality in sickle cell-β-thalassemia is ______(1) that in sickle cell-hemoglobin C disease and ______(2) that in sickle cell anemia.

a. Less than
b. Similar to
c. Greater than

28–33. Which of the following statements about prophylactic exchange transfusion for sickle hemoglobinopathies in pregnancy is correct?

a. Transfusions should be initiated as soon as pregnancy is confirmed.
b. Potential complications include hepatitis, iron overload, and alloimmunization.
c. Reduction of potentially adverse reactions is beyond the scope of present technology.

28–34. Which of the following characterizes sickle cell trait?

a. More S hemoglobin is produced than A hemoglobin.
b. Erythrocytes usually appear normal.
c. The frequencies of abortion and perinatal mortality are not increased.
d. There is an association with asymptomatic bacteriuria.
e. There is a higher incidence of pregnancy-induced hypertension.

Instructions for Items 28–35 to 28–38: Match the characteristic with the correct hemoglobin type.

a. Hemoglobin C
b. Hemoglobin E

28–35. Occurs in 2.5 percent of the black population
28–36. Presence of mild anemia
28–37. Folate and iron supplementation is needed in severe cases
28–38. Does not predispose to pathologic pregnancies

28–39. Hemolytic anemia characteristic of sickle cell anemia and sickle cell-hemoglobin C disease usually begins in utero.

a. True
b. False

28–40. If one parent has a hemoglobinopathy and the other parent has the trait, ______(1) percent of their offspring will have the disease and ______(2) percent will have the trait.

a. 0
b. 25
c. 50
d. 75
e. 100

28–41. What techniques have been utilized to identify a fetus genetically destined to develop sickle cell disease?

a. Fetoscopic collection of fetal red blood cells
b. Enzymatic treatment of amniocytes
c. Chorionic villus biopsy

28–42. Which of the following statements about hereditary spherocytosis is correct?

a. It may be transmitted as an autosomal dominant with variable penetrance.
b. Hemolysis depends on an intact, usually enlarged, spleen.
c. A previous normal pregnancy rules out the possibility of sudden anemia in a subsequent pregnancy.
d. A newborn who has inherited spherocytosis may or may not develop hyperbilirubinemia and anemia in the neonatal period.

28–43. What are thalassemias?

Instructions for Items 28–44 to 28–48: Match the α-thalassemia with the appropriate hemoglobin composition where (+) means the presence of a functioning globin chain gene.

a. Hemoglobin Bart's disease
b. Hemoglobin H disease
c. α-Thalassemia minor
d. Carrier state

28–44. – –/– –
28–45. – –/– +
28–46. – +/– +
28–47. – –/+ +
28–48. – +/+ +

28–49. Which of the following statements about α-thalassemia is correct?

a. In the fetus with hemoglobin Bart's disease there are four γ chains.
b. Homozygous α-thalassemia results in the clinical picture of nonimmune hydrops fetalis.
c. Hemoglobin H disease is incompatible with extrauterine life.
d. α-Thalassemia minor is characterized by mild to moderate microcytic anemia.
e. The simultaneous inheritance of sickle cell anemia and α-thalassemia results in a worse prognosis than that with sickle cell anemia alone.

28–50. Which of the following statements about β-thalassemia is correct?

a. The rate of hemoglobin synthesis is unchanged and the rate of red blood cell destruction increases.
b. β-Thalassemia minor is associated with intense hemolysis that is similar to that in the homozygous state.
c. A woman with β-thalassemia major is often sterile.
d. There is no specific therapy for β-thalassemia minor during pregnancy.
e. β-Thalassemia intermedia is actually a variation of sickle cell anemia.

28–51. Thrombocytopenia may be associated with

a. Aplastic anemia
b. Acquired hemolytic anemia
c. Eclampsia-severe preeclampsia
d. Consumptive coagulopathy
e. Lupus erythematosus
f. Megaloblastic anemia
g. Infections

28–52. Which of the following is a feature of immune idiopathic thrombocytopenia?

a. Presence of antiplatelet antibodies
b. Familial occurrence
c. Therapeutic response to splenectomy and/or corticosteroids
d. Ameliorated by pregnancy
e. Formation of IgG antibodies

28–53. Which of the following statements about the effects of maternal immune idiopathic thrombocytopenia on the fetus is correct?

a. There is a strong correlation between maternal and fetal platelet counts.
b. Administration of corticosteroids to the mother assures an adequate fetal platelet count.
c. Intrapartum platelet counts on fetal scalp blood may aid in patient management.
d. In a mother with severe thrombocytopenia, cesarean delivery is safest for both the mother and the fetus.

28–54. Which of the following is an effective treatment for immune idiopathic thrombocytopenia?

a. High doses of gamma globulin
b. Danazol (a synthetic weak androgen)
c. Estrogen plus progestin oral contraceptives

28–55. What are the principal findings in thrombotic thrombocytopenic purpura?

28–56. What pregnancy-related condition has been confused with thrombotic thrombocytopenic purpura?

28–57. What are effective treatment modalities for thrombotic thrombocytopenic purpura?

a. Exchange transfusion
b. Platelet transfusion
c. Plasmapheresis
d. Termination of pregnancy
e. Dextran 70

28–58. Obstetric hemorrhage is most commonly due to an inherited defect in the coagulation mechanism.

a. True
b. False

28–59. Which of the following is characteristic of hemophilia A?

a. It is less common in women than in men.
b. It is inherited as a sex-linked recessive trait.
c. Bleeding is dependent on the level of circulating Factor VIII:C.
d. Vaginal delivery is dangerous for the fetus with hemophilia A.
e. Prenatal diagnosis utilizing fetal plasma is possible near midpregnancy.

28–60. Antibodies to Factor VIII may be acquired and lead to life-threatening hemorrhage, especially in the puerperium.

a. True
b. False

28–61. Successful management of the pregnancy of a woman with hemophilia B requires the specific replacement of vitamin K.

a. True
b. False

28–62. Which of the following statements about von Willebrand's disease is correct?

a. It is a distinct clinical entity.
b. It is inherited only as an X-linked recessive trait.
c. It is characterized by easy bruising, mucosal hemorrhage, and excessive bleeding with trauma or surgery.
d. Bleeding time and partial thromboplastin time are prolonged.
e. The level of Factor VIII is decreased.
f. The hemostatic defects progressively worsen throughout pregnancy.

28–63. Which of the following is a relatively common disorder associated with pregnancy?

a. Factor IX deficiency
b. Familial hypofibrinogenemia
c. Congenital afibrinogenemia
d. Acquired hypofibrinogenemia

28–64. Which of the following statements about hematologic disorders in pregnancy is correct?

a. Pregnant women with leukemia may transmit the disease to their offspring.
b. Pregnancy adversely affects the course of Hodgkin's disease.
c. Polycythemia during pregnancy is usually secondary and related to hypoxia from cardiac or pulmonary disease.
d. Severe polycythemia is associated with poor pregnancy outcomes.
e. Serum erythropoietin may be helpful in differentiating secondary polycythemia from polycythemia vera.

28–65. Pregnancy usually predisposes to the development or exacerbation of diseases of the urinary tract.

a. True
b. False

28–66. Which of the following statements about urinary tract infections in pregnancy is correct?

a. Routine catheterization of the bladder at the time of delivery is recommended to prevent infection.
b. Bacteriuria is present in about 35 percent of pregnant women at the time of the first prenatal visit.
c. Asymptomatic bacteriuria need not be identified since it very rarely results in symptomatic urinary tract infections.
d. Acute pyelonephritis in pregnancy is commonly an ascending infection from the bladder.
e. Acute pyelonephritis is one of the most frequent complications of pregnancy.

28–67. Which of the following symptoms are typically associated with cystitis in pregnancy?

a. Dysuria
b. Urgency
c. Frequency
d. Fever
e. Hematuria

28–68. Symptoms of frequency, urgency, dysuria, and pyuria without bacteriuria may be due to what common pathogen of the genitourinary tract?

a. *Neisseria gonorrheae*
b. *Escherichia coli*
c. *Proteus mirabilis*
d. *Chlamydia trachomatis*

28–69. Which of the following statements about acute pyelonephritis in pregnancy is correct?

a. It is most frequent during the second trimester.
b. If unilateral, the disease is more common on the left side.
c. Signs and symptoms are usually very subtle.
d. The body temperature is always sharply elevated.
e. The causative agent is usually a gram-negative bacteria.

28–70. The differential diagnosis of acute pyelonephritis includes

a. Labor
b. Placental abruption
c. Appendicitis
d. Infarction of a myoma
e. Cystitis

28–71. What factors predispose the bacteriuric pregnant woman to acute pyelonephritis?

28–72. Which of the following puerperal factors predispose to acute pyelonephritis?

a. Anesthetic effects on bladder sensitivity
b. Pelvic discomfort
c. Antidiuretic effect of oxytocin
d. Bladder overdistention
e. Bladder catheterization

28–73. What is "asymptomatic bacteriuria?"

28–74. Which of the following statements about asymptomatic bacteriuria is correct?

a. The highest incidence is among black multiparas with sickle cell trait.
b. The condition is usually acquired in the second trimester.
c. A catheterized specimen is required to make the diagnosis.
d. Eradication of bacteriuria with antimicrobials prevents nearly all clinically evident infections.

28–75. Asymptomatic bacteriuria is not a prominent factor in the genesis of low birth weight or prematurity.

a. True
b. False

28–76. When should urologic evaluation be done in patients who do not respond to treatment of asymptomatic bacteriuria or who become reinfected after therapy?

a. As soon as possible
b. Immediately postpartum
c. After the puerperium

28–77. Which of the following statements about chronic pyelonephritis in pregnancy is correct?

a. It may be asymptomatic.
b. In advanced cases, the major symptoms are those of renal insufficiency.
c. Prior symptomatic urinary infections can be documented in most patients.
d. Fetal prognosis is uniformly poor.
e. There is an increased risk of superimposed acute pyelonephritis.

28–78. Which of the following statements about the management of urinary tract infections in pregnancy is correct?

a. Gentamicin is usually the treatment of choice.
b. Asymptomatic bacteriuria should be treated with the patient hospitalized.
c. Patients with acute pyelonephritis are at risk for bacterial shock.
d. Therapy for acute pyelonephritis should be continued for at least 10 days.
e. It is unnecessary to repeat urine cultures after treatment of a urinary tract infection if the patient's symptoms have disappeared within 2 days.

Instructions for Items 28–79 to 28–85: Match the antimicrobial therapy utilized for urinary tract infections with its potential side effects.

a. Sulfonamide
b. Nitrofurantoin
c. Tetracycline
d. Chloramphenicol
e. Gentamicin

28–79. Ototoxicity
28–80. Maternal hemolysis
28–81. Maternal jaundice
28–82. Infant tooth discoloration
28–83. Kernicterus
28–84. Nephrotoxicity
28–85. Aplastic anemia

28–86. In severely ill pregnant women, what drug regimen provides effective treatment for urinary tract infections while culture and sensitivity results are pending?

a. Sulfonamides
b. Nitrofurantoin
c. Tetracycline
d. Chloramphenicol
e. Ampicillin/gentamicin

28–87. After antimicrobial treatment for urinary tract infection, absence of pyuria is adequate evidence for cure.

a. True
b. False

28–88. A history of renal tuberculosis is an absolute contraindication to pregnancy.

a. True
b. False

28–89. Which of the following statements about urinary calculi during pregnancy is correct?

a. Pregnancy increases the risk of stone formation in women who have a history of renal stones.
b. There is an increased frequency of urinary tract infection among pregnant women with renal stones.
c. Surgical removal of stones should be accomplished as soon as they are discovered.
d. Renal calculi may be associated with hyperparathyroidism.

28–90. Which of the following statements about acute glomerulonephritis in pregnancy is correct?

a. The condition is rare in pregnancy.
b. It may be clinically indistinguishable from preeclampsia.
c. Management should consist of expectant observation.
d. Some cases may gradually turn into chronic glomerulonephritis.
e. Subsequent pregnancy is contraindicated.

28–91. Which of the following statements about chronic glomerulonephritis is correct?

a. It is characterized by progressive renal destruction.
b. Renal failure is almost always the first manifestation.
c. There is an increased rate of preeclampsia.
d. The prognosis for pregnancy outcome in cases of maternal azotemia or extreme hypertension is poor.
e. Renal plasma flow and glomerular filtration may increase during pregnancy.

28–92. Which of the following is found in nephrosis?

a. Edema
b. Massive proteinuria
c. Hypoalbuminemia
d. Hypercholesterolemia

28–93. Which of the following conditions is associated with the nephrotic syndrome?

a. Syphilis
b. Chronic glomerulonephritis
c. Lupus erythematosus
d. Diabetes
e. Amyloidosis
f. Renal vein thrombosis
g. Heavy metal poisoning

28–94. Since the advent of steroid therapy, all women with nephrosis should be able to undergo an uncomplicated pregnancy.

a. True
b. False

28–95. Which of the following statements about acute renal failure in pregnancy is correct?

a. The most common cause is acute pyelonephritis.
b. Diuretics should be instituted as soon as oliguria is identified.
c. A urine:plasma creatinine ratio of greater than 30 is suggestive of prerenal azotemia.
d. In prerenal azotemia, sodium readsorption is low.

28–96. Which of the following statements about acute tubular necrosis (ATN) is correct?

a. It is largely preventable.
b. Hemodialysis is warranted in cases of azotemia and persistent oliguria.
c. It is a progressive disease.
d. Future pregnancies are contraindicated in women with ATN.

28–97. What measures can help prevent acute tubular necrosis?

a. Vigorous blood replacement
b. Termination of pregnancies in the presence of severe preeclampsia or eclampsia
c. Early identification and treatment of septic shock
d. Aggressive use of potent diuretics
e. Early use of vasoconstrictors in cases of hypotension

28–98. Which of the following statements about renal cortical necrosis is correct?

a. It is more common than acute tubular necrosis.
b. Most cases in pregnant women have occurred after placental abruption, preeclampsia/eclampsia, or bacterial shock.
c. The condition usually improves spontaneously without treatment.
d. Renal cortical necrosis can be clinically distinguished from acute tubular necrosis during the early phase of the disease.
e. The prognosis depends on the extent of the necrosis.

28–99. The compression of the ureters by the large pregnant uterus commonly causes ureteral obstruction resulting in oliguria and azotemia.

a. True
b. False

28–100. Which of the following is characteristic of postpartum hemolytic uremic syndrome?

a. Necrosis and endothelial proliferation in glomeruli
b. Necrosis, thrombosis, and intimal thickening in renal arterioles
c. Necrosis, thrombosis, and intimal thickening in pulmonary arterioles
d. Microangiopathic hemolysis
e. Thrombocytopenia

28–101. There may be a normal pregnancy outcome in which of the following situations?

a. After renal transplantation
b. After unilateral nephrectomy
c. Orthostatic proteinuria
d. Polycystic kidney disease
e. Renal failure requiring hemodialysis during pregnancy

28–102. What are the two primary causes of cardiac disease in pregnancy?

a. Rheumatic heart disease
b. Myocarditis
c. Congenital heart disease
d. Kyphoscoliotic heart disease
e. Hypertensive heart disease

28–103. Which of the following statements about cardiac disease in pregnancy is correct?

a. It occurs in about 10 percent of pregnancies.
b. Prognosis is independent of the psychologic and socioeconomic situation of the patient and her family.
c. Cardiac decompensation seldom occurs after the 32nd week.
d. Cardiac failure can occur during the puerperium.

28–104. What physiologic changes of pregnancy may mask cardiac disease?

a. Systolic murmurs
b. Dyspnea
c. Changes simulating cardiac enlargement
d. Edema

28–105. Which of the following is confirmatory evidence for the diagnosis of heart disease in pregnancy?

a. Diastolic murmur
b. Continuous murmur
c. Cardiac enlargement
d. Severe arrhythmia
e. Loud, harsh systolic murmur associated with a thrill

Instructions for Items 28–106 to 28–109: Match the New York Heart Association classification with the corresponding limit on physical activity.

a. Class I
b. Class II
c. Class III
d. Class IV

28–106. Less than ordinary physical activity causes excessive fatigue
28–107. There is angina at rest
28–108. No limitation on physical activity
28–109. Ordinary physical activity causes dyspnea

28–110. Which of the following conditions may be especially hazardous for the pregnant patient with cardiac disease?

a. Excessive weight gain
b. Anemia
c. Abnormal retention of blood
d. Pregnancy-induced hypertension
e. Hypotension

28–111. Which of the following statements about the management of class I and class II cardiac disease in pregnancy is correct?

a. Most patients may be allowed to go through pregnancy.
b. Maximum rest and minimum work are important.
c. Cardiac failure can be precipitated by infection.
d. Vaginal delivery is associated with greater morbidity and mortality than cesarean delivery.
e. Hospitalization throughout pregnancy is necessary.

28–112. Which of the following are indications of heart failure during pregnancy?

a. Increased vital capacity
b. Persistent rales
c. Dyspnea on exertion
d. Hemoptysis
e. Progressive edema
f. Bradycardia

28–113. What is the major danger in the use of conduction anesthesia for delivery in a patient with cardiac disease?

28–114. Which of the following statements about the delivery of a patient with cardiac disease is correct?

a. Relief from pain and apprehension are particularly important.
b. The patient should be in the supine position.
c. Anesthesia for cesarean delivery should avoid succinylcholine.
d. Vital signs should be monitored more frequently in the second stage of labor than in the first stage.

28–115. At the first sign of cardiac failure during labor, delivery should be accomplished as quickly as possible.

a. True
b. False

28–116. Which of the following are important aspects of the medical treatment of heart failure in pregnancy?

a. Morphine
b. Oxygen
c. Intramuscular digitalis preparation
d. Oral diuretic
e. Fowler position

28–117. Which of the following statements about the management of patients with the potential for cardiac failure is correct?

a. Furosemide will reduce venous return and reduce pulmonary congestion.
b. Use of a Swan-Ganz catheter can aid in therapeutic decision making in cases of hypotension associated with cardiac failure.
c. Postpartum decompensation only occurs in those patients who suffered cardiac failure intrapartum.
d. In the absence of cardiac failure, breast feeding is not contraindicated.
e. Postpartum sterilization should be performed as soon after delivery as possible.

28–118. Which of the following statements about class III cardiac disease in pregnancy is correct?

a. Class III disease may be an indication for therapeutic abortion.
b. Unless preventive measures are taken, about one-third of patients will decompensate during pregnancy.
c. Hospitalization for the duration of pregnancy produces the best outcomes.
d. Cesarean section is the most appropriate delivery method.
e. Pregnancy has a long-term deleterious effect on the condition.

28–119. Prior to performing a therapeutic abortion on a patient in cardiac failure, what must be done to stabilize the patient?

28–120. What is the prime objective in treating a patient with class IV heart disease during pregnancy?

28–121. Severe maternal hypoxia predisposes to abortion, prematurity, and intrauterine death.

a. True
b. False

28–122. Which of the following statements about the effects of heart valve replacement on pregnancy is correct?

a. Valve replacements must not be done during pregnancy.
b. Women with artificial heart valves should take heparin during pregnancy.
c. Prolonged heparin administration during pregnancy may have adverse effects on the pregnancy outcome.
d. Complications with prosthetic valves include thrombosis and hemorrhage.
e. Spontaneous abortions and low birth weight infants are more common in women with a prosthetic valve.
f. Combination estrogen-progestin birth control pills are the contraceptive of choice for women with prosthetic valves.

28–123. If a woman with an artificial heart valve is taking heparin, how soon before delivery should it be stopped?

28–124. In the patient with a patent ductus arteriosus and pulmonary hypertension, what abnormality may develop if systemic blood pressure drops?

28–125. In pregnant patients with a very high hematocrit, spontaneous abortion will be the most likely pregnancy outcome.

a. True
b. False

28–126. Which of the following statements about cyanotic heart disease in pregnancy is correct?

a. There is no relation between polycythemia and the birth of underweight infants.
b. Maternal and fetal outcomes are both improved when defects are surgically corrected before pregnancy.
c. Women with tetralogy of Fallot that has been surgically corrected should still be counseled to have a therapeutic abortion.
d. Both maternal and perinatal mortality in Eisenmenger's syndrome is about 30 percent.
e. The prognosis for a pregnancy complicated by pulmonary hypertension from any cause is poor.

28–127. In what circumstances should future pregnancy probably be avoided?

a. If coronary angiography indicates severe disease in a patient who has suffered a myocardial infarction
b. If there is persistent cardiomegaly and heart failure in a patient who has had periportal cardiomyopathy
c. In patients requiring antibiotic prophylaxis for the prevention of bacterial endocarditis
d. In a patient with a documented mitral valve prolapse
e. In a patient with coarctation of the aorta

28–128. How does cor pulmonale develop in a patient with kyphoscoliotic heart disease?

28–129. Which of the following statements about kyphosis in pregnancy is correct?

a. Therapeutic abortion is indicated in women with marked degrees of kyphoscoliosis and markedly impaired pulmonary function.
b. Pelvic distortions may necessitate cesarean delivery.
c. Meperidine-induced respiratory depression is poorly tolerated.
d. Intermittent positive pressure breathing may be helpful.

28–130. Which of the following arrythmias is incompatible with a successful pregnancy outcome?

a. Complete heart block
b. Atrial fibrillation
c. Wolff-Parkinson-White's syndrome
d. Supraventricular tachycardia

Instructions for Items 28–131 to 28–137: Match the parameter with its change in pregnancy from the nonpregnant state.

a. Increases
b. Decreases

28–131. Transverse thoracic diameter
28–132. Vertical chest diameter
28–133. Residual volume
28–134. Respiratory rate
28–135. Tidal volume
28–136. Plasma carbon dioxide
28–137. Oxygen consumption

28–138. Which type of pneumonia, if untreated, may result in a loss of ventilatory capacity that may pose significant problems for mother and fetus?

a. *Streptococcus pneumoniae*
b. *Mycoplasma pneumoniae*
c. Aspiration pneumonia
d. Viral pneumonitis

28–139. Thromboembolism and pulmonary infarction are both more common in the puerperium than during pregnancy.

a. True
b. False

28–140. Which of the following statements about asthma in pregnancy is correct?

a. An elevated Pco_2 is an ominous sign.
b. Pregnancy exacerbates all asthmatic conditions.
c. Therapy for asthma during pregnancy is markedly different than that which is effective in the nonpregnant woman.
d. Oxygen therapy should be instituted when the Po_2 is less than 70 mm Hg.
e. Iodine-containing medications may induce a fetal goiter.

28–141. What therapeutic modalities can be helpful in managing the pregnant patient with asthma?

a. α-Adrenergic agents
b. Steroids
c. Theophyllines
d. Hydration

28–142. Which of the following statements about tuberculosis in pregnancy is correct?

a. Pulmonary resection for tuberculosis contraindicates future child bearing.
b. Chemotherapy that is effective when the woman is nonpregnant is also effective during pregnancy.
c. All positive skin tests should be immediately treated with isoniazid.
d. The infant should be isolated from a mother suspected of having acute disease.
e. Pelvic tuberculosis is usually fatal to the mother.

28–143. When isoniazid is used for tuberculosis in pregnancy, what other medication should be given to prevent fetal harm?

28–144. How should a pregnant woman be initially screened for tuberculosis?

a. Skin test
b. Chest x-ray
c. Physical examination
d. CT scan
e. Complete blood count

28–145. Corticosteroids should not be used to treat sarcoidosis in pregnancy.

a. True
b. False

28–146. Which of the following statements about cystic fibrosis and pregnancy is correct?

a. Cystic fibrosis is transmitted as an autosomal recessive trait.
b. The disease is more common in blacks than in whites.
c. Most females who survive to adulthood are infertile.
d. Pulmonary infection causes increased perinatal and maternal mortality.
e. Nutrition may be compromised in pregnant women with cystic fibrosis.

28–147. Diabetes mellitus is ______ (1) by pregnancy and ______ (2) the risk of a number of pregnancy complications.

a. Exacerbated
b. Improved
c. Increases
d. Decreases

28–148. Which of the following statements about diabetes in pregnancy is correct?

a. Before the discovery of insulin, diabetic women were most often too ill to conceive.
b. For most insulin dependent (type I) patients, there is no previous family history of diabetes.
c. Glycosuria usually reflects impaired glucose tolerance.
d. Lactose in the urine is definitive proof of diabetes.

28–149. The likelihood that a woman suffers from impaired carbohydrate metabolism is increased by

a. A strong family history of diabetes
b. The previous birth of a large infant
c. The presence of persistent glucosuria
d. An unexplained fetal loss

28–150. What is the criterion for the diagnosis of overt diabetes in pregnancy?

Instructions for Items 28–151 to 28–154: Select the minimum plasma glucose level that at the given time identifies the presence of class A diabetes in a glucose tolerance test during pregnancy.

a. 90 mg/dl
b. 105 mg/dl
c. 135 mg/dl
d. 145 mg/dl
e. 165 mg/dl
f. 175 mg/dl
g. 190 mg/dl

28–151. Fasting
28–152. 1 hour
28–153. 2 hours
28–154. 3 hours

28–155. Which of the following statements about the use of a glucose tolerance test to identify diabetes is correct?

a. The test is used to diagnose class A diabetes.
b. The patient should fast the day before the test.
c. The diagnosis of class A diabetes is made if two or more timed plasma glucose samples exceed expected values.
d. If early in pregnancy a woman has a normal fasting glucose level and an abnormal glucose tolerance test, she may later develop overt diabetes.
e. During pregnancy, the oral glucose tolerance test is more precise than in the non-pregnant patient.

28–156. Which of the following factors contributes to the final results of an oral glucose tolerance test?

a. Absorption of glucose from the intestinal tract
b. Uptake of glucose by tissues
c. Excretion of glucose in the urine
d. Stimulation of pancreatic insulin production

28–157. Which of the following contributes to impaired insulin action in pregnancy?

a. Placental lactogen
b. Estrogen
c. Progesterone
d. Placental insulinase

28–158. Which of the following statements about the effects of pregnancy on diabetes is correct?

a. The worsening of diabetes seen during pregnancy usually disappears after delivery.
b. Nausea and vomiting during pregnancy may result in either insulin shock or insulin resistance.
c. Hypoglycemia may occur during labor, unless insulin levels are adjusted.
d. Pregnancy provides resistance to the ketoacidosis that might otherwise result from a severe infection.
e. There is less likelihood of developing metabolic acidosis during pregnancy complicated by diabetes than during normal pregnancy.

28–159. Which of the following are adverse maternal effects caused by diabetes during pregnancy?

a. Increased risk of preeclampsia/eclampsia
b. Greater frequency and severity of infections
c. Greater risk of maternal birth trauma from delivery of a large fetus
d. Risks from cesarean delivery
e. Risks from hydramnios and its effects
f. Increased frequency of postpartum hemorrhage

28–160. The potential adverse fetal effects resulting from maternal diabetes include an increased risk of

a. Perinatal death
b. Birth injury
c. Respiratory distress
d. Hypoglycemia
e. Hypocalcemia
f. Congenital anomalies
g. Diabetes

28–161. Which of the following statements about fetal effects of diabetes in pregnancy is correct?

a. In cases of macrosomia, the brain is affected more than any other organ.
b. Babies of diabetic mothers are always macrosomic.
c. Maternal hypoglycemia is the cause of compensatory fetal macrosomia.
d. In the infants of diabetic mothers, the islets of Langerhans are frequently hypertrophic and hyperplastic.

28–162. Inclusion of which of the following principles of management will result in the best outcome in cases of pregnancy complicated by diabetes?

a. Identification of the presence of abnormal carbohydrate metabolism
b. Control of blood sugar levels
c. Antepartum care by experienced providers
d. Perinatal and neonatal care by experienced providers

28–163. Which of the following statements about the management of class A diabetes in pregnancy is correct?

a. The patients may usually be successfully managed by diet alone.
b. Delivery should be induced at 36 weeks.
c. An adequate diet should provide about 35 calories per kilogram per day.
d. Even with experienced health care providers, perinatal mortality is still about four times that in the general population.
e. Ten to fifteen percent of class A diabetics develop overt diabetes during pregnancy.

28–164. Which of the following statements about the management of overt diabetes during pregnancy is correct?

a. Successful outcome is based solely on the control of blood sugar levels.
b. With proper care, perinatal mortality can approximate that in the general population.
c. Congenital malformations may be related to diabetes that was poorly controlled before conception and early in pregnancy.
d. Maternal glucose levels should be kept as close to normal as possible.
e. Pregnancy should always continue until pulmonary maturity is achieved.

28–165. Which of the following can help to achieve improved outcomes in pregnancies complicated by diabetes?

a. Frequent meals
b. Appropriate administration of insulin
c. Frequent measurement of plasma glucose levels
d. Precise knowledge of gestational age
e. Prenatal counseling

28–166. Insulin dosage in a pregnancy complicated by diabetes should be adjusted to eliminate glucosuria.

a. True
b. False

28–167. What management should follow the identification of acetonuria in a pregnancy complicated by diabetes?

28–168. Which of the following drugs is recommended for use in pregnancy complicated by diabetes?

a. Tolbutamide
b. Estradiol
c. Stilbestrol with progesterone
d. Stilbestrol with ethisterone
e. Estradiol with 17-hydroxyprogesterone caproate

28–169. Which of the following parameters presently offers the most information about fetal well-being near term in a woman with diabetes?

a. 24-Hour urinary estriol
b. Plasma estriol
c. Nonstress test/fetal heart reactivity test
d. Glycosylated hemoglobin A

28–170. What criteria must be met in order to safely begin induction of labor in a pregnancy complicated by diabetes?

a. The fetus must not be excessively large
b. The pelvis must not be contracted
c. Parity must not be great
d. The cervix must be favorable
e. There must be a vertex presentation
f. The presenting part must be fixed in the pelvis

28–171. Which of the following statements about delivery in a pregnancy complicated by diabetes is correct?

a. Cesarean delivery can avoid trauma to the fetus and the mother.
b. Long-acting insulin should be used on the day of delivery.
c. Plasma glucose levels should be checked frequently.
d. Postpartum insulin requirements are easily predictable based on maternal weight.
e. Postpartum starvation and infection pose significant maternal risks.

28–172. Which of the following are sources of significant perinatal morbidity in infants from pregnancies complicated by diabetes?

a. Congenital malformations
b. Hyperglycemia
c. Hypocalcemia
d. Hyperbilirubinemia
e. Idiopathic respiratory distress

28–173. In infants from pregnancies complicated by diabetes, organ system maturity is directly proportional to birth weight.

a. True
b. False

28–174. Which of the following reversible contraceptive methods is the best choice for women with overt diabetes?

a. Intrauterine device
b. Estrogen-progestin oral contraceptives
c. Contraception, barrier methods
d. Rhythm method

28–175. What normal pregnancy-induced changes mimic the signs and symptoms of thyroid dysfunction?

a. Increased cutaneous blood flow
b. Increased heart rate
c. Elevated free thyroxine
d. Increased thyroid uptake of radioiodine
e. Decreased thyroid-binding globulin

28–176. Which of the following is a helpful sign for identifying hyperthyroidism during pregnancy?

a. Excessive tachycardia
b. Elevated pulse rate during sleep
c. Enlarged thyroid gland
d. Exophthalmos
e. Failure to gain weight normally

28–177. Which of the following statements about the diagnosis of hyperthyroidism during pregnancy is correct?

a. The level of thyroxine in plasma is usually elevated.
b. The decreased uptake of triiodothyronine seen in normal pregnancy does not occur.
c. A normal plasma thyroxine level rules out hyperthyroidism.
d. A definitive diagnosis requires measuring thyroid uptake of radioactive iodine.
e. Management for a successful pregnancy outcome is primarily dependent on measurement of serial levels of thyroxine and triiodothyronine.

28–178. Which of the following statements about the medical treatment of hyperthyroidism in pregnancy is correct?

a. Medical management is primarily utilized to prepare the patient for definitive surgical treatment.
b. Fetal goiter and hypothyroidism may be induced by maternal ingestion of propylthiouracil.
c. Thyroid supplementation is often necessary when propylthiouracil is administered during pregnancy.
d. Propranolol is contraindicated during pregnancy.
e. Iodine should only be utilized for long-term therapy during pregnancy.

28–179. How is the proper dosage of propylthiouracil determined during pregnancy?

28–180. What adverse fetal effects may be associated with the use of propranolol for the treatment of hyperthyroidism during pregnancy?

a. Intrapartum fetal distress
b. Intrauterine growth retardation
c. Hypoglycemia
d. Hyperbilirubinemia
e. Low Apgar scores

28–181. Where drug therapy is toxic or the patient cannot adhere to the medical treatment plan, subtotal thyroidectomy after medical control has been achieved may be the treatment of choice for hyperthyroidism.

a. True
b. False

28–182. Antithyroid drugs ingested by the mother ______________ appear in breast milk.

a. Do
b. Do not

28–183. What mechanism causes a woman with Grave's disease who is not hyperthyroid to give birth to an infant with manifestations of thyrotoxicosis?

28–184. A woman treated with propylthiouracil during pregnancy may give birth to an infant who is initially euthyroid but becomes hyperthyroid several days later.

a. True
b. False

28–185. Though thyroid storm may occur during pregnancy, women are resistant during the puerperium.

a. True
b. False

28–186. Which of the following statements about hypothyroidism and pregnancy is correct?

a. The rates of infertility and spontaneous abortion are higher in women with hypothyroidism.
b. Untreated congenital hypothyroidism is associated with mental retardation.
c. The infant of a patient with severe hypothyroidism may be a cretin if radioactive iodine therapy was utilized during pregnancy.
d. Simple maternal thyroid goiter results in congenital hypothyroidism in greater than 90 percent of cases.

28–187. Which of the following statements about parathyroid disease is correct?

a. Hyperparathyroidism in pregnancy is rare.
b. Neonatal tetany may be associated with maternal hyperparathyroidism.
c. Hypoparathyroidism is much more common than hyperparathyroidism.
d. Hypoparathyroidism usually leads to fetal demise.

28–188. Which of the following statements about adrenal dysfunction in pregnancy is correct?

a. Due to advances in therapy, pregnancy has become more common in women with adrenocortical hypofunction.
b. The level of steroid replacement required in patients with Addison's disease approximately doubles each trimester.
c. Pregnancy associated with Cushing's disease is rare.
d. Primary aldosteronism in pregnancy is usually life threatening for the mother.
e. Pheochromocytoma in pregnancy is potentially associated with high fetal and maternal mortality rates.

28–189. Which of the following statements about pituitary disease in pregnancy is correct?

a. Diabetes insipidus in pregnancy is rare.
b. Pregnancies associated with diabetes insipidus should be terminated.
c. A pituitary adenoma during pregnancy predisposes to fetal acromegaly.
d. Bromocriptine in pregnancy has been shown to cause significant fetal skeletal deformities.

28–190. Which of the following statements about epilepsy in pregnancy is correct?

a. The condition of a woman with well-controlled seizures before conception will deteriorate significantly during pregnancy.
b. Anticonvulsant medication may not be absorbed as well in the pregnant patient.
c. Protein binding of drugs decreases in pregnancy.
d. Doses of phenytoin administered during pregnancy should be at least one-third higher than in the nonpregnant state.

28–191. What fetal anomalies have been associated with maternal ingestion of phenytoin during pregnancy?

a. Craniofacial anomalies
b. Distal limb dysmorphosis
c. Mental deficiency
d. Cleft lip/palate
e. Congenital heart lesions
f. Hemorrhagic disease of the newborn

Instructions for Items 28–192 to 28–195: Match the anticonvulsant medication with its potential fetal effects.

a. Carbamazepine (Tegretol)
b. Valproic acid

28–192. Craniofacial anomalies
28–193. Small head size
28–194. Neural tube defects
28–195. Facial, digital, and skeletal malformations

28–196. All women should cease taking anticonvulsant medications prior to conceiving.

a. True
b. False

28–197. What type of anemia has been reported to be aggravated by anticonvulsant medications?

28–198. Parenteral administration of ________________ will often control the convulsions of epilepsy as well as those of eclampsia.

28–199. Which of the following statements about intracranial hemorrhage in pregnancy is correct?

a. Hemorrhage can be readily identified by CT scan.
b. There are minimal fetal risks from surgical repair.
c. Therapeutic abortion may be indicated if the hemorrhage occurs early in pregnancy.
d. All patients who survive the hemorrhage should undergo elective cesearean delivery.

28–200. Presence of which of the following maternal conditions is a strong indication for therapeutic abortion?

a. Ventriculoperitoneal shunt
b. Maternal brain death
c. Pseudotumor cerebri
d. Spinal cord lesion
e. Multiple sclerosis
f. Guillain-Barre's syndrome
g. Myasthenia gravis
h. Huntington's chorea
i. Chorea gravidarum
j. Bell's palsy

28–201. Which of the following may complicate pregnancy in a woman with a spinal cord lesion?

a. Urinary tract infections
b. Pressure necrosis of the skin
c. Autonomic hyperreflexia
d. Painless, precipitous labor
e. Prolonged second stage labor

28–202. Exacerbation of multiple sclerosis in the first few months postpartum is relatively common.

a. True
b. False

28–203. Which of the following statements about myasthenia gravis in pregnancy is correct?

a. The primary therapy is thymectomy.
b. Pregnancy and labor usually occur without difficulty.
c. The second stage of labor may be prolonged because of impaired expulsive effects.
d. The fetus seems to be protected against the disease while in utero.
e. Neonatal myasthenia has been reported in greater than 90 percent of infants of myasthenic mothers.
f. With proper treatment, neonatal myasthenia usually subsides completely within 5 to 6 weeks.

28–204. What characterizes neonatal symptomatic myasthenia gravis?

a. Feeble cry
b. Poor suckling
c. Respiratory distress
d. Response to parenteral neostigmine

28–205. What drugs may be potentially dangerous to patients with myasthenia gravis?

a. Quinine
b. Magnesium sulfate
c. Kanamycin
d. Gentamicin

28–206. Patients who often have migraine headaches tend to improve dramatically during pregnancy until the onset of labor.

a. True
b. False

28–207. Which of the following statements about the treatment of psychosis in pregnancy and the puerperium is correct?

a. Electroshock therapy is incompatible with normal pregnancy outcome.
b. The use of therapeutic lithium carbonate may be associated with fetal cardiac anomalies.
c. Tricyclic antidepressants may be safely administered as they have no adverse fetal or neonatal effects.
d. Bottle feeding is recommended when a woman is ingesting lithium carbonate.

28–208. What are the physiologic changes in pregnancy related to liver function?

a. Decreased serum albumin
b. Increased plasma urea nitrogen
c. Increased alkaline phosphatase activity
d. Delayed excretion of sulfobromophthalein
e. Palmar erythema
f. Spider angiomata

28–209. What liver-related diseases are induced by pregnancy?

28–210. Which of the following are synonomous terms?

a. Recurrent jaundice of pregnancy
b. Idiopathic cholestasis of pregnancy
c. Cholestatic hepatosis
d. Icterus gravidarum

28–211. What are the two main clinical characteristics of intrahepatic cholestasis?

28–212. Which of the following statements about intrahepatic cholestasis is correct?

a. It is more common in people of Asian extraction.
b. Bile acids accumulate in the plasma.
c. Ultrasonography may aid in establishing the diagnosis by ruling out the presence of gallstones.
d. The use of cholestyramine is associated with the possibility of impaired coagulation.
e. Intrahepatic cholestasis does not result in increased prematurity or pregnancy wastage.

28–213. What are the prominent histologic findings in acute fatty liver?

a. Swollen hepatocytes
b. Centrally placed hepatocyte nuclei
c. Microvesicular fat droplets in hepatocyte cytoplasm
d. Periportal sparing
e. Liver necrosis

28–214. Which of the following statements about acute fatty liver is correct?

a. The histology is similar to that seen in Reye's syndrome.
b. The most usual onset is in the second trimester.
c. The onset of clinical symptoms is usually insidious.
d. Delivery is essential for cure.
e. Subsequent pregnancy should be avoided as the disease tends to recur in most cases.

28–215. What symptom signals potentially life-threatening liver involvement in pregnancy-induced hypertension?

28–216. Which of the following statements about hyperemesis gravidarum is correct?

a. The differential diagnosis includes cholecystitis, hepatitis, peptic ulcer, gastroenteritis, and pyelonephritis.
b. Jaundice and elevation of SGOT may result from hyperemesis.
c. Social and psychological factors may play a contributing role.
d. Treatment includes fluid and electrolyte replacement.
e. Pregnancy termination is often necessary.

28–217. In rare circumstances, which of the following can result from hyperemesis?

a. Weight loss
b. Dehydration
c. Starvation acidosis
d. Alkalosis due to hydrochloric acid loss in vomitus
e. Hypokalemia

28–218. Which of the following statements about viral hepatitis A is correct?

a. Feces, secretions, and bed pans from hepatitis A patients should be handled while wearing gloves.
b. The incubation period is from 2 to 7 weeks.
c. Spread is by ingestion of contaminated water and blood.
d. Diagnosis is confirmed by the appearance of hepatitis A antibody.
e. Treatment should consist of a nutritious diet and sedentary living.
f. Hepatitis A is teratogenic.
g. Risk of transmission to the fetus is greater than 50 percent.

28–219. A pregnant woman who has been exposed to hepatitis A should not receive prophylactic gamma globulin.

a. True
b. False

28–220. Which of the following statements about hepatitis B is correct?

a. The disease is most often found among intravenous drug users, homosexuals, health care personnel, and individuals frequently treated with blood products.
b. Only one immunologic marker for the disease has been identified.
c. The infectious state is characterized by the presence of E antigen.
d. The disease can be vertically transmitted.
e. An infant can obtain the virus through breast feeding.
f. Newborns can be effectively protected prophylactically with hepatitis B immune globulin and vaccine.

Instructions for Items 28–221 to 28–223: Match the type of hepatitis in pregnancy with its potential effects.

a. Hepatitis A
b. Hepatitis B

28–221. Disease course is not appreciably affected by pregnancy
28–222. There is an increased risk of prematurity
28–223. Antigenic screening of high-risk pregnant women should be carried out

28–224. What is the significance of the presence of E antigen in cases of hepatitis B during pregnancy?

28–225. What type of hepatitis most commonly develops after a blood transfusion?

a. Hepatitis A
b. Hepatitis B
c. non-A–non-B hepatitis
d. Cytomegalovirus hepatitis
e. Epstein-Barr virus hepatitis

28–226. Immune serum globulin for prophylaxis against non-A–non-B hepatitis should be administered to the newborn of a mother with active disease.

a. True
b. False

28–227. Which of the following statements about chronic active hepatitis in pregnancy is correct?

a. The disease can progress to hepatic failure.
b. Fetal loss is increased.
c. There is no effective therapy.
d. Therapeutic abortion is usually necessary to save the mother.
e. There is a markedly increased rate of fetal malformations in those pregnancies that are maintained.

28–228. There is high morbidity and appreciable mortality in pregnancies complicated by cirrhosis of the liver.

a. True
b. False

28–229. Which of the following statements about the origin and management of gallbladder disease in pregnancy is correct?

a. There is usually incomplete emptying of the gallbladder during pregnancy.
b. The incidence of gallstones is higher than in the nonpregnant state.
c. Surgical management of gallbladder disease should be avoided during pregnancy.
d. Cholecystectomy is contraindicated during pregnancy.

28–230. What factors can mask the diagnosis of appendicitis in pregnancy?

28–231. Which of the following statements about appendicitis in pregnancy is correct?

a. Pregnancy predisposes to appendicitis.
b. Appendicitis has no effect on the likelihood of abortion or preterm labor.
c. The prognosis is worse if the disease occurs late in gestation.
d. Appendicitis-related mortality is most often related to surgical delay.
e. Cesarean delivery is usually indicated at the time of appendectomy.
f. Appendicitis is rare during the puerperium.

28–232. Which of the following statements about abdominal pain during pregnancy is correct?

a. Right upper quadrant pain or epigastric pain may be a sign of severe preeclampsia.
b. Peptic ulcer symptoms usually improve during pregnancy.
c. Tetracycline and diuretics have been implicated in the occurrence of pancreatitis during pregnancy.
d. Intestinal obstruction during pregnancy is most commonly associated with the presence of a malignancy.

28–233. Which of the following statements about chronic inflammatory bowel disease in pregnancy is correct?

a. Therapeutic abortion should be offered in most cases.
b. Pregnancy exacerbates regional enteritis.
c. Ulcerative colitis predisposes to congenital malformations.
d. Exacerbation of ulcerative colitis during pregnancy may be induced by psychogenic factors.

28–234. What are the complications of pregnancy that are likely to develop in obese patients?

a. Hypertension
b. Diabetes
c. Aspiration of gastric contents during anesthesia
d. Wound complications
e. Thromboembolism

28–235. Weight reduction during pregnancy should be recommended for the markedly obese patient.

a. True
b. False

28–236. For a successful pregnancy outcome after a patient has undergone gastric or jejunoileal bypass surgery for obesity, conception should be postponed until after the period of rapid postoperative weight loss.

a. True
b. False

28–237. List the criteria that may be utilized for the diagnosis of systemic lupus erythematosus.

28–238. A diagnosis of lupus may be made when ______________ of the possible criteria are present, either serially or simultaneously.

a. 2
b. 4
c. 6
d. 8
e. 10

28–239. Which of the following statements about lupus in pregnancy is correct?

a. The major nonrenal manifestations of lupus are not induced by pregnancy unless immunosuppressive therapy is discontinued.
b. Renal function usually remains good during pregnancy.
c. An increase in the dosage of glucocorticosteroids and azathioprine may be advisable during labor and the puerperium.
d. Maternal diabetes may be a complication of steroidal therapy during pregnancy.

28–240. What laboratory tests are helpful in monitoring the activity of lupus during pregnancy?

a. Sedimentation rate
b. c3 and c4 Complement levels
c. Hematologic evaluations
d. Liver function tests
e. Renal function tests

28–241. What similar manifestations may occur in severe preeclampsia/eclampsia and systemic lupus erythematosus?

28–242. Which of the following are possible fetal effects of maternal systemic lupus erythematosus?

a. Stillbirth
b. Intrauterine growth retardation
c. Prematurity
d. Congenital heart block
e. Anemia
f. Transient discoid lupus
g. Positive LE factor in the infant's blood

28–243. Asymptomatic mothers of infants with isolated complete heart block should be evaluated for possible systemic lupus erythematosus.

a. True
b. False

28–244. Which of the following statements about lupus and reproduction is correct?

a. Drug-induced lupus is lifelong.
b. Pregnancy should be undertaken when the disease is in remission.
c. Limitation of family size may be warranted due to the possible poor prognosis in lupus.
d. Oral contraceptives are the method of choice for patients with lupus who wish to reversibly limit child bearing.

28–245. What is lupus anticoagulant and what is its significance for fetal outcome?

28–246. Which of the following statements about connective tissue diseases in pregnancy is correct?

a. Rheumatoid arthritis usually worsens during pregnancy.
b. Medical therapy for rheumatoid arthritis has no adverse fetal effects.
c. Dermatomyositis in pregnancy is an indication for therapeutic abortion.
d. Scleroderma markedly increases perinatal mortality.
e. Polyarteritis nodosa is associated with an unfavorable maternal outcome.

28–247. Due to the risk of dissecting aortic aneurysm, patients with Marfan's syndrome should be delivered by elective cesarean section.

a. True
b. False

28–248. Pregnancy makes the woman immune to several of the more common sexually transmitted diseases.

a. True
b. False

28–249. Which of the following is characteristic of syphilis?

a. It is readily preventable.
b. It is not susceptible to therapy.
c. There is a 3-day incubation period.
d. The primary lesion lasts from 1 to 5 weeks.
e. Secondary syphilitic lesions may go unnoticed.

28–250. The raised lesions of secondary syphilis are known as ______________________.

28–251. The first suggestion of syphilitic disease in many women is the birth of a stillborn infant or a liveborn infant with congenital syphilis.

a. True
b. False

28–252. Which of the following statements about the diagnosis of syphilis in pregnancy is correct?

a. A VDRL screening test is a necessary part of the prenatal laboratory work-up.
b. Serologic tests for syphilis are positive from 2 weeks of contracting the disease.
c. A treponemal test is used to confirm a positive reagin test.
d. For high-risk patients, repeat screening should be done in the third trimester and testing of cord blood is indicated.

Instructions for Items 28–253 to 28–259: Match the CDC recommended treatments of syphilis with the appropriate clinical situation.

a. Benzathine penicillin G: 2.4 million units, IM
b. Benzathine penicillin G: 2.4 million units weekly for 3 weeks, IM
c. Crystalline penicillin G: 2 to 4 million units every 4 hours for 10 days, IV; then benzathine penicillin G: 2 to 4 million units weekly for 3 weeks, IM
d. Erythromycin: 500 mg four times daily for 15 days, orally
e. Tetracycline: 500 mg four times daily for 15 days, orally

28–253. Incubating syphilis
28–254. Culture proven gonorrhea present
28–255. Pregnant woman who is allergic to penicillin
28–256. Pregnant woman who is not allergic to penicillin
28–257. Persistent or recurrent signs of syphilis
28–258. Initial antibody titer is greater than 1:8
28–259. Neurosyphilis

28–260. If spinal fluid was positive for syphilis, at what intervals should repeat testing be done?

28–261. Which of the following statements about the treatment of syphilis in pregnancy is correct?

a. For pregnant patients not allergic to penicillin, the optimal treatment is the same as for nonpregnant women.
b. Women with a penicillin allergy can be desensitized.
c. Tetracycline use during pregnancy can cause the staining of the child's permanent teeth.
d. Women treated for syphilis should be monitored by monthly spinal fluid titers.
e. The sexual partner of an infected woman should also be treated.

28–262. Which of the following statements about congenital syphilis is correct?

a. Every infant suspected of having syphilis should have a cerebrospinal fluid examination before treatment.
b. The drug of choice for symptomatic infants is erythromycin.
c. Asymptomatic seropositive infants with a negative cerebrospinal fluid examination need not be treated.
d. Infants born of mothers treated with erythromycin for syphilis during pregnancy should be treated as if they have congenital syphilis.

28–263. Why is gonococcal salpingitis not a problem after the 3rd month of pregnancy?

28–264. Which organs of the lower genital tract may be affected by gonorrhea?

a. Cervix
b. Urethra
c. Bartholin glands
d. Periurethral glands

28–265. What clinical outcomes may result from gonorrhea in pregnancy?

28–266. Asymptomatic gonorrhea should be identified and treated during pregnancy.

a. True
b. False

28–267. Which of the following is recommended for the treatment of all forms of uncomplicated gonorrhea during pregnancy?

a. Aqueous procaine penicillin plus probenecid
b. Ampicillin
c. Amoxicillin
d. Spectinomycin
e. Tetracycline

Instructions for Items 28–268 to 28–271: Match the treatment for gonorrhea during pregnancy with the appropriate situation.

a. Erythromycin
b. Spectinomycin
c. Aqueous crystalline penicillin
d. Ampicillin
e. Tetracycline
f. Aqueous procaine penicillin

28–268. Penicillinase-producing gonococci
28–269. Coexistent chlamydial infection
28–270. Disseminated gonococcal infection
28–271. Infants of mothers with gonorrhea

28–272. What three drugs are recommended in the treatment of penicillinase-producing gonococci?

28–273. How should gonococcal ophthalmia be treated?

28–274. Which of the following statements about chlamydial infections in pregnancy is correct?

a. One specific serotype causes lymphogranuloma venereum.
b. Culture techniques for *Chlamydia trachomatis* are readily available.
c. The treatment of choice during pregnancy is tetracycline.
d. There is no known deleterious effect of the disease on pregnancy.

28–275. Which type of herpes simplex virus is recovered almost exclusively from the genital tract?

28–276. Which of the following statements about herpes infections is correct?

a. The incubation period for primary infections is 2 to 3 weeks.
b. The cervix is the most common site of genital tract infection.
c. Involvement of the cervix and the vagina is usually asymptomatic.
d. Vulvar lesions are likely to be tender and easily traumatized.
e. The virus is harbored in nerve ganglia.

28–277. Recurrent herpes infections can be prevented by treatment with acyclovir (Zovirax).

a. True
b. False

28–278. Which of the following statements about the identification of genital herpes is correct?

a. Cervical smears usually contain large multinucleate cells with eosinophilic viral inclusion bodies.
b. Monoclonal antibodies are available to identify herpes simplex virus.
c. Women with herpes should undergo annual Pap smears to screen for cervical neoplasia.

28–279. Which of the following statements about herpes infection and the neonate is correct?

a. The incidence of neonatal herpes has been slowly decreasing over the past 10 years.
b. The morbidity rate, but not the mortality rate, is high in cases of neonatal herpes.
c. The fetus is usually infected prior to rupture of the membranes.
d. Infection in the newborn may be asymptomatic.
e. Central nervous system and ocular involvement have been commonly reported in infected infants.

28–280. What is the rationale for advocating cesarean delivery for infants of mothers with suspected or documented herpes?

28–281. Which of the following statements about delivery and postpartum care in cases of maternal herpes is correct?

a. All women with a history of herpes must undergo cesarean delivery.
b. If the membranes have already been ruptured, cesarean delivery provides no protection to the fetus.
c. The neonate must be monitored more closely than usual.
d. Breast feeding by infected mothers should not be allowed.

Instructions for Items 28–282 to 28–288: Match the infection with the appropriate statement.

a. Chancroid
b. Granuloma inguinale

28–282. Caused by *Haemophilus ducreyi*
28–283. Caused by *Donovania granulomata*
28–284. Painful nonindurated genital ulcers
28–285. Multiple, large, foul-smelling ulcerations
28–286. Painful inguinal lymphadenopathy
28–287. Diagnosis by culture of the infecting organism from lesions
28–288. Diagnosis by identification of Donovan bodies in smears

28–289. Which of the following statements about varicella in pregnancy is correct?

a. The disease is uncommon in adults.
b. Varicella pneumonia may prove fatal.
c. Acyclovir may be useful in preventing and treating varicella pneumonitis.
d. Administration of immune globulin should be considered for exposed nonimmune pregnant women.
e. Transplacental passage of the virus with fetal infection may occur.
f. Exposure of the fetus during delivery may result in visceral and central nervous system disease.

Instructions for Items 28–290 to 28–297: Match the infection with the appropriate statement.

a. Increases risk of abortion
b. Increases risk of prematurity
c. Vaccination during pregnancy is helpful
d. Vaccination in pregnancy is contraindicated
e. May result in pneumonia
f. Pregnant women more susceptible to the infection

28–290. Mumps
28–291. Rubeola
28–292. Influenza
28–293. Common cold
28–294. Poliomyelitis
28–295. Scarlet fever
28–296. Typhoid fever
28–297. Malaria

28–298. Which of the following diseases indicates therapeutic abortion?

a. Coxsackie virus
b. Erysipelas
c. Malaria
d. Poliomyelitis
e. Amebiasis
f. Coccidioidomycosis
g. Hansen's disease (leprosy)

28–299. Which of the following characterizes herpes gestationis?

a. Increased perinatal mortality
b. Caused by herpes virus I
c. Involvement of abdomen and extremities
d. Relieved by prednisone
e. IgG serum factor identifiable

28–300. Which of the following statements about diseases of the skin during pregnancy is correct?

a. Acne in pregnancy should be treated with retinoic acid isotretinoin.
b. Papular dermatitis can be controlled by steroids.
c. Chloasma and melasma gravidarum usually recede before delivery.
d. Postpartum loss of hair is usually a temporary phenomenon.

28–301. Which of the following statements about melanoma in pregnancy is correct?

a. Benign nevi do not become malignant during pregnancy.
b. Melanoma may grow rapidly and spread widely.
c. The prognosis for the pregnant woman with the disease is good.
d. Melanoma is the most common tumor metastatic to the placenta.
e. Melanoma is the most common disease metastatic to the fetus.

28–302. Delivery improves the prognosis in which of the following conditions?

a. Carpal tunnel syndrome
b. Extensive burns
c. Hiatal hernia
d. Symphyseal separation

28–303. Which of the following statements about breast carcinoma and pregnancy is correct?

a. Therapeutic abortion improves the prognosis.
b. Breast cancer prognosis in pregnancy depends on fetal gestational age at the time of diagnosis.
c. Mastectomy adversely affects subsequent pregnancy outcomes.
d. Chemotherapy cannot be administered during pregnancy.

Instructions for Items 28–304 to 28–318: Match the classification of diabetes according to White with the appropriate description.

a. Type A
b. Type B
c. Type C_1
d. Type C_2
e. Type D_1
f. Type D_2
g. Type D_3
h. Type D_4
i. Type D_5
j. Type E
k. Type F
l. Type G
m. Type H
n. Type R
o. Type T

28–304. Proliferating retinopathy
28–305. Neuropathy
28–306. Age 10 to 19 years at onset
28–307. Over 20 years' duration
28–308. Chemical diabetes

28–309. Calcified vessels of legs
28–310. Ten to nineteen years' duration
28–311. Hypertension
28–312. Maturity onset, duration under 10 years, no vascular lesions
28–313. Under 10 years at onset
28–314. Benign retinopathy
28–315. No longer sought
28–316. Cardiomyopathy
28–317. Renal transplant
28–318. Many failures

29. DYSTOCIA CAUSED BY ANOMALIES OF THE EXPULSIVE FORCES

29–1. List the four distinct abnormalities that, alone or in combination, cause dystocia.

29–2. The most common cause of dystocia is __________.

29–3. As a generalization, uterine dysfunction is common whenever there is disproportion between the presenting part of the fetus and the birth canal.

a. True
b. False

Instructions for Items 29–4 to 29–5: Match the stage of labor with the appropriate cervical changes.

a. Latent phase
b. Active phase

29–4. Cervix undergoes softening and effacement
29–5. Rapid cervical dilation occurs

29–6. Complete the following table characterizing contractions during labor using the following descriptors: strong, mild, irregular, regular, long or short.

	Latent Phase	Active Phase
Strength	(1)	(2)
Duration	(3)	(4)
Frequency	(5)	(6)

29–7. Which of the following statements about lack of progress in labor is correct?

a. Lack of progress in the first stage of labor presents no real danger to the mother or fetus.
b. Prolongation of the latent phase of labor is defined as 20 hours in both nulliparas and multiparas.
c. A protracted active phase is defined as cervical dilation of less than 1.2 cm per hour in nulliparas.
d. A protracted active phase is defined as cervical dilation of less than 1.5 cm per hour in multiparas.

Instructions for Items 29–8 to 29–14: Match the type of uterine dysfunction with the appropriate description.

a. Hypotonic uterine dysfunction
b. Hypertonic (incoordinate) uterine dysfunction

29–8. Basal hypertonus may be present
29–9. No basal hypertonus
29–10. There is a normal uterine pressure gradient during a contraction
29–11. The uterine pressure gradient during a contraction may be distorted
29–12. Occurs during the active phase of labor after the cervix has dilated to more than 4 cm
29–13. Contractions are especially painful but ineffective
29–14. Contractions become less frequent and intense during labor

29–15. Complete the following table that describes the diagnostic criteria for abnormal labor patterns (according to Friedman)

Labor Pattern	Diagnostic Criteria: Nulligravida	Diagnostic Criteria: Multigravida
Prolongation disorder:		
Prolonged latent phase	>20 hr	(1)
Protraction disorder:		
Protracted active phase dilation	(2)	<1.5 cm/hr
Protracted descent	<1 cm/hr	(3)
Arrest disorder:		
Prolonged deceleration phase	(4)	>1 hr
Secondary arrest of dilation	(5)	>2 hr
Arrest of descent	>1 hr	(6)
Failure of descent	(7)	No descent in the deceleration phase or in the second stage

29–16. According to Cohen and Friedman, in a prolonged latent phase the preferred treatment is ______ (1) and the exceptional treatment is ______ (2). In cases of protracted active phase or protracted descent, the preferred treatment is ______ (3) and the exceptional treatment is ______ (4).

29–17. The most common cause of dystocia associated with uterine dysfunction is the presence of a cervix too rigid to dilate.

a. True
b. False

29–18. Which of the following is a potential complication of prolonged dysfunctional labor?

a. Intrauterine infection
b. Maternal exhaustion
c. Psychological effects on mother
d. Fetal or neonatal death

29–19. What two general conditions must be met before treatment of hypotonic uterine dysfunction with intravenous oxytocin may be initiated?

29–20. Why is uterine rupture not a common outcome in cases of cephalopelvic disproportion?

29–21. Which of the following factors contribute to the decision to augment labor in cases of hypotonic uterine dysfunction?

a. Fetal size
b. Presentation
c. Position
d. Parity
e. Pelvic size

29–22. Describe the characteristics of a noncontracted pelvis.

29–23. If the criteria for a noncontracted pelvis are not met, oxytocin stimulation should not be utilized.

a. True
b. False

29–24. What potential problem is associated with the infusion of dextrose in water during oxytocin stimulation?

29–25. In which of the following situations at Parkland Memorial Hospital is the use of oxytocin to stimulate labor generally be avoided?

a. High parity
b. Oligohydramnios
c. Uterine overdistention
d. Presence of a dead fetus
e. Presence of a uterine scar

29–26. Which of the following statements about the use of oxytocin to stimulate labor is correct?

a. A dilute solution of 10 units of oxytocin in 1 liter of balanced salt solution should be utilized.
b. The infusion rate of oxytocin may be increased every 10 minutes until a clinically adequate labor pattern is established.
c. Infusion rates of more than 10 mU/min for augmentation or 30 to 40 mU/min for induction are rarely needed.
d. The mean half-life of oxytocin is about 30 minutes.
e. Continuous clinical monitoring of the patient during oxytocin stimulation is necessary.
f. The hypotonic uterus often requires 4 to 5 hours to respond to oxytocin.

29–27. If oxytocin fails to stimulate labor within a few hours, cesarean delivery should be performed.

a. True
b. False

29–28. Prolonged latent phase is always due to either injudicious use of analgesics or anesthetics, false labor or hypertonic uterine dysfunction.

a. True
b. False

29–29. Which of the following statements about the use of prostaglandins in the stimulation of labor is correct?

a. Prostaglandins $F_2\alpha$ and E_2 have been approved by the FDA for use in the United States.
b. Prostaglandins are capable of augmenting but not inducing labor.
c. Prostaglandins have been shown to be effective in ripening the cervix preparatory to the induction of labor.
d. Use of prostaglandins has been associated with a higher rate of cesarean deliveries.

29–30. Hypertonic uterine dysfunction

a. Is characterized by pain that is more severe than expected for the intensity of the contractions
b. Characteristically appears after the cervix is dilated 4 cm or more
c. Is relatively infrequent compared to hypotonic uterine dysfunction
d. Is best treated by dilute oxytocin infusion to create a more rhythmic uterine contraction pattern

29–31. Which of the following statements about inadequate voluntary expulsive force is correct?

a. Conduction anesthesia may reduce the reflex to "push."
b. Conduction anesthesia may impair a woman's ability to contract her abdominal muscles sufficiently to generate the needed force.
c. Insufficient expulsive forces may be the consequence of longstanding paralysis of the abdominal muscles.
d. Nitrous oxide may be used with women who cannot bear down with each contraction due to great discomfort.

29–32. Precipitate labor

a. May result from low resistance of the cervix and birth canal
b. May result from abnormally strong contractions
c. May cause amnionic fluid embolism, especially if there is resistance from the cervix and birth canal
d. Does not affect perinatal mortality or morbidity rates because of the shortened time the fetus is exposed to the stresses of labor
e. May be effectively treated by β-mimetic tocolytics
f. Is associated with an increased incidence of postpartum hemorrhage

29–33. Which of the following statements about localized abnormalities of the uterus is correct?

a. Prolonged labor may result in localized rings or contractions of the uterus.
b. The pathologic retraction ring of Bandl is the most common type of retraction ring.
c. In modern obstetrics, pathologic contraction rings are rarely seen because prolonged labor is relatively uncommon.
d. The most likely time for the occurrence of a contraction ring is after the delivery of the first of twins.

29–34. Describe the circumstances surrounding missed labor.

30. DYSTOCIA CAUSED BY ABNORMALITIES IN PRESENTATION, POSITION, OR DEVELOPMENT OF THE FETUS

30–1. About ________ (1) percent of singleton pregnancies are breech at the start of the second half of pregnancy, whereas at term the incidence of breech presentations is ________ (2).

30–2. Which of the following conditions is associated with an increased incidence of breech presentation?

a. Grand multiparity
b. Multifetal pregnancy
c. Hydramnios
d. Contracted pelvis
e. Hydrocephalus
f. Protracted labor
g. Anencephalus
h. Oligohydramnios
i. Previous breech delivery
j. Uterine anomalies
k. Uterine tumors
l. Cornual-fundal placental implantation
m. Placenta previa
n. Abruptio placentae

30–3. List the complications that occur with increased frequency in association with a breech delivery.

Instructions for Items 30–4 to 30–6: Match the type of breech presentation with the appropriate description.

a. Frank breech
b. Complete breech
c. Incomplete breech

30–4. Lower extremities flexed at the hips; one or both knees are flexed

30–5. Lower extremities flexed at the hips and extended at the knees; the feet lie in close proximity to the head

30–6. One or both hips are not flexed and one or both feet or knees lie below the breech

30–7. The most common breech presentation near term is the

a. Frank breech
b. Complete breech
c. Incomplete breech

30–8. In cases of breech presentation, the maneuvers of Leopold are ineffective for determining fetal presentation and position.

a. True
b. False

30–9. In a breech presentation, the location where fetal heart sounds are usually best heard is ______ (1), whereas with a cephalic presentation the fetal heart sounds are loudest ______ (2).

30–10. Which of the following statements about the vaginal examination in cases of breech presentation is correct?

a. The ischial tuberosities, the sacrum, and the anus are usually palpable.
b. The diagnosis of position and variety are based on the location of the sacrum and its spinous processes.
c. In footling presentations, the feet may be felt alongside the buttocks.
d. Due to swelling caused by prolonged labor, it may be hard to differentiate the fetal buttocks and face.

30–11. Sonography is better than x-ray for identifying the relationship of the lower extremities to the fetal pelvis.

a. True
b. False

30–12. Which of the following contributes to the increased maternal morbidity and mortality for pregnancies complicated by persistent breech presentation?

a. Greater frequency of operative delivery
b. Greatly prolonged labor
c. Increased incidence of preeclampsia-eclampsia

30–13. List the main contributing factors to the increased perinatal morbidity and mortality in breech presentation.

30–14. Which organ is most frequently found to be injured during traumatic vaginal deliveries of breech presentations?

a. Liver
b. Adrenal glands
c. Spleen
d. Spinal cord
e. Brain

30–15. Use of cesarean delivery in all breech presentations reduces the risk of neonatal mortality to approximately that of the overall population.

a. True
b. False

30–16. Which of the following statements about breech presentation in mature fetuses (>2500 g) is correct?

a. The overall perinatal mortality rate for breech presentation is about equal to that for cephalic presentations.
b. Major congenital anomalies are more frequent in breech than in vertex presentations.
c. The incidence of fetal distress of undetermined cause is greater in breech than in vertex presentations.
d. The incidence of overt prolapse of the umbilical cord is approximately equal in frank breech and in vertex presentations.

30–17. In cases of breech presentation in mature fetuses (>2500 g), the mortality and morbidity rates from delivery trauma are ______ to fetal weight.

a. Directly proportional
b. Inversely proportional
c. Unrelated

30–18. Perinatal mortality associated with vaginal delivery as a breech in premature infants is ______ in term breech infants.

a. Greater than
b. The same as
c. Less than

30–19. Which of the following statements about external version in a breech presentation is correct?

a. External version is more readily accomplished in multiparous women.
b. Conduction, or occasionally general, anesthesia should be used to relax the abdominal walls.
c. External version is more likely to be successful early in the third trimester than later.
d. Attempts at external version may be complicated by antepartum hemorrhage, premature labor, fetal death, and fetomaternal hemorrhage.

30–20. Which of the following problems is associated with the vaginal delivery of breech presentations?

a. Delivery of the breech draws the cord into the pelvis, which can lead to cord compression.
b. Once the breech has passed the vaginal introitus, the parts still to be delivered are readily compressible.
c. The time required for accommodation of the fetal head may lead to fetal acidosis and hypoxia.
d. With a premature fetus, the disparity between the size of the head and the buttocks is less than with a larger fetus.

30–21. List the clinical circumstances where cesarean delivery of breech presentations is recommended.

30–22. Which of the following pelvic shapes is unfavorable for vaginal delivery of breech presentations.

a. Gynecoid
b. Android
c. Anthropoid
d. Platypelloid

30–23. Vaginal delivery in cases of hyperextension of the fetal head may lead to what injury?

30–24. Vaginal delivery should be relatively safe for a frank breech presentation if

a. A previous cephalic delivery was successful
b. The fetus is judged to weigh less than 8 pounds
c. Orderly effacement and dilation of the cervix and descent of the breech occurs
d. Individuals skilled in breech delivery are available

30–25. In face presentations, the fetal head is

a. Hyperflexed
b. Hyperextended

30–26. Which of the following factors is associated with face presentations?

a. Contracted pelvis
b. Small fetus
c. Pendulous maternal abdomen
d. Anencephalic fetus

30–27. Face presentation

a. Has a reported incidence of <1 percent
b. Generally starts as a brow presentation with extension of the head as descent occurs during labor
c. Cannot be easily confirmed by roentgenogram because of interference from the maternal pelvic bones
d. Is usually best managed by cesarean delivery because of its association with pelvic contraction

30–28. Which of the following statements about brow presentation is correct?

a. The fetal head occupies a position midway between full flexion and full extension.
b. Except where the head is small or the pelvis is large, vaginal delivery is difficult.
c. Brow presentation is usually unstable and in a majority of cases converts to occiput or face presentations.
d. Caput succedaneum may be so extensive over the forehead that identification of the brow by palpation is difficult.

Instructions for Items 30–29 to 30–30: Match the type of presentation with the features that can be felt on vaginal examination.

a. Face presentation
b. Brow presentation

30–29. Frontal sutures, large anterior fontanel, orbital ridges, and eyes can be felt but the mouth and chin cannot

30–30. Mouth and nose, malar bones, and orbital ridges can be felt

Instructions for Items 30–31 to 30–32: Match the type of shoulder presentation with the appropriate description.

a. Transverse lie
b. Oblique lie

30–31. Fetal long axis forms an acute angle with the maternal long axis

30–32. Fetal long axis is approximately perpendicular to the maternal long axis

30–33. Shoulder presentation

a. Is designated as right or left depending on the orientation of the fetal acromion to the maternal pelvis
b. Occurs in <1 percent of singleton pregnancies
c. Is suspected when the abdomen is wide from side to side and the uterine fundus does not extend much above the umbilicus
d. Is associated with an increased incidence of prolapse of the hand and arm, especially as labor progresses

30–34. Shoulder presentation (and transverse lie) is more common in

a. Nulliparous patients
b. Grand multiparity
c. Postmature gestations
d. Premature gestations
e. Placental abruption
f. Placenta previa
g. Women with a large pelvis
h. Women with a contracted pelvis

30–35. Most maternal deaths associated with shoulder presentation occur in neglected cases from ________.

30–36. Even with appropriate care, the reasons for increased maternal morbidity and mortality in shoulder presentation include

a. Association with placenta previa
b. Increased incidence of cord accidents
c. Necessity for major operative procedures
d. Likelihood of sepsis associated with extrusion of the arm into the vagina

30–37. Shoulder presentation

a. Does not allow vaginal delivery except in the case of conduplicato corpore
b. Is usually managed by external version although this is difficult after 8 cm dilation
c. Is usually managed by lower segment transverse cesarean section
d. Is best treated by including antibiotic therapy after delivery, whether or not there are signs of infection

30–38. In cases of shoulder presentation, if the fetus is dead and the cervix fully dilated, fetal decapitation with vaginal delivery presents less risk than cesarean delivery.

a. True
b. False

30–39. Compound presentation

a. Occurs when an extremity prolapses alongside the presenting part
b. Is more common in premature pregnancies
c. Is associated with a reported 25 percent perinatal loss rate
d. Is best managed by cesarean section

30–40. The persistent occiput posterior position

a. Undergoes spontaneous anterior rotation in about 65 percent of cases
b. Rarely results in spontaneous vaginal delivery
c. May in most instances be managed by forceps delivery under local anesthesia with a midline episiotomy
d. May be managed by forceps rotation (Scanzoni maneuver)

30–41. In persistent occiput posterior position as compared to occiput anterior position

a. Labor is usually prolonged
b. The perinatal mortality rate is increased threefold
c. Significantly lower Apgar scores are common
d. Extended episiotomies are required

30–42. The persistent occiput transverse position

a. Usually converts spontaneously to occiput anterior position when pelvic anatomy is normal
b. May remain persistent in cases of hypotonic uterine dysfunction
c. May remain persistent because of pelvic contraction
d. May take the form of deep transverse arrest, requiring cesarean delivery in most cases

30–43. Describe deep transverse arrest as it occurs in persistent occiput transverse presentations.

30–44. Fetal macrosomia is defined as an infant weighing ____________________.

30–45. Fetal macrosomia is associated with

a. A large mother
b. A large father
c. Multiparity
d. Primaparity
e. Maternal diabetes
f. Maternal obesity
g. Prolonged gestation
h. Previous delivery of a large infant

30–46. Which of the following statements about fetal macrosomia is correct?

a. It occurs in about 5 percent of newborns.
b. It cannot be diagnosed clinically.
c. Sonographic evaluation of the dimensions of the head, thorax, and abdomen provides a fairly accurate estimate of fetal size.
d. Fetal macrosomia is associated with increased perinatal morbidity and mortality.

30–47. The incidence of shoulder dystocia is ____________ to fetal weight.

a. Directly proportional
b. Inversely proportional

30–48. Describe the danger to the fetus associated with shoulder dystocia.

30–49. Which of the following statements about the prevention and management of shoulder dystocia is correct?

a. There is an increased likelihood of shoulder dystocia following a prolonged second stage of labor managed by instrumental vaginal delivery of the head from the midpelvis.
b. Comparison of chest and head circumference measurements reveal situations where there is a high likelihood of shoulder dystocia.
c. Cesarean delivery is required in cases of shoulder dystocia.

30–50. Describe the sequence of maneuvers described by Benedetti and Gabbe for the management of shoulder dystocia.

30-51. Internal hydrocephalus

a. Occurs in about 1 in every 2000 fetuses and accounts for about 12 percent of all severe fetal malformations found at birth
b. Is associated with spina bifida in about all cases
c. Involves excessive accumulation of cerebrospinal fluid (500 to 1500 cc) in the fetal brain ventricles
d. Is associated with breech presentation in about one-third of cases
e. Is associated with severe dystocia in most cases

30-52. Which of the following statements about internal hydrocephalus is correct?

a. Internal hydrocephalus is best diagnosed radiographically by the appearance of an enlarged fetal head of a fetus in the breech position.
b. Diagnosis is confirmed by ultrasonographic demonstration of enlarged fetal ventricles and decreased brain cortex.
c. Internal hydrocephalus is associated with an increased danger of uterine rupture.
d. Aspiration of excess cerebrospinal fluid can be accomplished by transvaginal or transabdominal puncture.
e. The intrapartum use of a ventricular "shunt" is now widely possible.

30-53. Which of the following criteria aid the roentgenographic identification of hydrocephalus?

a. The face is small in relation to the head.
b. The hydrocephalic cranium tends to be ovoid rather than globular.
c. The shadow of the hydrocephalic cranium is often thin or scarcely visible.

30-54. Which of the following can enlarge the fetal abdomen enough to potentially cause dystocia?

a. Greatly distended bladder
b. Ascites
c. Enlarged kidneys
d. Enlarged liver

30-55. In general, after excess fluid is removed from the abdomen the prognosis for the fetus is good regardless of the route of delivery.

a. True
b. False

31. DYSTOCIA CAUSED BY PELVIC CONTRACTION

31-1. Contraction of which of the following pelvic diameters may cause dystocia?

a. The pelvic inlet
b. The midpelvis
c. The pelvic outlet

31-2. The pelvic inlet is considered to be contracted when the

a. Shortest anteroposterior diameter is less than 10 cm
b. Greatest transverse diameter is less than 12 cm
c. Diagonal conjugate is less than 11.5 cm

31-3. The incidence of obstetric difficulty when either the anteroposterior or the transverse diameters of the pelvic inlet is contracted is ________ when both diameters are contracted.

a. Greater than
b. The same as
c. Less than

31-4. Maternal size is ________ (1) related to pelvic size and ________ (2) related to fetal size.

a. Directly
b. Inversely

31-5. Which of the following statements about attempts to determine fetal head size in relation to the size of the pelvic inlet is correct?

a. Inability to push the fetal head into the pelvis by abdominal pressure indicates that vaginal delivery is impossible.
b. A flexed fetal head that overrides the symphysis pubis is indicative of disproportion.
c. Very precise measurements of the fetal head can be made by roentgenographic techniques.
d. A fetal head that is elongated in the occipitofrontal diameter (dolichocephaly) may lead to the underestimation of fetal weight and gestational age.

31-6. A fetal head that is elongated in the occipitofrontal diameter is associated with

a. Breech presentation
b. Multifetal gestation
c. Oligohydramnios

31-7. Which of the following statements about fetal presentations associated with a contracted pelvic inlet is correct?

a. When the pelvic inlet is contracted, descent into the pelvic cavity does not usually begin until after the onset of labor.
b. Vertex presentations occur in about one-third of cases.
c. Face and shoulder presentations are three times more frequent in women with contracted pelves.
d. Prolapse of the umbilical cord and of the extremities occurs four to six times more frequently in women with contracted pelves.

31-8. Contraction of the pelvic inlet is associated with

a. Precipitate labor and delivery
b. Early spontaneous rupture of the membranes
c. Slow or absent dilation of the cervix during labor
d. An increased incidence of vesicovaginal, vesicocervical, or rectovaginal fistulas
e. An increased incidence of intrapartum infection
f. The possibility of uterine rupture

31-9. The appearance of a pathologic retraction ring in a laboring patient with a clinically contracted pelvic inlet is indication for immediate cesarean delivery.

a. True
b. False

31-10. Which of the following statements about the fetal head in labors associated with a contracted pelvis is correct?

a. A large caput succedaneum may develop, causing diagnostic error from overestimation of the degree of fetal descent.
b. Pressure from uterine contractions may cause overlapping of the fetal skull bones at their sutures (molding).
c. Fetal tentorial tears and intracranial hemorrhage may result from molding that reduces the biparietal diameter more than 0.2 cm.
d. Accommodation of the fetal head to a contracted pelvis is easier when the bones of the head are completely ossified.

Instructions for Items 31-11 to 31-18: Determine the effects of the following situations on the prognosis for vaginal delivery in a patient with a borderline contracted pelvic inlet (anteroposterior diameter only slightly below 10 cm).

a. Favorable prognosis for vaginal delivery
b. Unfavorable prognosis for vaginal delivery

31-11. Occiput presentation
31-12. Breech presentation
31-13. Large fetus
31-14. Android pelvis
31-15. Orderly progression of cervical dilation
31-16. Uterine dysfunction
31-17. Previous difficult labor
31-18. Asynclitism

31-19. In the management of a contracted pelvic inlet,

a. A trial of labor is always indicated
b. Conduction anesthesia is preferred because of the anticipitated protracted extent of labor
c. Close monitoring of the mother and fetus for signs of impending uterine rupture is essential
d. The infusion of dilute oxytocin solution may facilitate molding and engagement of the fetal head

31-20. Describe the anatomic constituents that make up the plane of the obstetric midpelvis.

31-21. A transverse line connecting the ____________ divides the midpelvis into fore and hind portions.

31-22. Supply the following average measurements of the diameters of the midpelvis.

Transverse (interspinous) diameter: ____________ cm
(1)
Anteroposterior diameter: ____________ cm
(2)
Posterior sagittal diameter: ____________ cm
(3)

31-23. The midpelvis should be considered contracted when the sum of the interischial spinous and the posterior sagittal diameters falls at or below ____________.

a. 10.5 cm
b. 11.5 cm
c. 12.5 cm
d. 13.5 cm
e. 14.5 cm

31-24. There is reason to suspect the existence of midpelvic contraction whenever the interischial spinous diameter is less than

a. 8 cm
b. 9 cm
c. 10 cm
d. 11 cm
e. 12 cm

31-25. Midpelvic contraction may be precisely diagnosed by a combination of x-ray and ultrasonographic evaluations.

a. True
b. False

31-26. Midpelvic contraction is probably ____________ inlet contraction.

a. More common than
b. As common as
c. Less common than

31–27. Which of the following statements about the treatment of labor complicated by midpelvic contraction is correct?

a. Use of forceps before the head has passed the contracted midpelvis facilitates flexion.
b. Early use of forceps reduces the space available for the fetal head.
c. Midforceps delivery is contraindicated in cases where the biparietal diameter of the fetal head has not passed beyond the level of contraction.
d. Vacuum extraction may be useful after complete cervical dilation.
e. Oxytocin should not be used in the treatment of dystocia caused by pelvic contraction.

31–28. Contraction of the pelvic outlet is defined as ________________.

31–29. Supply the anatomic constituents of the two triangles that comprise the pelvic outlet.

	Triangles	
	Anterior	**Posterior**
Base	(1)	(2)
Sides	(3)	(4)
Apex	(5)	(6)

31–30. Outlet contraction without simultaneous contraction of the midpelvis occurs in about 50 percent of cases.

a. True
b. False

31–31. What is a possible complication of a contracted pelvic outlet when disproportion with the fetal head is not sufficiently great to cause serious dystocia?

31–32. Previous history of pelvic fracture is an automatic indication for cesarean delivery.

a. True
b. False

31–33. Complete the following table by listing the complications of labor associated with the kyphotic patient.

Gibbus Location	**Common Complication**
Thoracic	(1)
Lumbar	(2)
Thoracolumbar	(3)

31–34. Which of the following statements concerning the effects of an anatomically deformed bony pelvis is correct?

a. Unilateral lameness will often result in an asymmetric deformity of the pelvis that may cause dystocia.
b. Bilateral lameness is more likely than unilateral lameness to be associated with pelvic contraction sufficient to cause dystocia.
c. All dwarf pelves are characterized by incomplete ossification and the presence of varying amounts of cartilage.
d. All patients with bony abnormalities of the pelvis should be delivered by cesarean section.

32. DYSTOCIA FROM OTHER ABNORMALITIES OF THE REPRODUCTIVE TRACT

32–1. Which of the following statements about dystocia associated with abnormalities of the vulva is correct?

a. Complete vulvar atresia is usually incompatible with conception unless it is surgically corrected.
b. Incomplete vulvar atresia resulting from adhesions or scars may allow vaginal delivery at the cost of deep perineal tears.
c. When the vulvovaginal outlet is small, rigid, and inelastic, adequate episiotomy will usually prevent dystocia and lacerations.
d. An extremely edematous vulva commonly results in dystocia.
e. Presence of *Condylomata acuminata* is an absolute indication for cesarean delivery.

32–2. Which of the following statements about dystocia associated with abnormalities of the vagina is correct?

a. Both complete and incomplete vaginal septa usually do not cause dystocia.
b. Annular stricture of the vagina usually causes significant dystocia that requires cesarean delivery.
c. Transverse vaginal septa do not allow a normal course of labor.
d. The softening of tissues in pregnancy usually overcomes the obstruction caused by vaginal scarring.
e. Gartner duct cysts seldom cause dystocia, but may have to be asceptically aspirated during vaginal delivery.
f. Tetanic contraction of the levator ani muscle usually responds to anesthesia, thus allowing vaginal delivery.

32–3. Which of the following can cause cervical stenosis?

a. Conization
b. Cauterization
c. Corrosives used to induce abortion
d. Cervical amputation
e. Infection and tissue destruction

32–4. Which of the following statements about atresia or stenosis of the cervix is correct?

a. Complete cervical atresia prevents the possibility of future conception.
b. Normal tissue softening during pregnancy usually reduces stenosis sufficiently to allow cervical dilation during labor.
c. Conglutination of the cervical os usually causes dystocia severe enough to require cesarean delivery.
d. Congenital abnormalities of the cervix that cause dystocia are frequently associated with other abnormalities of the genital and urinary tracts.

32–5. Extensive invasion of the cervix by carcinoma will usually impede dilation.

a. True
b. False

Instructions for Items 32–6 to 32–9: Match the type of extreme uterine displacement with the circumstances with which it is associated.

a. Anteflexion
b. Retroflexion

32–6. Associated with diastasis recti and a pendulous abdomen
32–7. Associated with spontaneous abortion in the first half of pregnancy
32–8. Associated with sacculation and a risk of uterine rupture
32–9. Associated with impeded cervical dilation

32–10. Which of the following statements about the management of uterine displacement is correct?

a. Marked anteflexion of the uterus may be corrected by use of a properly fitting abdominal binder.
b. Persistent retroflexion of the uterus requires cesarean delivery.
c. Operative shortening of the round ligaments to affect uterine suspension does not adversely influence labor in a subsequent pregnancy.
d. Pregnancy after fixation of the uterine fundus to the anterior abdominal wall may be complicated by considerable discomfort.

Instructions for Items 32–11 to 32–14: Match the type of uterine myoma with the appropriate description.

a. Submucous myoma
b. Subserous myoma
c. Intramural myoma
d. Pedunculated myoma

32–11. Confined to the myometrium
32–12. Located immediately beneath the uterine serosa
32–13. Located immediately beneath the endometrial or decidual surface
32–14. Attached to the uterus by a stalk

32–15. Which of the following statements about uterine myomas is correct?

a. Uterine myomas increase greatly in size during pregnancy and remain large thereafter.
b. Implantation over the site of a submucous myoma is either unsuccessful or leads to faulty placentation and abortion.
c. Hemorrhagic infarction of myomas ("red" degeneration) is usually life threatening for the mother.
d. With a submucous myoma, pregnancy occasionally progresses to term, with the myoma then prolapsing through the cervix at delivery.

32–16. The signs and symptoms of hemorrhagic infarction may make it difficult to distinguish from

a. Appendicitis
b. Placental abruption
c. Placenta previa
d. Ureteral stone
e. Pyelonephritis

32–17. Which of the following statements about the treatment of uterine myomas in pregnancy is correct?

a. Complications of the antepartum or intrapartum periods are common in women with uterine myomas.
b. While dystocia from fundal myomas is uncommon, postpartum hemorrhage is a frequent and serious complication.
c. Uterine myomas shown by ultrasonography to be in the lower uterine segment require cesarean delivery because of the dystocia that they will cause.
d. Myomectomy during pregnancy should be limited to tumors with discrete pedicles.

32–18. Which of the following statements about ovarian tumors in pregnancy is correct?

a. The two most common ovarian tumors in pregnancy are cystic teratoma and mucinous cystadenoma.
b. About one-quarter of ovarian tumors in pregnancy are malignant.
c. The most common complication of ovarian tumors in pregnancy is rupture of a cystic ovarian mass.
d. Torsion of an ovarian tumor is most common in the first trimester.
e. Most ovarian tumors during pregnancy are symptomatic.
f. It is almost always possible to make the diagnosis of an ovarian tumor clinically.

32–19. Which of the following statements about treatment of ovarian tumors in pregnancy is correct?

a. The safest time to perform laparotomy is the fourth month of gestation.
b. When the diagnosis of a benign ovarian tumor is made late in pregnancy, it is best to delay laparotomy until the fetus is mature.
c. With all ovarian tumors, cesarean delivery is usually preferable to vaginal delivery.

32–20. Which of the following statements about pelvic masses causing dystocia is correct?

a. A distended bladder, with or without cystocele, will not delay the normal course of labor.
b. Pelvic kidneys, either natural or transplanted, usually necessitate cesarean delivery.
c. Enteroceles frequently cause dystocia.
d. Bladder tumors rarely cause dystocia severe enough to require cesarean delivery.
e. Tumors or inflammation in the lower part of the rectum or the pelvic connective tissue may cause dystocia.

33. INJURIES TO THE BIRTH CANAL

33–1. In cases of deep perineal laceration, suturing of the external integuments without repair of underlying fascia and muscle may contribute to

a. Relaxation of the vaginal outlet
b. Rectocele
c. Cystocele
d. Uterine prolapse

33–2. Which of the following statements about obstetric injuries to the vagina is correct?

a. Isolated lacerations unassociated with lacerations of the perineum or cervix are equally likely in the lower, middle, and upper thirds of the vagina.
b. Lacerations of the anterior vaginal wall in close proximity to the urethra are relatively common.
c. Laceration in the periurethral area may cause difficulty in voiding, a complication that should be treated by intermittent catheterization.
d. Injuries to the levator ani as a result of birth canal overdistention may interfere with the function of the pelvic diaphragm.
e. The likelihood of urinary incontinence resulting from injury to the pubococcygeus muscle is minimized by appropriate use of episiotomy.

33–3. Bleeding while the uterus is firmly contracted is evidence of

a. A genital tract laceration
b. Retained placental fragments
c. The presence of a uterine tear

33–4. Which of the following statements about obstetric injury to the cervix is correct?

a. Extensive lacerations of the cervix and/or the upper vagina are usually associated with difficult forceps deliveries.
b. Any cervical laceration greater than 1 cm should be considered to be the result of improper obstetric management.
c. Operative forceps deliveries should be followed by extensive inspection of the cervix only when there is profuse bleeding immediately after delivery.
d. Annular cervical detachment is associated with difficult midforceps deliveries.
e. Persistent leukorrhea sometimes results from cervical laceration.

33–5. Which of the following statements about the management of cervical lacerations is correct?

a. Postpartum digital examination of the cervix is usually sufficient.
b. To ensure correct anatomic approximation of cervical lacerations, suturing is best started from the distal end.
c. Packing as a treatment for cervical lacerations generally results in a poorer outcome than surgical repair.
d. Treatment of extensive cervical lacerations includes evaluation of extension superiorly and laterally, by laparotomy if needed.
e. Persistent leukorrhea associated with cervical lacerations may be treated by cautery or cryotherapy.

33–6. The nontraumatized, normally laboring uterus rarely undergoes spontaneous rupture.

a. True
b. False

33–7. List the causes of uterine rupture associated with injury before the current pregnancy that are related to: (1) surgery involving the myometrium and (2) coincidental trauma to the uterus.

33–8. List the causes of uterine rupture associated with injury during the current pregnancy that can occur: (1) before delivery and (2) during delivery.

33–9. Which of the following uterine defects is least likely to lead to uterine rupture?

a. Pregnancy in an incompletely developed uterus or uterine horn
b. Placenta increta
c. Placenta percreta
d. Placenta accreta
e. Choriocarcinoma
f. Sacculation of an adherent retroverted uterus

Instructions for Items 33–10 to 33–11: Match the type of uterine rupture with the correct definition.

a. Incomplete
b. Complete

33–10. Laceration communicates directly with the peritoneal cavity

33–11. Laceration is separated from the peritoneal cavity by the uterine or broad ligament peritoneum

33–12. Incomplete uterine ruptures rarely become complete.

a. True
b. False

33–13. Which of the following statements about scars from a previous cesarean section is correct?

a. Rupture of a cesarean section scar is defined as the separation of the old incision throughout most of its length without accompanying rupture of the fetal membranes.
b. In the dehiscence of a cesarean section scar, the fetal membranes are usually ruptured and all or part of the fetus is extruded into the peritoneal cavity.
c. The degree of obstetric hemorrhage in rupture or dehiscence is approximately equal.
d. Dehiscence usually occurs gradually, while rupture of a previous scar is a more rapid process.

33–14. A classical cesarean section scar is derived from an incision made in what location?

33–15. Which of the following statements about cesarean section scars is correct?

a. In the rupture of a classical cesarean section scar, the maternal mortality rate is about 25 percent and the perinatal mortality rate is about 50 percent.
b. The probability of rupture of a classical cesarean section scar is several times greater than the probability of rupture of a lower segment scar.
c. About two-thirds of classical cesarean section scars that will rupture do so before labor begins.
d. Early repeat cesarean section of patients with classical cesarean section scars will prevent most ruptures.
e. In patients with lower segment uterine scars, dehiscence is much more frequent than rupture.

33–16. Cesarean section scars show evidence of healing by scar tissue formation.

a. True
b. False

33–17. Which of the following statements about the rupture of the unscarred uterus is correct?

a. During pregnancy, uterine rupture is more commonly caused by blunt trauma to the abdomen than by placental abruption.
b. Oxytocin should probably not be administered antepartum to women of high parity because of their increased risk of spontaneous uterine rupture.
c. Excessive stretching of the lower uterine segment with the formation of a pathologic contraction ring is highly associated with spontaneous uterine rupture.
d. Formation of a retroperitoneal hematoma is equally likely with complete and incomplete uterine rupture.
e. Development of a uteroabdominal pregnancy is a rare outcome of uterine rupture.

33–18. Spontaneous uterine rupture during labor may be associated with

a. Cessation of most labor pain
b. Abrupt shock
c. Severe immediate vaginal hemorrhage
d. Massive hemoperitoneum formation

33–19. Which of the following statements about the detection of a uterine rupture during labor is correct?

a. When the fetus is totally extrauterine, abdominal palpation or vaginal examination are helpful in identifying fetal parts.
b. A contracted uterus may be felt alongside the fetus.
c. Failure to detect a tear on vaginal examination means that uterine rupture has not occurred.
d. Abdominal paracentesis or culdocentesis may be employed to detect hemoperitoneum.

133–20. The perinatal mortality rate associated with uterine rupture is between ____________________.

33–21. Which of the following statements about the management of a uterine rupture is correct?

a. Surgical control of bleeding and treatment of hypovolemia and shock are the critical components of immediate management.
b. Hysterectomy is usually required, although uterine repair may be possible in selected cases.
c. Oxytocin administration should be avoided in all cases because it extends the uterine laceration.
d. Antibiotic therapy is only indicated in cases where there is antecedent chorioamnionitis.
e. Ligation of the hypogastric arteries to control bleeding interferes with subsequent reproductive function.

33–22. A ________________ fistula is the most frequent type formed as a result of obstructed labor.

34. ABNORMALITIES OF THE THIRD STAGE OF LABOR

34–1. Postpartum hemorrhage has most often been defined as the loss of more than ________________ ml of blood during the first 24 hours after delivery.

34–2. Delayed postpartum hemorrhage is defined as ________________.

34–3. The most common cause of serious blood loss in obstetrics is

a. A low implanted placenta
b. Postpartum hemorrhage
c. Placental abruption
d. Ectopic pregnancy
e. Uterine rupture
f. Hemorrhage from abortion

34–4. Which of the following may contribute to the development of uterine atony?

a. Prolonged labor
b. Very rapid labor
c. High parity
d. An overdistended uterus
e. Use of general anesthesia
f. Use of vigorous oxytocin stimulation
g. Uterine infection

34–5. Which of the following are the two most common causes of immediate postpartum hemorrhage?

a. Coagulation defects
b. A large episiotomy
c. Lacerations of the vagina and cervix
d. A hypotonic myometrium
e. Retained placental tissue

34–6. Retention of part or all of the placenta may cause

a. Immediate postpartum hemorrhage
b. Delayed postpartum hemorrhage

34–7. Which of the following is characteristic of postpartum hemorrhage?

a. It is usually difficult to predict in advance of delivery which women will hemorrhage.
b. There is usually a sudden massive hemorrhage.
c. The effects of the hemorrhage depend on the nonpregnant blood volume, the degree of pregnancy-induced hypervolemia, and the presence of anemia at the time of delivery.
d. Pulse and blood pressure may only undergo moderate alterations until a large amount of blood has been lost.

34–8. Kneading and squeezing of a contracted uterus aids the mechanism of placental separation and shortens the third stage of labor.

a. True
b. False

34–9. The determination of whether postpartum hemorrhage is the result of uterine atony or genital tract lacerations begins with an examination of __________.

Instructions for Items 34–10 to 34–13: Match the clinical situation with the appropriate postpartum management to prevent hemorrhage.

a. Inspection of the cervix
b. Inspection of the vagina
c. Examination of the uterine cavity

34–10. After a breech extraction
34–11. After every delivery
34–12. After internal podalic version
34–13. After a vaginal delivery in a woman with a previous cesarean delivery

34–14. Describe the clinical picture of complete Sheehan's syndrome that follows severe intrapartum or early postpartum hemorrhage.

34–15. The incidence of Sheehan's syndrome in the United States is about 1 in ______________ deliveries.

a. 5,000
b. 10,000
c. 20,000
d. 40,000
e. 80,000

Instructions for Items 34–16 to 34–17: Match the type of third stage bleeding with the mechanism of placental separation.

a. Mechanism of Duncan
b. Mechanism of Schultze

34–16. Immediate escape of blood into the vagina
34–17. Blood concealed behind the placenta and fetal membranes until the placenta is delivered

34–18. Which of the following statements about the management of the placenta in the third stage of labor is correct?

a. Uterine massage is indicated when external hemorrhage precedes the expulsion of the placenta.
b. Uterine massage and gentle traction will often result in placental separation and expulsion.
c. Placental separation is usually first recognized by a slackening of the umbilical cord or a gush of blood.
d. Manual removal of the placenta is mandatory in the case of continued third stage bleeding.
e. Manual placental removal is accomplished by inserting a gloved hand into the uterine cavity and gently peeling the placenta from its attachment, then grasping it with the hand, which is gradually withdrawn.
f. The membranes should not be removed during the process of manual placental removal.

34–19. Which of the following statements about management after the delivery of the placenta is correct?

a. Palpation of the uterine fundus is only necessary when hemorrhage persists after the delivery of the placenta.
b. Ergonovine (Ergotrate) or methylergonovine (Methergine) should be administered only if vigorous fundal massage and the intravenous infusion of dilute oxytocin solution do not result in a firm, contracted uterus.
c. Bimanual compression of the uterus is often effective in the management of postpartum bleeding after the removal of all placental remnants.
d. Uterine packing is often effective in the management of postpartum bleeding after the removal of all placental remnants.
e. Prostaglandins have proved effective in the management of postpartum bleeding after the removal of all placental remnants.

34–20. Describe the technique of bimanual compression.

34–21. Describe the essential steps in the management of postpartum hemorrhage that is not controlled by uterine massage or oxytocics.

34–22. Lacerations of the vagina and cervix are repaired by interrupted single or figure-of-eight sutures starting ______________ the apex of the laceration.

a. Just above
b. At
c. Just below

34–23. What should be done to stabilize the patient prior to performing a therapeutic hysterectomy for the treatment of postpartum hemorrhage?

Instructions for Items 34–24 to 34–26: Match the type of abnormally adherent placenta with the appropriate description.

a. Placenta increta
b. Placenta percreta
c. Focal placenta accreta
d. Partial placenta accreta
e. Total placenta accreta

34–24. Placental villi penetrate through the myometrium
34–25. Placental villi invade the myometrium
34–26. Several cotyledons are firmly attached to the myometrium

34–27. The direct attachment of placental villi to the myometrium occurs because of what abnormal events in placental development?

34–28. The incidence of abnormally adherent placenta is about 1 in every 55 deliveries.

a. True
b. False

34–29. Which of the following is associated with placenta accreta in approximately one-quarter or more of cases?

a. Placenta previa
b. Previous cesarean delivery
c. Previous uterine curretage
d. Grand multiparity
e. Maternal age greater than 35 years

34–30. The clinical characteristics of placenta accreta include

a. Frequent antepartum bleeding, usually due to associated placenta previa
b. An increased incidence of uterine rupture, especially over a uterine scar
c. A high incidence of dysfunctional labor
d. An inverse relationship between the extent of the placenta accreta and the extent of obstetric hemorrhage, before manual placental removal is attempted

34–31. Which of the following statements about the management of an abnormally adherent placenta is correct?

a. Placenta increta may be identified ultrasonographically by the absence of a subplacental sonolucent area.
b. Hysterectomy is usually necessary in all types of placenta accreta.
c. Manual removal is often possible in both partial and total placenta accreta.
d. Conservative management of abnormally adherent placentas (by packing) is as effective as hysterectomy in preventing maternal mortality.

34–32. Uterine inversion is

a. Almost always the consequence of strong traction on the umbilical cord of a fundally implanted placenta
b. Almost always associated with some degree of placenta accreta
c. Associated with massive blood loss, the extent of which is often underestimated
d. Associated with shock disproportionate to the degree of blood loss
e. Associated with inexperienced personnel performing the delivery

34–33. Outline in sequential order the major steps in the management of uterine inversion.

34–34. If transvaginal reposition of the uterus is not possible, laparotomy should be performed so that the fundus can both be pushed upward from below and pulled from above.

a. True
b. False

35. PUERPERAL INFECTION

35–1. Puerperal infection is defined as_______________.

35–2. Puerperal morbidity

a. Is defined as a temperature of at least 38.0 °C, occurring on any 2 of the first 10 postpartum days (exclusive of the first 24 hours), when measured by a standard technique at least four times daily
b. Is used as an estimate of the incidence of puerperal infection
c. Only includes infectious causes of temperature elevation

35–3. What causes other than infection of the reproductive tract may result in a temperature elevation during the puerperium?

a. Pyelonephritis
b. Thrombophlebitis
c. Upper respiratory infection
d. Breast engorgement
e. Postpartum hemorrhage

35–4. The general factors that are associated with a likelihood of serious postpartum infection include

a. The amount of time the amnionic sac was ruptured prior to delivery
b. The length of labor
c. The number of vaginal examinations that were performed
d. The extent of intrauterine manipulations that were required during delivery
e. The number and size of obstetric incisions and lacerations

35–5. Which of the following statements about antepartum factors that may predispose to puerperal infection is correct?

a. Maternal anemia of any cause is associated with a twofold increase in the incidence of serious puerperal infection.
b. Transferrin may decrease maternal resistance to infection.
c. Poor nutrition decreases cell-mediated immunity, causing a significant increase in the incidence of infection.
d. Sexual intercourse in the 6 weeks before the onset of labor causes a significantly increased incidence of infection.

35–6. Which of the following statements about intrapartum factors that may predispose to puerperal infection is correct?

a. Iatrogenic introduction of bacteria into the upper genital tract through intrapartum vaginal examination is a major factor causing infection.
b. Significant sources of infection are the bacteria already present on the pudenda or vagina and nasopharyngeal droplet contamination from obstetric personnel.
c. Trauma that destroys and devitalizes tissue predisposes to puerperal infection.
d. Obstetric hemorrhage of greater than 1200 ml is a predisposing factor.

35–7. Explain the statement that puerperal infection is basically a wound infection.

35–8. Which of the following statements about puerperal infection associated with lesions of the perineum, vulva, vagina, and cervix is correct?

a. In the localized infection of a repaired laceration or episiotomy, the wound edges become necrotic and pus may exude from the opening created.
b. Infection in lacerations of the vagina is more likely to remain localized than infection in deep lacerations of the cervix.
c. Dysuria, with or without urinary retention, is an indication of severe infection.
d. The first treatment for puerperal infections of the lower genital tract is antibiotic therapy, followed after 48 hours by surgical drainage if no improvement has occurred.

35–9. Which of the following statements about puerperal metritis (endometritis) is correct?

a. Metritis refers to infection of the decidua and adjacent myometrium.
b. True metritis involves a uniform infection of the entire decidual surface.
c. Metritis is characterized by a profuse, foul, bloody, and sometimes frothy discharge.
d. β-Hemolytic streptococci are most often associated with the foul, profuse discharge of metritis.
e. Metritis is always characterized by a spiking high fever associated with chills, tachycardia, and uterine tenderness.
f. In severe cases, breast feeding should be discontinued.
g. All patients with metritis should be treated with intravenously administered broad-spectrum antibiotics.

Instructions for Items 35–10 to 35–12: Match the vessels initially involved in thrombophlebitis with the sites to which infection may spread.

a. Right ovarian vein
b. Left ovarian vein
c. Uterine veins

35–10. Involvement of the renal vein and kidneys
35–11. Extension to the inferior vena cava
35–12. Extension to the common iliac veins

35–13. Which of the following statements about puerperal thrombophlebitis is correct?

a. Anaerobic bacteria can exist and grow in venous thrombi.
b. In almost all cases, the sole method for the spread of puerperal infection is along the veins.
c. The uterine veins are usually involved bilaterally, whereas the right ovarian vein is more commonly involved than the left ovarian vein.
d. The most frequent occurrence is the development of large emboli which reach the pulmonary artery.

35-14. Multiple small septic thromboemboli are more often associated with cor pulmonale and sepsis, whereas large emboli are more frequently associated with sudden death.

a. True
b. False

35-15. Venous thrombi associated with metritis may

a. Block the spread of infection along venous routes
b. Suppurate, causing the vascular wall to become edematous and necrotic
c. Reach the terminal branches of pulmonary vessels, resulting in pleurisy, pneumonia, pulmonary infarcts, and abscesses
d. Lead to septic shock through the release of bacterial products into the circulation

Instructions for Items 35-16 to 35-18: Select the appropriate treatment for the following conditions.

a. Broad-spectrum antibiotic therapy
b. Anticoagulation (usually heparinization)
c. Ligation of the ovarian veins and/or the inferior vena cava

35-16. Pelvic thrombophlebitis
35-17. Recurrent pulmonary emboli
35-18. Septic pulmonary embolization

35-19. Puerperal infection may extend to either the peritoneum, causing ________ (1) or to the loose connective tissue between the layers of the broad ligament, causing ________ (2).

a. Pelvic cellulitis (parametritis)
b. Peritonitis

35-20. In pelvic peritonitis, which of the following is a common site for abscess formation?

a. The cul-de-sac
b. The subdiaphragmatic space
c. Folds between the infundibulopelvic and broad ligaments
d. The space of Retzius

35-21. Describe the ways that infection of the retroperitoneal connective tissue in pelvic cellulitis (parametritis) can occur.

35-22. Lymphatic transmission of infection from the ________ is commonly associated with the development of pelvic cellulitis (parametritis).

a. Uterus
b. Cervix
c. Vagina
d. Perineum

35-23. Which of the following statements about pelvic cellulitis (parametritis) is correct?

a. Pelvic cellulitis is more often unilateral.
b. Direct extension of pelvic cellulitis may ultimately cause a pointing abscess along the upper border of Poupart's ligament.
c. Retrocervical extension of pelvic cellulitis may result in localized abscess formation in the cul-de-sac of Douglas.
d. After cesarean section, infection of the tissue anterior to the cervix results in cellulitis in the space of Retzius.

35-24. Which of the following statements about the bacteriology of puerperal infections is correct?

a. Most puerperal infections result from contamination with organisms that normally exist in the bowel and lower genital tract.
b. Iatrogenic infection with organisms carried to the patient by obstetric staff is relatively uncommon, although β-hemolytic streptococcal infections sometimes occur.
c. Anaerobic and aerobic cultures of the infection site are more likely to be of diagnostic benefit than blood cultures.
d. Only anaerobic bacteria are involved in puerperal infections.
e. Usually only one species of bacteria is involved in a given case of puerperal infection.

35-25. It is usually possible to precisely identify the bacterial species responsible for any given puerperal infection.

a. True
b. False

35-26. Which of the following statements about the clinical course of pelvic cellulitis (parametritis) is correct?

a. The condition should be suspected when persistent, steady elevations of temperature occur in the puerperium.
b. Unilateral or bilateral abdominal tenderness and tenderness on vaginal examination are common.
c. The uterus may become fixed due to the parametrial exudate.
d. Rectovaginal examination may help to identify a posterior extension of the exudate into the broad ligament along the sacrouterine folds.
e. Suppuration of the parametrial mass occurs in the majority of patients.
f. Adhesion and abscess formation are common and serious complications.

35–27. Which of the following statements about the clinical course of peritonitis is correct?

a. Pelvic and surgical peritonitis are clinically indistinguishable.
b. Marked bowel distention and paralytic ileus are more common in surgical than in pelvic peritonitis.
c. Due to antibiotic therapy, the duration of the disease and the mortality rate have both decreased.
d. The most common cause of death before the advent of antibiotic therapy was pulmonary involvement.

35–28. Toxic shock syndrome is

a. An acute febrile illness confined to the lower reproductive tract
b. Characterized by fever, headache, mental confusion, scarlatiniform rash, subcutaneous edema, nausea, vomiting, watery diarrhea, marked hemoconcentration, oliguria, and renal failure
c. Associated with *Staphylococcus* species and their endotoxin
d. Best treated with broad-spectrum antibiotics

35–29. List the most common extragenital causes of puerperal fever.

35–30. Which of the following statements about causes of fever in the puerperium is correct?

a. Respiratory complications, especially atelectasis, are most commonly seen in the first 24 hours after delivery.
b. The first sign of pyelonephritis is usually costovertebral angle pain and tenderness.
c. The late signs of pyelonephritis include nausea and vomiting.
d. Pyelonephritis should be confirmed with a catheterized urine culture and sensitivity.
e. Breast engorgement usually causes a moderate temperature rise that lasts not more than 24 hours, whereas fever in true mastitis is usually sustained and greater than 38.5 °C.
f. Wound abscess is usually obvious on close inspection of the wound site.

35–31. A painful swollen leg, femoral triangle tenderness, or pain with dorsoflexion of the foot associated with significant fever is consistent with the diagnosis of thrombophlebitis.

a. True
b. False

35–32. Which of the following statements about antibiotic therapy utilized for puerperal infections at Parkland Memorial Hospital is correct?

a. The first-line treatment is usually one of the second generation cephalosporins such as cefoxitan or cefamandole.
b. If there is evidence of severe infection associated with bacterial shock or hemolysis, or if the febrile course continues in the face of single agent therapy, clindamycin and gentamicin should be added.
c. Chloramphenicol may be substituted for clindamycin and gentamicin in patients with impaired renal function.
d. Ileus may be an indication for the use of chloramphenicol rather than clindamycin and gentamicin.
e. Pseudomembranous colitis is associated with *Clostridium difficile,* which is best treated by the addition of vibramycin to the treatment regimen.
f. Metronidazole is the agent of choice for all anaerobic infections of the upper genital tract.

35–33. Pelvic cellulitis (parametritis) must be treated by antibiotic therapy and may require surgical drainage of abscesses.

a. True
b. False

35–34. Which of the following statements about the treatment of generalized peritonitis is correct?

a. The treatment of peritonitis that begins in the uterus is generally medical.
b. The treatment of peritonitis that begins with a bowel lesion is generally surgical.
c. Clindamycin and gentamicin plus cephalosporin or penicillin are usually effective against the organisms causing the infection.
d. Fluid and electrolyte therapy is extremely important.
e. Treatment of paralytic ileus should include gastric decompression and the use of drugs to stimulate peristalsis.

36. OTHER DISORDERS OF THE PUERPERIUM

36–1. Deep venous thrombosis and thromboembolism are limited to the puerperium.

a. True
b. False

36–2. The strongest single predisposing factor to deep vein thrombosis is ________________________.

36–3. The increasing incidence of venous thromboembolic disease during the puerperium is due to increases in the use of oral contraceptives before conception and in the number of women who work at sedentary jobs.

a. True
b. False

36–4. Puerperal thromboembolic disease can be decreased by

a. Early ambulation
b. Prohibition of ambulation

Instructions for Items 36–5 to 36–6: Match the type of venous thrombosis with the appropriate description.

a. Thrombophlebitis
b. Phlebothrombosis

36–5. Venous thrombosis associated with an inflammatory response
36–6. Venous thrombosis without evidence of inflammation

36–7. Deep and superficial venous thrombosis of the legs have an equal potential for generating pulmonary emboli.

a. True
b. False

36–8. Superficial venous thrombosis of the legs is treated solely with analgesia, elastic support, and rest.

a. True
b. False

36–9. Which of the following statements about deep venous thrombosis of the legs is correct?

a. It is sometimes called phlegmasia alba dolens or "milk leg."
b. It is characterized by an abrupt onset of swelling and pain in one or both extremities, usually with the demonstration of a positive Homan sign.
c. It may be definitively identified by doppler and impedance plethysmography.
d. Puerperal deep vein thrombosis is treated with antibiotics (if there is associated fever), anticoagulation, bed rest, and analgesia.
e. Antepartum deep venous thrombosis is treated by prolonged anticoagulation.

Instructions for Items 36–10 to 36–14: Match the drug utilized for anticoagulation therapy with the appropriate statement.

a. Heparin
b. Warfarin (coumadin)

36–10. Inhibits the synthesis of vitamin K-dependent coagulation factors
36–11. May result in congenital malformations if administered early in pregnancy
36–12. May produce maternal thrombocytopenia
36–13. Crosses the placenta
36–14. Does not cross the placenta

36–15. Which of the following statements about the anticoagulant therapy of deep venous thrombosis is correct?

a. In pregnancy, warfarin (coumadin) is as effective as heparin in the long-term treatment of deep venous thrombosis.
b. Thrombosis with embolization is less likely to recur after heparin therapy than after warfarin therapy.
c. Warfarin is the drug of choice for long-term prophylaxis in the absence of pregnancy.
d. Aspirin and other drugs that impair platelet function are useful adjuvants to low dose heparinization.

36–16. Which of the following statements about pelvic venous thrombosis is correct?

a. Pelvic vein thrombosis, which occurs very infrequently, is characterized by the acute onset of deep pelvic pain.
b. Ovarian vein thrombophlebitis rarely occurs in the left vein.
c. Ovarian vein thrombophlebitis is characterized by the acute onset of pain, with or without fever, in the 2nd or 3rd postpartum day.
d. Optimal therapy for ovarian vein thrombophlebitis is operative removal of the firm tumefaction of the ovarian vein and the overlying inflamed peritoneum, ligation of the inferior vena cava, followed in 48 hours by heparinization.

36–17. Which of the following statements about delivery in the presence of anticoagulation therapy is correct?

a. Treatment with warfarin continued until just before delivery may result in fetal hemorrhage.
b. Slow intravenous administration of 10 mg of vitamin K, increases the levels of vitamin K-dependent coagulation factors to safe levels in both the mother and fetus in about 8 hours.
c. Infusion of plasma or plasma fractions rich in Factors II, VII, IX, and X results in immediate reversal of low levels in both mother and fetus.
d. In most cases, heparin therapy may be continued during labor and delivery.
e. Protamine sulfate will promptly neutralize the effect of heparin.
f. Given in excess, protamine has an anticoagulant effect.

36–18. List the variables that influence the risk of excessive blood loss/hematoma formation during labor and delivery for a patient undergoing therapy with heparin.

36–19. If a woman who has recently suffered a pulmonary embolism must be delivered by cesarean, ligation of the inferior vena cava above the insertion of the right renal vein and of the left ovarian vein near its insertion into the renal vein will yield the most favorable outcome.

a. True
b. False

36–20. The incidence of pulmonary embolism associated with pregnancy has been reported to be between ________________.

36–21. Which of the following signs and symptoms are characteristic of puerperal pulmonary embolism?

a. Chest discomfort
b. Shortness of breath
c. Respiratory rate <16 per minute
d. Air hunger
e. Obvious apprehension

36–22. Which of the following statements about the diagnosis of pulmonary embolism is correct?

a. Physical examination of the chest characteristically identifies an accentuated pulmonic valve second sound, rales, and friction rub.
b. Right axis deviation may or may not be observed in an electrocardiogram.
c. The classic triad of hemoptysis, pleuritic chest pain, and dyspnea are present in over 80 percent of patients.
d. A combination of ventilation-perfusion scintigraphy and pulmonary angiography is required for an accurate diagnosis to be made.

36–23. Which of the following statements about heparin therapy for pulmonary embolism during pregnancy is correct?

a. Treatment with heparin, either 5000 to 7500 units intravenously every 4 hours or by a constant infusion pump at a rate of approximately 1 IU/ml of estimated blood volume every 4 hours, is effective.
b. Measurement of the whole blood clotting time and the plasma partial thromboplastin time are useful for monitoring the effectiveness of heparin therapy.
c. Frequent measurement of the hematocrit is useful to detect hemorrhage during heparin therapy.
d. Heparin therapy may be discontinued in 10 days to 2 weeks if the disease process has abated and factors predisposing to recurrence are absent.
e. If anticoagulation with warfarin is desired, therapy with it should overlap the therapy with heparin for about 6 days until the prothrombin time has reached therapeutic levels.

36–24. What is the treatment of choice when heparin therapy fails to prevent recurrent pulmonary embolism from the pelvis or legs?

36–25. Which of the following statements about problems of the puerperium involving the uterus is correct?

a. Unless therapy is instituted, subinvolution of the uterus is always associated with leukorrhea followed by hemorrhage.
b. The diagnosis of subinvolution is made by bimanual examination.
c. Subinvolution is associated with retained placental fragments and pelvic infection (metritis).
d. Subinvolution is treated with ergonovine or methylergonovine in addition to antibiotics if there is associated metritis.

36–26. Cervical erosions or eversions, a complication of the early puerperium, can best be treated by cone biopsy.

a. True
b. False

36–27. What are the possible causes of hemorrhage that occurs late in the puerperium?

36–28. Hemorrhage late in the puerperium is best treated by

a. Prompt curettage
b. Oxytocics
c. Hysterectomy

36–29. Which of the following statements about puerperal hematomas is correct?

a. Hematomas of the genital tract are characterized by the acute onset of a painful, swollen mass in the vulva or vagina.
b. Hematomas may infrequently be located above the pelvic fascia and may progress by a retroperitoneal route all the way to the diaphragm.
c. Vulvar hematomas, even those that are subperitoneal, ultimately cause external bleeding, which may take the form of hemorrhage or the discharge of large clots.
d. Vulvar hematomas should be incised, the bleeding points ligated, and the remaining cavity obliterated with mattress sutures.
e. Broad-spectrum antibiotics are of value in the treatment of vulvar hematomas.
f. The blood loss in vulvar hematomas is usually slight.

36–30. Which of the following statements about urinary tract disease in the puerperium is correct?

a. The puerperal bladder is less sensitive to intravesical pressure than the bladder in a nonpregnant woman.
b. In most patients, there is postpartum bladder distention and overflow incontinence of small amounts of urine.
c. The distended bladder and/or residual urine may serve as a site for bacterial infection, requiring antibiotic therapy.
d. If there is continued overdistention of the bladder, 24 hours of continuous catheter drainage is the appropriate initial therapy.
e. Catheterization should be reinitiated if a woman cannot void within 4 hours after removal of the catheter or if there is more than 200 ml of urine in her bladder.

36–31. Which of the following statements about breast engorgement in the puerperium is correct?

a. For the first 24 to 48 hours after the development of lacteal secretion, it is not uncommon for the breasts to become distended, firm, and nodular.
b. Engorged or "caked breasts" are the result of overdistention of the lacteal system with milk.
c. Fever is uncommon with simple breast engorgement.
d. The treatment of breast engorgement is support with a binder or brassiere, ice packs, and analgesics as needed.

36–32. Which of the following statements about the suppression of lactation is correct?

a. Suppression may be accomplished by support with a comfortable binder, application of cold, and administration of mild analgesics.
b. If the breasts are not stimulated by pumping, signs and symptoms disappear after several weeks.
c. Some estrogens used to suppress lactation may predispose to venous thrombosis and thromboembolism.
d. Bromocriptine is an effective but expensive method to suppress lactation.

36–33. Mastitis

a. Is as common antepartum as in the puerperium
b. Usually becomes symptomatic in the puerperium during the third or fourth weeks
c. Is characterized by breast engorgement followed by inflammation, fever, tachycardia, and discomfort
d. Always pursues an acute course
e. Is most commonly caused by *Staphylococcus aureus*

36–34. The immediate cause of mastitis is usually the introduction of bacteria from the nursing infant's nose and throat through a fissure or abrasion in the nipple.

a. True
b. False

36–35. Which of the following statements about the prevention of mastitis is correct?

a. Careful screening of infants in the newborn nursery for bacterial infection and frequent handwashing by personnel will reduce the risk of iatrogenic infection.
b. Bacterial interference techniques have not proven effective for control of staphylococcal epidemics in the newborn nursery.
c. Nasopharyngeal cultures with phage typing of nursery personnel to identify asymptomatic carriers is useful in a suspected outbreak of staphylococcal infection.
d. Suppurative mastitis outbreaks in the postpartum ward are often associated with staphylococcal infections in the nursery.

36–36. Describe the process of bacterial interference.

36–37. Which of the following statements about the treatment of mastitis is correct?

a. Culture of milk expressed from the breast will usually identify the responsible organism and its sensitivities.
b. Prompt antibiotic therapy (with either penicillin G or a penicillinase-resistant compound) will usually prevent a suppurative infection.
c. Nursing should be discontinued when the diagnosis of suppurative mastitis is confirmed.
d. Antibiotic therapy may be discontinued as soon as the patient has been asymptomatic for 24 hours.
e. An abscess should be treated by a radial incision and drainage followed by packs in decreasing sizes.

36–38. Galactocele results from ________________.

36–39. Which of the following statements about puerperal breast disorders is correct?

a. Supernumary breasts (polymastia) occur in about 1 in 10,000 women.
b. Supernumary breasts have little obstetric significance apart from sometimes becoming enlarged and mildly painful at the start of nursing.
c. Some nipples are depressed, not allowing suckling.
d. Fissures of the nipple cause pain and harbor infection.

36–40. Galactorrhea, amenorrhea, and evidence of estrogen deficiency (formerly referred to as Chiari-Frommel's syndrome) is most often associated with a pituitary adenoma.

a. True
b. False

36–41. Which of the following statements about obstetric paralysis is correct?

a. Obstetric paralysis is characterized by intense neuralgia or cramp-like pain extending into one or both legs.
b. Obstetric paralysis is caused by pressure on the sacral plexus branches by the fetal head during descent in labor.
c. Obstetric paralysis/pain rarely continues into the puerperium.
d. Footdrop usually results from improper positioning of the patient in stirrups or leg holders.

36–42. Labor-associated separation of the symphysis pubis or one of the sacroiliac synchondroses is usually not associated with difficulties in the puerperium.

a. True
b. False

37. PRETERM AND POSTTERM PREGNANCIES AND FETAL GROWTH RETARDATION

37–1. Determination of the appropriateness of fetal growth depends on knowledge of what important factor?

Instructions for Items 37–2 to 37–4: Match the term with the appropriate interval following the LMP (when ovulation and fertilization occurred 2 weeks later).

a. Fetus (infant) at term
b. Preterm infant
c. Premature infant
d. Postterm infant

37–2. An infant born before the 38th week

37–3. An infant born between the 38th and 42nd weeks

37–4. An infant born at or after 42 completed weeks

Instructions for Items 37–5 to 37–7: Match the term with the correct definition.

a. Appropriately grown, preterm fetus
b. Growth-retarded, term fetus
c. Growth-retarded, preterm fetus

37–5. A shortened gestation and an impaired rate of growth

37–6. A shortened gestation and a normal rate of growth

37–7. A gestation of normal duration and an impaired rate of growth

37–8. An infant whose birth weight is below the ________ (1) percentile is defined as small for gestational age, while an infant above the ________ (2) percentile is categorized as large for gestational age.

37–9. It is useful in obstetric practice to exactly equate fetal size with level of fetal maturity.

a. True
b. False

37–10. In utero fetal growth is somewhat retarded in infants who are born prematurely.

a. True
b. False

37–11. Which of the following factors influences birth weight in term pregnancies?

a. Sex of the infant
b. Parity
c. Race
d. Maternal age

37–12. The mean birth weight in the United States at 40 weeks of gestation is reported as ________ (1) g with a range of ________ (2) g.

37–13. According to Hendricks, the mean daily fetal growth in grams during the previous week of gestation increases until about the ________ week and then begins to decline.

a. 31st
b. 34th
c. 37th
d. 40th

37–14. High-risk pregnancy refers to a situation where the fetus may not be liveborn, may not survive after birth, or may suffer physical, intellectual, or emotional impairment as the consequence of a hostile antepartum, intrapartum, or neonatal environment.

a. True
b. False

37–15. Fetal distress refers to the acute situation where compromise of the fetal unit is discovered by electronic fetal monitoring or direct blood gas sampling.

a. True
b. False

37–16. Which of the following statements about intensive neonatal care is correct?

a. Advances in intensive care have lowered the neonatal death rate by nearly 100 percent in the last quarter century.
b. All hospitals providing maternity care should have all facilities for neonatal intensive care available.
c. Maternal or infant transportation to well-equipped intensive care facilities are equally acceptable in terms of cost, safety, and logistics.
d. With modern neonatal care facilities, there are no demonstrable differences in long-term outcome of term and preterm infants (excluding infants with congenital anomalies or severe birth trauma).
e. Most infants weighing more than 1000 g or born after 27 weeks of gestation and who are not malformed will survive with appropriate intensive care.
f. Much of the cost of prematurity could be avoided by appropriate levels of antepartum care.

37–17. Complete the following table by supplying the outcome of preterm deliveries (according to Walker and associates).

Birthweight (g)	Neonatal Mortality (%)	Frequency of Severe Handicaps Among Survivors (%)
500–599	(1)	(2)
600–699	(3)	(4)
700–799	(5)	(6)
800–899	(7)	(8)
900–999	(9)	(10)

37–18. What is the first question to be answered when preterm labor is diagnosed?

37–19. Until term, the intrauterine environment is safer for the fetus than extrauterine existence, unless the mother is mortally ill.

a. True
b. False

37–20. Which of the following statements about conditions that predispose to preterm labor is correct?

a. The onset of labor remote from term is commonly preceded by rupture of the membranes.
b. Cervical incompetency is a common predisposing factor to preterm labor.
c. Uterine anomalies are a relatively rare predisposing factor.
d. Overdistention of the uterus, as with severe hydramnios or multifetal pregnancy, is associated with an increased incidence of preterm labor.
e. Anomalies of the fetus or placenta predispose to preterm labor.
f. Faulty placentation is associated with preterm labor.

37–21. A woman who previously gave birth to a preterm infant is at no higher risk for a subsequent delivery remote from term than the general population.

a. True
b. False

37–22. What are the signs generally used to identify preterm labor?

37–23. In essentially all cases of preterm labor, the good of the fetus requires that an attempt be made to inhibit the labor.

a. True
b. False

37–24. Which of the following statements about the treatment of preterm labor is correct?

a. Bed rest alone never provides a satisfactory outcome.
b. The administration of progestational agents (especially 17α-hydroxyprogesterone or Delalutin) has proven effective in inhibiting labor.
c. Ethanol inhibits endogenous oxytocin formation, which results in successful inhibition of labor.

37–25. Which of the following statements about the use of magnesium sulfate in the treatment of preterm labor is correct?

a. Ionic magnesium in high enough concentrations alters myometrial activity.
b. Magnesium is presumed to act as an antagonist of calcium in the process of muscle contraction.
c. Magnesium toxicity can be a problem for the mother but not for the fetus-infant.
d. The possibility of hypermagnesemia is monitored by checking the patellar reflex and monitoring respiration.
e. Magnesium sulfate is clearly an effective long-term inhibitor of preterm labor.

Instructions for Items 37–26 to 37–27: Match the β-receptor with the appropriate cell type.

a. β_1 receptor
b. β_2 receptor

37–26. Heart and intestine
37–27. Myometrium, blood vessels, bronchioles

37–28. Which of the following statements about the use of β-Adrenergic receptor stimulants in the treatment of preterm labor is correct?

a. Epinephrine in low doses is an effective and long-acting depressant of myometrial activity.
b. β-Adrenergic agonists act by coupling with adrenergic receptors located on the myometrial cell membrane, ultimately resulting in the reduction of intracellular calcium ions.
c. The ideal β-agonist would stimulate only β-adrenergic receptors on myometrial cells without stimulation of β-receptors on other cell types.
d. None of the compounds similar in structure to epinephrine that have been evaluated to date has been found to be ideal in the inhibition of preterm labor.

37–29. Which of the following β-adrenergic agonists is approved for use by the FDA?

a. Isoxuprine
b. Ritodrine
c. Terbutaline
d. Salbutamol
e. Fenoterol

Instructions for Items 37–30 to 37–32: Match the β-adrenergic receptor stimulant with its significant potential side effects.

a. Isoxuprine
b. Ritodrine
c. Terbutaline
d. Salbutamol
e. Fenoterol

37–30. Maternal pulmonary edema
37–31. Maternal tachycardia and hypotension
37–32. Hypoglycemia in the infant after delivery

37–33. Which of the following statements about the management of preterm labor is correct?

a. Combined therapy with ritodrine and magnesium sulfate has proved especially effective in refractory cases.
b. While some antiprostaglandins seem to be effective in the arrest of preterm labor, their use is discouraged because they may cause cardiovascular problems such as premature closure of the ductus arteriosus.
c. Narcotics and sedatives have little efficacy in inhibiting preterm labor and they may depress the preterm infant.
d. Diazoxide is safe and effective since its side effects are uncomfortable but not dangerous.

Instructions for Items 37–34 to 37–35: Match the term with the correct definition.

a. Preterm rupture of the membranes
b. Premature rupture of the membranes

37–34. Rupture of the membranes at any time before the onset of labor

37–35. Rupture of the membranes remote from term

37–36. In most cases, premature rupture of the membranes is followed within a few days by labor and delivery.

a. True
b. False

37–37. Describe the management of rupture of the membranes remote from term that is utilized at Parkland Memorial Hospital.

37–38. Prolonged rupture of the membranes is defined as ______________________________.

37–39. Prophylactic antibiotics should be administered to infants in all cases of prolonged rupture of the membranes.

a. True
b. False

37–40. In which of the following situations is there the possibility of accelerated surfactant production in an infant remote from term?

a. Maternal chronic renal or cardiovascular disease
b. Sickle cell disease
c. Heroin addiction
d. Hyperthyroidism
e. Chorionamnionitis
f. Placental infarction

37–41. Even though rupture of the membranes remote from term is associated with accelerated fetal lung maturation, the risk of infection makes deliberate delay in delivery poor obstetric practice.

a. True
b. False

37–42. Glucocorticoid therapy for preterm rupture of the membranes

a. Has been clearly shown to accelerate the production of pulmonary surfactant
b. Has a transient effect of about 7 days in humans
c. Is associated with an increased risk of maternal and fetal infection
d. May intensify the metabolic derangements of diabetes and worsen severe pregnancy-induced hypertension
e. May result in long-term risks for the fetus-infant

37–43. Which of the following statements about the management of preterm labor and delivery is correct?

a. The more premature the fetus, the greater the risk, especially in the breech position.
b. Significant birth passage resistance is uncommon in preterm labor.
c. Cord compression is relatively common with premature rupture of the membranes.
d. The fragile preterm head is best protected during vaginal delivery by the application of outlet forceps.
e. A liberal episiotomy is advantageous in the vaginal delivery of a preterm infant.

37–44. For any gestational age, as weight decreases below the ______________ percentile, the risk of fetal death increases greatly.

a. 10th
b. 20th
c. 30th

37–45. A small for gestational age fetus born of a small woman is more likely to be growth retarded than if the mother were of normal size.

a. True
b. False

37–46. If a mother is large and otherwise healthy, below average weight gain in the absence of disease is ______________ to be associated with appreciable fetal growth retardation.

a. Likely
b. Less likely

37–47. Which of the following situations is associated with fetal growth retardation?

a. Chronic maternal vascular disease complicated by superimposed preeclampsia and proteinuria
b. Late occurring pregnancy-induced hypertension
c. Chronic maternal renal disease
d. Maternal anemia of any cause
e. Maternal cyanotic heart disease
f. Smoking
g. Alcoholism
h. Maternal residence at high altitude
i. Cytomegalic inclusion disease
j. Rubella

Instructions for Items 37–48 to 37–53: Match the placental abnormality with the likelihood of fetal growth retardation.

a. Commonly associated with fetal growth retardation
b. Not commonly associated with fetal growth retardation

37–48. Chronic focal placental abruption
37–49. Extensive placental infarction
37–50. Placenta previa
37–51. Chorioangioma
37–52. Circumvallate placenta
37–53. Velamentous insertion of the umbilical cord

37–54. Fetal growth retardation is usually not a repetitive event.

a. True
b. False

37–55. Growth retardation is common with

a. Multifetal pregnancy
b. Chronic fetal infection
c. Prolonged pregnancy
d. Extrauterine pregnancy
e. High maternal hemoglobin concentrations

37–56. A careful medical history including factors predisposing to fetal growth retardation and careful serial measurements of uterine fundal height reinforced by ultrasonography are sufficient to diagnose fetal growth retardation in essentially all cases of singleton pregnancy.

a. True
b. False

37–57. Which of the following statements about the types of fetal growth retardation is correct?

a. In asymmetrical growth retardation, the head is of relatively normal size.
b. Symmetrical growth retardation is often difficult to distinguish from erroneous determination of gestational age.
c. Sonographic measurement of the biparietal diameter and head circumference at the level of the third ventricle will detect both symmetrical and asymmetrical growth retardation.
d. Normally, the head and abdominal circumferences are about equal between 32 and 36 weeks of gestation.
e. After 36 weeks of gestation, the head circumference normally exceeds the abdominal circumference.

37–58. Evidence of both oligohydramnios and fetal growth retardation is usually an indication for delivery.

a. True
b. False

37–59. Prompt delivery is the best management for a severely growth retarded fetus at or near term.

a. True
b. False

37–60. Which of the following statements about the management of fetal growth retardation remote from term is correct?

a. The risk of preterm labor is virtually eliminated by strict bed rest.
b. The demonstration of an L/S ratio <2 means that respiratory distress will most likely occur upon delivery.
c. Worsening maternal disease that has contributed to the growth retardation is an indication for delivery only if the L/S ratio is >2.
d. When the estimated fetal weight is below the 10th percentile for a given gestational age and remains static, continued intrauterine time does not decrease perinatal mortality.

37–61. Intrapartum fetal distress is more common when there is fetal growth retardation than when there is none.

a. True
b. False

37–62. Compared to a normal infant, the growth retarded infant is

a. At increased risk of being born hypoxic
b. More likely to require cesarean delivery
c. More likely to show intrapartum evidence of uteroplacental insufficiency
d. More susceptible to hypothermia
e. More likely to become hyperglycemic

Instructions for Items 37–63 to 37–65: Match the following situations with the subsequent development of the growth retarded infant.

a. Likely to attain normal growth and/or to catch up
b. Likely to remain small or slow growing

37–63. Symmetrical growth retardation
37–64. Asymmetrical growth retardation
37–65. Normal length at birth

37–66. In most cases, growth retardation is associated with subsequent neurologic and intellectual problems.

a. True
b. False

37–67. Fifteen percent of all pregnancies eventually become postterm.

a. True
b. False

37–68. The reported incidence of postterm pregnancies may be inaccurate because of ________________.

37–69. Postterm pregnancy is associated with

a. Anencephaly
b. A history of previous postterm pregnancy
c. A history of previous preterm pregnancy
d. Placental sulfatase activity
e. Extrauterine pregnancy
f. Multifetal pregnancy

37–70. The in utero postterm fetus

a. May continue to grow, with an increased risk of fetopelvic disproportion
b. May suffer an arrest of growth
c. May experience umbilical cord compression and fetal distress, especially when there is associated oligohydramnios
d. Is often at increased risk for meconium defecation and aspiration

37–71. Outline the management of postterm pregnancy utilized at Parkland Memorial Hospital.

37–72. What are the most dangerous times for the postterm fetus?

37–73. A cesarean delivery should be strongly considered in a woman in early labor who has hypotonic uterine dysfunction and thick meconium in her amnionic fluid.

a. True
b. False

37–74. There is no convincing evidence that the serial use of either nonstress or contraction stress tests improves the outcome in postterm pregnancies.

a. True
b. False

37–75. The presence of scant amnionic fluid is the most ominous sign of impending fetal distress in postterm pregnancy.

a. True
b. False

38. OTHER DISEASES OF THE FETUS AND NEWBORN INFANT

38–1. What is the function of the surfactant synthesized by the type II pneumocytes of the fetal lung?

38–2. What are the characteristics of respiratory distress that develops in the neonate?

a. Formation of hyaline membrane in the distal bronchioles and alveoli
b. Cardiopulmonary shunting of blood
c. Hypoxia
d. Metabolic and respiratory alkalosis

38–3. Which of the following statements about hyaline membrane disease is correct?

a. It is more common in female than in male newborns.
b. It is more common in black than in white newborns.
c. It accounts for about one-third of all neonatal deaths in the United States.

38–4. Hyaline membrane disease

a. Requires that the newborn exert more effort to overcome the low compliance of its atelectatic lungs
b. Is characterized by an increased respiratory rate
c. Is associated with a grunting tachypnea
d. Is often associated with poor peripheral circulation and systemic hypotension
e. Is identified by an x-ray pattern of diffuse reticulogranular infiltrates throughout the lung fields and an air-filled tracheobronchial tree

38–5. Which of the following causes of respiratory insufficiency may be confused with idiopathic respiratory distress (hyaline membrane disease)?

a. Pneumonia
b. Sepsis
c. Aspiration
d. Pneumothorax
e. Diaphragmatic hernia
f. Heart failure
g. Patent ductus arteriosus
h. Primary myocardial disease

38–6. Which of the following statements about the treatment of hyaline membrane disease is correct?

a. An arterial Po_2 of less than 40 mm Hg indicates the need for oxygen therapy.
b. Humidified oxygen should be administered to maintain an arterial Po_2 tension of 50 to 70 mm Hg.
c. It is important to keep the neonate warm to reduce oxygen consumption.
d. The administration of oxygen-rich air under pressure prevents the collapse of unstable alveoli.

38–7. The establishment of appropriately staffed and equipped neonatal intensive care units has served to dramatically reduce the number of deaths from idiopathic respiratory distress, even in very small infants.

a. True
b. False

Instructions for Items 38–8 to 38–11: Match the complication associated with the treatment of hyaline membrane disease with the appropriate cause.

a. Persistent hyperoxia
b. Prolonged endotracheal intubation
c. Prolonged high oxygen tension therapy

38–8. Neonatal pulmonary hypertension
38–9. Retrolental fibroplasia
38–10. Tracheal abrasion
38–11. Bronchopulmonary dysplasia

38–12. Bronchopulmonary dysplasia is characterized by

a. Hypoxia
b. Hypercarbia
c. Bronchiolar epithelial damage
d. Peribronchial and interstitial fibrosis

38–13. Which of the following statements about meconium aspiration is correct?

a. Aspiration of small amounts of meconium is a normal event that occurs in most pregnancies.
b. Aspiration causes both mechanical obstruction of the airways and chemical pneumonitis.
c. Aspiration may be associated with atelectasis, consolidation, pneumothroax, and pneumomediastinum.
d. It often occurs as a consequence of fetal distress.

38–14. In the newborn who has suffered meconium aspiration, the initial chest x-ray is useful for predicting outcome.

a. True
b. False

38–15. List the steps that should be taken at the time of delivery when meconium is identified in the amnionic fluid.

38–16. At present, the largest single cause of blindness in the United States is retrolental fibroplasia.

a. True
b. False

38–17. Retrolental fibroplasia

a. Occurs when air enriched with more than 30 percent oxygen is administered to a newborn
b. Results from vascular damage to the developing eye with subsequent adhesion, scar formation, and retinal detachment
c. May be prevented by the administration of vitamin E

38–18. In the hours after delivery, neonatal hematocrit values may

a. Rise
b. Fall

38–19. Which of the following statements about fetal to maternal bleeding is correct?

a. The severely anemic fetus may demonstrate an ominous heart rate pattern.
b. A large fetal to maternal hemorrhage is usually due to a placental lesion.
c. Placental abruption commonly leads to severe fetal to maternal hemorrhage.
d. A large fetal to maternal hemorrhage may cause a transfusion reaction in the mother.
e. The majority of stillbirths are caused by a massive in utero fetal to maternal hemorrhage.

38–20. Why does severe hemolytic disease occur in only a few pregnancies when the potential exists in a great many more?

38–21. Which of the following statements about Rh antigens is correct?

a. They are usually inherited independently from other blood group antigens.
b. The distribution of Rh antigens varies with regard to sex.
c. American Indians and Asiatics are almost all Rho(D) positive.
d. Black and white Americans both average about 25 percent Rho(D) negative
e. Most Rh antigens are moderately to strongly immunogenic.

38–22. All pregnant women should be routinely tested for the presence or absence of Rho(D) antigens.

a. True
b. False

38–23. Which of the following statements about the factors influencing the perinatal mortality rate in cases of Rho(D) hemolytic disease is correct?

a. The number of perinatal deaths from Rho(D) hemolytic disease has dropped dramatically in recent times.
b. Pregnant women who are Rho(D) negative and possess antibody to Rho(D) antigen can be readily identified.
c. It is difficult to accurately determine hemolysis in the fetus of a Rho(D)-negative woman.
d. Administration of Rho(D) immune globulin to the Rho(D)-negative woman during or immediately after pregnancy has eliminated most, but not all, cases of isoimmunization.

38–24. Rho(D) immune globulin should be administered to previously unsensitized Rho(D)-negative women in which of the following situations?

a. Abortion
b. Ectopic pregnancy
c. Hydatidiform mole
d. Amniocentesis
e. Vaginal bleeding during pregnancy

38–25. Rho(D)-negative women who receive transfusions of blood or blood products should be given Rho(D) immune globulin only if there is evidence of maternal hemolysis.

a. True
b. False

38–26. As a general rule, when in doubt about whether or not to administer Rho(D) immune globulin, the rule of thumb should be to give it.

a. True
b. False

38–27. Describe the recommended procedure for treating the Rho(D)-negative nonsensitized pregnant woman with immune globulin.

38–28. The administration of prophylactic Rho(D) immune globulin to an Rho(D)-negative woman will, in about 90 percent of cases, result in a weakly positive direct Coombs test on cord and infant blood.

a. True
b. False

38–29. Which of the following statements about maternal-fetal bleeds is correct?

a. A maternal-fetal bleed must have occurred sometime before the clamping of the umbilical cord for an Rho(D)-negative woman to have become sensitized in utero to Rho(D) antigen.
b. A major blood group incompatibility does not offer appreciable protection against Rho sensitization.
c. Studies suggest that about 2 percent of Rho(D)-negative women with Rho(D)-positive mothers will have been sensitized in utero.
d. Rho(D) immune globulin prophylaxis should be instituted for all Rho(D)-negative female neonates born to Rho(D)-positive mothers.

38–30. When an acid elution test is performed, fetal red cells are ________ (1) stained and maternal red cells are ________ (2) stained.

a. Darkly
b. Lightly

38–31. In cases of fetal to maternal hemorrhage, sensitization of the mother can be prevented by injecting sufficient Rho(D) immune globulin intramuscularly to provide demonstrable free antibody in the maternal serum.

a. True
b. False

38–32. In the absence of intervention, the perinatal mortality in the case of a Rho(D)-negative sensitized woman with an Rho(D)-positive fetus will be about ________ percent.

a. 10
b. 30
c. 50
d. 70
e. 90

38–33. Optimal outcome of cases involving Rho(D) isoimmunization requires the individualization of management based on information about what factors?

38–34. Which of the following statements about the use of antibody measurement in the management of the Rho(D)-negative sensitized mother is correct?

a. An indirect Coombs test is utilized to assess antibody titer.
b. A titer no higher than 1:64 almost always assures that the fetus will not die in utero from hemolytic disease.
c. A titer higher than 1:64 assures that severe, often fatal, hemolytic disease will occur in utero.
d. If the fetus is Rho(D) negative, the titer will never be above 1:16.

38–35. Appropriately timed amniocentesis is indicated when an antibody titer of ________ is found in suspected cases of Rho(D) isoimmunization.

a. 1:8
b. 1:16
c. 1:32
d. 1:64

38–36. For any gestational age, the intensity of hemolytic disease correlates well with the absorbance of amnionic fluid supernatant at a wavelength of 450 nm.

a. True
b. False

Instructions for Items 38–37 to 38–39: Match the severity of the hemolytic disease as determined by absorbance of amnionic fluid at 450 nm (Liley zones) with the appropriate prognosis.

a. Zone 1
b. Zone 2
c. Zone 3

38–37. Fetus will be unaffected or will have mild hemolytic disease
38–38. Fetal death will most likely occur within 10 days
38–39. Prognosis inaccurate; requires further measurements to determine trends

38–40. Which of the following statements about hemolytic disease of the newborn associated with Rho(D) isoimmunization is correct?

a. Antibodies to fetal Rho(D)-positive erythrocytes produced by the Rho(D)-negative mother are both adsorbed onto fetal red cells and exist free in the infant's serum.
b. The adsorbed antibodies act as hemolysins, accelerating the rate of red cell destruction.
c. Maternal antibodies in the infant circulation disappear by 3 weeks after birth.
d. An indirect Coombs test will definitively determine whether antibodies are adsorbed on infant red cells.
e. The severity of Rho(D) isoimmune hemolytic disease depends on the duration of exposure to antibodies and the intensity of the immunologic reaction.

38–41. Which of the following statements about immune hydrops is correct?

a. Hydrops fetalis is characterized by the accumulation of ascites, both subcutaneous and effusive, in the serous cavities.
b. The diagnosis of hydrops fetalis can only be made by examining the infant after delivery.
c. Immune hydrops is associated with a small, atrophic placenta and chronic uteroplacental insufficiency.
d. Extramedullary hematopoiesis is a common finding.
e. Heart failure associated with severe fetal anemia is the main cause of the ascites seen in immune hydrops.
f. Ascites and hepatosplenomegaly may be severe enough to cause dystocia.
g. Hydropic infants usually survive until after birth.

38–42. What are the clinical signs of kernicterus?

38–43. The anemia associated with neonatal hemolytic disease is due to low production of erythropoietin.

a. True
b. False

38–44. The preterm infant with hemolytic disease from maternal Rh isoimmunization is at ________ risk of developing hyaline membrane disease.

a. Increased
b. Decreased

38–45. Intrauterine transfusion of blood into the fetal peritoneal cavity for the management of Rho(D) isoimmunization

a. Should be limited to cases between 23 and 32 weeks of gestation, where the likelihood of in utero death is high
b. Is associated with a 20 percent overall survival rate
c. Is more likely to be successful if the fetus is not hydropic
d. Is associated with an approximately 75 percent incidence of mild to moderate neurologic disease

38–46. Which of the following modalities has proved to be an acceptable method to minimize fetal hemolysis?

a. Plasmapheresis
b. Promethazine (Phenergan) in large doses
c. Rho(D)-positive erythrocyte membrane in enteric capsules
d. Corticosteroids

38–47. A sinusoidal fetal heart rate and repetitious decelerations in the presence of Rh isoimmunization is often indicative of severe fetal anemia.

a. True
b. False

38–48. Cesarean delivery should be employed in all cases of hemolytic disease caused by Rh isoimmunization.

a. True
b. False

38–49. Which of the following statements about exchange transfusion for hemolytic disease of the newborn is correct?

a. If the infant is overtly anemic, the initial exchange should be carried out promptly.
b. If the infant is not overtly anemic, the rate of bilirubin increase, the maturity of the infant, and the presence of other complications determine whether an exchange transfusion should be performed.
c. Excluding moribund, hydropic, and kernicteric infants, the mortality rate for exchange transfusions is about 15 percent.

38–50. Which of the following statements about ABO incompatibility is correct?

a. The major blood group factors A and B are the most common, although not the most serious, cause of hemolytic disease.
b. About 20 percent of infants have an ABO incompatibility that results in some degree of hemolytic disease.
c. There are no racial differences in the incidence or severity of hemolytic disease associated with ABO incompatibility.
d. Like Rho(D) disease, the stillbirth rate is increased in the presence of ABO isoimmune disease.
e. ABO-associated isoimmune disease is very rarely seen in primigravidas.
f. ABO disease is likely, but not certain, to recur.

38–51. List the usual criteria utilized for the diagnosis of hemolysis associated with ABO incompatibility.

38–52. Which of the following statements about the evaluation and treatment of ABO incompatibility is correct?

a. There are no adequate antenatal diagnostic methods.
b. Like Rho(D) disease, the Coombs antiglobulin test is always positive in ABO isoimmune disease.
c. Infants affected by ABO isoimmune disease deal with their residual bilirubin more efficiently than do infants with Rho(D) isoimmune disease.
d. Simple or exchange transfusion with group O blood is the basic treatment of choice.

38–53. Rho(D) incompatibility and ABO heterospecificity are the causes of about 98 percent of all neonatal hemolytic disease.

a. True
b. False

38–54. Nonimmune hydrops fetalis occurs ________ ________ frequently than hydrops fetalis associated with isoimmune fetal red cell destruction.

a. More
b. Less

38–55. Unconjugated or free bilirubin is readily transferred across the placenta from the fetus to the mother, but not from the mother to the fetus.

a. True
b. False

38–56. Which of the following factors may contribute to the development of kernicterus?

a. A level of unconjugated bilirubin above 18 to 20 mg/dl
b. Hypoxia and acidosis
c. Hyperthermia
d. Hyperglycemia
e. Sepsis

38–57. Administration of which of the following drugs may contribute to or cause hyperbilirubinemia/kernicterus?

a. Sulfonamides
b. Salicylates
c. Sodium benzoate in injectable diazepam
d. Furosemide
e. Gentamicin
f. Vitamin K analogs

38–58. Breast milk jaundice

a. May be caused by the presence in breast milk of the steroid pregnane-3 (alpha), 20 (beta)-diol, which blocks bilirubin conjugation
b. May be caused by the inability of milk from certain mothers to block bilirubin reabsorption
c. Is associated with bilirubin levels that rise from the 4th day to the 15th day, and then slowly decline over the next few weeks
d. Will persist in all cases if breast feeding is continued
e. Results in kernicterus and encephalopathy in about 5 percent of cases

38–59. Which of the following statements about neonatal physiologic jaundice is correct?

a. It is the most common form of unconjugated nonhemolytic jaundice.
b. In mature infants, bilirubin increases to levels of about 10 mg/dl and then falls rapidly.
c. Jaundice is often more prolonged and severe in premature infants.
d. It almost never requires therapy, since the resolution is usually rapid.

38–60. The mechanisms involved in physiologic jaundice of the newborn include a

a. Normally increased rate of erythrocyte destruction and bilirubin production
b. Decreased rate of uptake of free bilirubin by hepatic cells
c. Decreased rate of bilirubin conjugation in the liver
d. Reduced conversion of bilirubin to urobilinogen by intestinal bacteria

38–61. Which of the following statements about the treatment of hyperbilirubinemia in the neonate is correct?

a. Exchange transfusion is indicated in severe cases.
b. The sole mechanism by which phototherapy decreases hyperbilirubinemia is through the photooxidation of unconjugated bilirubin.
c. Serum bilirubin levels should continue to be monitored for at least 24 hours after phototherapy is discontinued.
d. Phenobarbital may increase the conjugation and excretion of bilirubin through an increase in liver microenzymes.

38–62. Which of the following is characteristic of hemorrhagic disease of the newborn?

a. Spontaneous internal or external bleeding
b. Hypoprothrombinemia
c. Low levels of vitamin K-dependent coagulation factors
d. Bleeding usually beginning 2 to 6 hours after birth
e. Prolonged prothrombin and partial thromboplastin times

38–63. Which diseases are included in the differential diagnosis of hemorrhagic disease of the newborn?

38–64. The physiologic hypoprothrombinemia in the neonate is a consequence of poor placental transport of vitamin K_1 to the fetus.

a. True
b. False

38–65. Hemorrhagic disease of the newborn may be treated

a. Prophylactically by the intramuscular injection of 1 mg of vitamin K_1 just after birth
b. By intravenous administration of vitamin K_1
c. With intravenous heparin
d. By breast feeding the affected infant

Instructions for Items 38–66 to 38–71: Match the type of immune thrombocytopenia with the appropriate statement.

a. Autoimmune (idiopathic) thrombocytopenia purpura
b. Isoimmune thrombocytopenia

38–66. Antiplatelet IgG transferred from mother to fetus
38–67. Maternal isoimmunization exists against fetal platelet antigens
38–68. Infant but not maternal thrombocytopenia is present
38–69. Treatment includes corticosteroid therapy for the infant

38–70. Treatment includes transfusion of maternal platelets to the infant

38–71. Cesarean delivery is of benefit to the fetus and of little added risk to the mother

38–72. Which of the following statements about polycythemia and hyperviscosity syndrome is correct?

a. The viscosity of neonatal blood rises remarkably as the hematocrit reaches 50.
b. Polycythemia and hyperviscosity are associated with the various transfusion syndromes and with chronic hypoxia.
c. Signs and symptoms include plethora, cyanosis, and neurologic aberrations.
d. Laboratory findings include hyperbilirubinemia, thrombocytosis, erythrocyte fragmentation, and hypoglycemia.
e. Partial exchange transfusion with plasma is the immediate treatment.

38–73. Which of the following statements about infections in the newborn is correct?

a. Active immunologic capacity is impaired in the neonate as compared with an older child.
b. Passive immunity is temporarily provided by maternal IgM transferred across the placenta.
c. Early infection in the neonate may be difficult to recognize because the signs are often vague and nonspecific.
d. In general, infection occurring within 72 hours of birth was acquired in utero.
e. Infection manifesting after 72 hours was most likely acquired after birth.

Instructions for Items 38–74 to 38–76: Match the organism to the time period when it was the major cause of neonatal infection in the United States.

a. Group A β-hemolytic streptococci
b. Group B β-hemolytic streptococci
c. Staphylococci

38–74. 1930s to 1940s

38–75. 1950s

38–76. 1970s

38–77. Which of the following statements about neonatal staphylococcal infection is correct?

a. Penicillin-sensitive staphylococcal disease, while uncommon, represents a significant but usually preventable neonatal infection.
b. Infection may become epidemic when contamination from infected or carrier staff or from infant to infant occurs.
c. The risk of infection may be eliminated by careful handwashing and child handling by nursery staff.
d. Continuous epidemiologic surveillance in the nursery is only necessary when there has been an outbreak of infection within the past 6 months.
e. Routine care of the umbilical cord with the use of triple dye is important to prevent infection.

38–78. Currently, gram-negative organisms are the most common neonatal pathogens.

a. True
b. False

38–79. Which of the following statements about group B β-hemolytic streptococcal infection in the newborn is correct?

a. About 10 percent of women harbor group B β-hemolytic streptococci in their genital tracts during pregnancy.
b. About 5 percent of newborns are colonized with the bacteria.
c. About 1 percent of newborns develop serious clinical infections.
d. In utero infection is possible but very rare.

Instructions for Items 38–80 to 38–85: Match the type of group B β-hemolytic infection with the appropriate statement.

a. Early onset disease
b. Late onset disease

38–80. Disease usually develops within 48 hours of birth

38–81. There is usually prolonged rupture of the membranes before delivery

38–82. Serotype III is most common

38–83. Signs include respiratory distress, apnea, and shock

38–84. Disease becomes evident as meningitis

38–85. The mortality rate is between 30 and 90 percent

38–86. Administering penicillin to the mother (in the late third trimester) but not to the newborn has proved effective in preventing infection with group B β-hemolytic streptococci.

a. True
b. False

38–87. Diarrhea of the newborn

a. Is often associated with pathogenic strains of *Escherichia coli*
b. Is usually caused by contact with an infected infant or by transmission from infected nursery staff
c. Is characterized by loose, watery, greenish stools; lethargy; dehydration; unstable temperature; and anorexia
d. Is rarely associated with a mortality rate greater than 0.5 percent
e. Should be controlled by closure of the nursery until all exposed infants have been treated or released

38–88. Which of the following statements about necrotizing enterocolitis is correct?

a. Necrotizing enterocolitis is characterized clinically by abdominal distention, ileus, and bloody stools.
b. It is characterized radiologically by pneumotosis intestinalis and bowel perforation.
c. Premature and mature infants are equally likely to contract necrotizing enterocolitis.
d. It has a virtually 100 percent mortality rate.
e. Treatment consists of resection of the affected bowel segments before perforation occurs.

38–89. Susceptible women should be vaccinated against rubella as part of their routine medical and gynecologic care.

a. True
b. False

38–90. Which of the following statements about the diagnosis of rubella is correct?

a. Absence of maternal rubella antibodies indicates the absence of immunity.
b. The presence of maternal rubella antibody in a nonvaccinated woman indicates that rubella infection has occurred within the last 6 to 8 months.
c. A woman with rubella antibodies has little chance of infection if exposed to rubella while pregnant.
d. Peak antibody levels are seen 1 to 2 weeks after the onset of rash, and 2 to 3 weeks after the onset of viremia.
e. An antibody titer done 10 days after the onset of a rash can differentiate between the presence of the disease and a previously acquired immunity.
f. The presence of specific IgM indicates a primary infection has occurred within the previous month.

38–91. Rubella occurring in the 1st month of pregnancy probably causes serious defects in about ________ (1) percent of infants who survive; in the 2nd month the incidence of defects is ________ (2) percent, and in the 3rd month the incidence is ________ (3) percent.

38–92. List the abnormalities that may form part of the congenital rubella syndrome.

38–93. There may be a relationship between congenital rubella and juvenile diabetes.

a. True
b. False

38–94. Rubella vaccine is an attenuated live virus, which can cross the placenta and cause fetal infection and defects.

a. True
b. False

38–95. List ways that humans may be infected by *Toxoplasma gonadii.*

38–96. Which of the following statements about toxoplasmosis is correct?

a. For congenital toxoplasmosis to occur, the mother must have acquired the infection during pregnancy.
b. Maternal toxoplasmosis is always characterized by fatigue, muscle pain, and lymphadenopathy.
c. Virulence of the fetal infection is increased if it occurs late in pregnancy.
d. Chorioretinitis occurs in those infants who develop symptoms in the neonatal period but not in those who develop neurologic disease later in life.
e. The Sabin-Feldman dye test, IgM fluorescent antibody test, and the indirect fluorescent antibody test are screening blood tests for toxoplasmosis.

38–97. Which of the following statements about cytomegalovirus infection is correct?

a. It is the most common type of congenital infection, occurring in about 0.5 to 2.0 percent of births.
b. Fifty percent of infected infants will be permanently affected.
c. Infection may lead to abortion or to a wide variety of abnormalities, some of which are fatal.
d. Specific IgM antibody is present in all affected infants.
e. There is no effective treatment.

38–98. Which of the following neonatal abnormalities can be associated with cytomegalovirus infection?

a. Microcephaly
b. Hydrocephaly
c. Mental retardation
d. Cerebral palsy
e. Epilepsy
f. Deafness
g. Chorioretinitis
h. Blindness
i. Hemolytic anemia
j. Thrombocytopenia
k. Hepatosplenomegaly

38–99. The use of the TORCH screening test series has proven to be of significant value in reducing neonatal morbidity and mortality.

a. True
b. False

38–100. Which of the following statements about *Chlamydia trachomatis* infection is correct?

a. *Chlamydia trachomatis* has been cultured from the cervices of up to 13 percent of pregnant women.
b. Neonates can acquire infection, including conjunctivitis and pneumonia, from transvaginal delivery.
c. Erythromycin is effective for treatment of maternal but not neonatal infections.
d. Chlamydial infection is a major cause of spontaneous abortion and premature labor.

38–101. Which of the following statements about syphilis is correct?

a. Even in recent years, syphilis remains a major cause of fetal and neonatal death.
b. Common neonatal syphilitic lesions include interstitial changes in the lungs, liver, spleen, and pancreas.
c. Osteochondritis is especially noticeable in the lower ends of the femur, tibia, and radius.
d. Intrauterine syphilis is characterized by uteroplacental insufficiency associated with a small, infarcted placenta.

38–102. Which of the following is characteristic of the pregnancies of drug-addicted women?

a. Low birth weight infants
b. Fetal growth retardation
c. Pregnancy-induced hypertension
d. Respiratory distress syndrome
e. Neonatal withdrawal symptoms

38–103. The infants born of mothers under methadone treatment rarely demonstrate withdrawal symptoms.

a. True
b. False

39. INJURIES AND MALFORMATIONS OF THE FETUS AND NEWBORN INFANT

39–1. The reduction of birth injuries in recent years is in large part the result of what changes in obstetric practice?

39–2. Which of the following statements about intracranial hemorrhage is correct?

a. Most cases of intracranial hemorrhage are the result of inappropriate obstetric management.
b. Severe molding is sometimes associated with rents in the veins entering the sagittal sinus from the cortex.
c. Essentially all intracranial hemorrhages occur in the subarachnoid area.
d. Compression of the fetal skull may be associated with tears in the vein of Galen and/or tentorial stretching.

39–3. In most cases, intracranial hemorrhage secondary to birth trauma results in a rapidly deteriorating clinical status that begins just after birth.

a. True
b. False

39–4. Which of the following signs and symptoms may be associated with neonatal intracranial hemorrhage?

a. Drowsiness
b. Apathy
c. Feeble cry
d. Pallor
e. Dyspnea
f. Cyanosis
g. Vomiting
h. Convulsions

39–5. List the conditions that are included in the differential diagnosis of intracranial hemorrhage in the newborn.

39–6. What sites of intracranial hemorrhage are more common in premature infants?

39–7. Which of the following statements about the management of intracranial hemorrhage in the newborn is correct?

a. Oxygen should be administered to correct associated dyspnea and cyanosis.
b. Sedation is administered to control associated convulsions.
c. Needle aspiration of the accumulated blood to relieve intracranial pressure should be performed in all types of intracranial hemorrhage.
d. Plasma-clotting factors should be infused to decrease bleeding.
e. Intramuscular injection of vitamin K is indicated for all newborn infants.

39–8. Cerebral palsy is a specific clinical syndrome arising solely from birth injury/asphyxia.

a. True
b. False

Instructions for Items 39–9 to 39–13: Match the clinical condition with the appropriate description.

a. Caput succedaneum
b. Cephalohematoma

39–9. The effusion consists of blood
39–10. Fluid accumulation overlies the periosteum
39–11. Fluid accumulation lies under the periosteum
39–12. Is at maximum size at birth, and subsequently grows smaller
39–13. Appears after birth and grows larger

39–14. Extensive cephalohematoma warrants evaluation of the newborn for coagulation defects and the possibility of extensive intracranial injury.

a. True
b. False

Instructions for Items 39–15 to 39–19: Match the type of brachial plexus injury with the appropriate statement.

a. Duchenne's or Erb's paralysis
b. Klumpke's paralysis

39–15. Arises from injury to the upper roots of the brachial plexus
39–16. Arises from injury to the lower roots of the brachial plexus
39–17. Paralysis of the arm excluding the fingers
39–18. Paralysis of the hand
39–19. Results from pulling on the head, sharply flexing it toward a shoulder

39–20. Which of the following statements about brachial plexus injuries at birth is correct?

a. Brachial plexus injury is always associated with difficult deliveries.
b. Brachial plexus injury in a cephalic presentation is usually associated with an unusually large fetus.
c. To prevent brachial plexus injury in breech presentations, the extension of the arms over the head should be prevented.
d. With appropriate physiotherapy, the prognosis for most brachial plexus injuries is good.

39–21. Facial paralysis is almost always associated with forceps deliveries.

a. True
b. False

39–22. Which of the following statements about neonatal fractures at the time of birth is correct?

a. Fractures of the clavicle are usually associated with shoulder dystocia.
b. Fractures of the humerus are much less common than fractures of the clavicle.
c. Fractures of the femur are uncommon and usually associated with vaginal breech delivery.
d. Crepitation or unusual irregularity on palpation of the bony skeleton is an indication for further evaluation by x-ray.
e. Fracture of the skull is usually associated with forcible attempts at delivery.

39–23. As a child grows, progressive turning of the head toward the side of the sternocleidomastoid muscle that was injured at birth is called ______________.

39–24. Which of the following statements about constricting bands and congenital amputations is correct?

a. Focal constrictions of the extremities are relatively common.
b. Premature rupture of the amnion with subsequent formation of tough, adherent bands may cause constriction of an extremity.
c. Actual amputation of an extremity by an amnionic band is quite rare.
d. Lesser degrees of constriction may result in edema.

39–25. Which of the following deformities may result from oligohydramnios and the presence of a small, inappropriately shaped uterine cavity?

a. Talipes
b. Scoliosis
c. Hip dislocation
d. Limb reduction
e. Polydactyly
f. Body wall deficiency

39–26. Maternal trauma is relatively unlikely to result in trauma to the fetus because of ________.

39–27. In cases of severe maternal trauma, the major risks to the fetus are indirect, through the effect of the maternal injuries on maternal cardiac output, maternal blood oxygenation, and uteroplacental perfusion.

a. True
b. False

39–28. Congenital malformations are the leading cause of death in infants under 1 year of age.

a. True
b. False

39–29. What percent of deaths in infants less than 1 year of age are due to congenital malformations?

a. 9
b. 18
c. 28
d. 47
e. 69

39–30. The incidence of severe developmental defects among aborted fetuses and stillbirths is ________ than the incidence in liveborn infants.

a. Higher
b. Lower

39–31. A minority of congenital malformations are directly caused by environmental influences and the majority are due to genetic causes.

a. True
b. False

39–32. Susceptibility to teratogenic agents ________ after organs and organ systems become fully developed.

a. Increases
b. Decreases

39–33. Which of the following statements about the etiology of congenital malformations is correct?

a. A given teratogenic agent acts on a specific aspect of cell metabolism, producing the same effect regardless of the stage of embryonic development.
b. In many malformations, both a genetic predisposition and a teratogenic agent are required to produce the anomaly.
c. Most teratogenic agents are also seriously deleterious to the mother.
d. Agents tend to be teratogenic across species, causing the same malformations in animal models and in man.
e. Many substances that cause congenital malformations also cause an increase in embryonic/fetal mortality rates.

39–34. The fact that supernumerary digits are more common in black than in white infants demonstrates the genetic basis of some congenital malformations.

a. True
b. False

Instructions for Items 39–35 to 39–38: Match the syndrome with the signs that are recognizable at birth.

a. Turner's
b. Klinefelter's
c. Triple X
d. Down's trisomy 21
e. Trisomy 13–15
f. Trisomy 16–18

39–35. Cleft palate, harelip, eye defects, polydactyly
39–36. Lymphangiectatic edema of hands and feet
39–37. Mongoloid facies, simian line
39–38. No signs recognizable at birth

39–39. The estimated incidence of chromosomal abnormalities in liveborn infants is ________ (1) percent, in stillborn infants it is ________ (2) percent, and in spontaneous early abortions it is ________ (3) percent.

39–40. If nondisjunction occurs during gamete formation, the resulting embryo may be ________ (1), while if nondisjunction occurs during the mitoses after fertilization the embryo is ________ (2).

a. Mosaic
b. Trisomic

39–41. In mosaicism, the major phenotypic defects are usually obvious.

a. True
b. False

39–42. Which of the following statements about the chromosomal defects that give rise to Down's syndrome is correct?

a. It is the most common defect detectable by early second trimester amniocentesis.
b. It is most commonly caused by the presence of an extra chromosome.
c. It may result from the translocation of part of a chromosome.
d. A female carrier with a 13 to 15/21 translocation has a 50 percent chance of having a Down's syndrome child.
e. A 21/21 translocation in either parent will always result in a Down's syndrome infant.
f. The presence of a 21/22 translocation can only be distinguished from a 21/21 translocation by the birth of a normal child.

39–43. Which of the following statements about Down's syndrome is correct?

a. Down's syndrome is an infrequent cause of spontaneous abortion.
b. Karyotype evaluation of a bone marrow aspirate may be used postpartum to confirm the diagnosis of Down's syndrome.
c. There is a 50 percent reduction in fertility of both males and females affected with Down's syndrome.
d. Paternal age is not a risk factor.

39–44. What is the frequency of Down's syndrome in infants born to mothers of the following ages?

30 ______ (1)
35 ______ (2)
40 ______ (3)
45 ______ (4)

39–45. Which of the following statements about phenylketonuria is correct?

a. Individuals with phenylketonuria cannot metabolize phenylalanine to tyrosine.
b. The specific defect is abnormal phenylalanine hydroxylase activity.
c. The disease is inherited as an autosomal recessive.
d. It is more common in black infants than in white ones.
e. The condition results in mental retardation if untreated.
f. The disease manifestations can be controlled by a diet low in phenylalanine.
g. Affected women may have poor pregnancy outcomes.

39–46. Phocomelia is

a. Characterized by defects in or absence of the radius, ulna, and/or humerus
b. Associated with mental retardation in about 50 percent of cases
c. Associated with perinatal death in about one-third of cases
d. Associated with the prenatal ingestion of the tranquilizer thalidomide

39–47. Which of the following statements about anencephaly is correct?

a. Anencephaly is characterized by rudimentary or absent cerebral hemispheres and the absence of overlying skull.
b. The pituitary gland is either absent or hypoplastic.
c. The facies are characteristic, with prominent bulging eyes and protruding tongue.
d. The adrenal glands are usually diminished in size.
e. Male and female fetuses are equally likely to be anencephalic.

39–48. Which of the following statements about the diagnosis of anencephaly is correct?

a. Anencephaly is probably caused by a combination of genetic and environmental factors.
b. Failure to palpate a fetal head is suggestive of anencephaly, but the diagnosis must be confirmed by x-ray or ultrasonography.
c. Gross hydramnios is very commonly associated with anencephaly.
d. Breech and face presentations are most common with anencephalic fetuses.
e. The levels of α-fetoprotein are usually below normal in amnionic fluid.

39–49. Preterm labor is very common in pregnancies with an anencephalic fetus.

a. True
b. False

39–50. Which of the following statements about the management of pregnancies with an anencephalic fetus is correct?

a. The uterus containing an anencephalic fetus may be somewhat refractory to oxytocin.
b. Amniocentesis to relieve excessive hydramnios may help to avoid placental abruption after rupture of the membranes and rapid decompression of the uterus.
c. Delivery may often be accomplished by cervical dilation with laminaria followed by the administration of prostaglandins.

39–51. Which of the following statements about spina bifida is correct?

a. Spina bifida is a hiatus, usually lumbosacral, in the vertebral column through which a meningeal sac protrudes.
b. If the meningeal sac contains spinal cord, the defect is termed a meningomyelocele.
c. The defect is slight in cases of spina bifida occulta.
d. If the meningeal sac includes brain tissue, the defect is termed meningoencephalocele.
e. Commonly associated malformations include hydrocephaly, anencephaly, and talipes.

39–52. Hydrocephalus is

a. Associated with dystocia
b. Associated with uterine rupture
c. Associated with spina bifida
d. Identified by ultrasonographic recognition of dilation of the lateral ventricles

Instructions for Items 39-53 to 39-56: Match the developmental abnormality of the urinary tract with the appropriate statement.

a. Renal agenesis
b. Persistent urinary tract obstruction

39-53. Accompanied by oligohydramnios
39-54. The infant characteristically has prominent epicanthal folds, a flattened nose, and large, lowset ears
39-55. Associated with pulmonary hypoplasia
39-56. Occurs more frequently in male infants

39-57. What problem should be suspected in the mature infant who appears normal at birth and then develops tachypnea, cyanosis, marked tachycardia, and hepatomegaly in the next few hours or days?

39-58. Clubfoot (talipes equinovaris) occurs with what frequency?

39-59. Which of the following statements about congenital dislocation of the hip is correct?

a. The malformation is more frequent in males than in females.
b. The frequency of the defect varies geographically.
c. The defect is more common in breech than in vertex deliveries.
d. The cause of the problem is defective formation of the acetabulum.
e. The displacement does not usually begin until after birth.

39-60. What is the appropriate treatment for polydactyly?

39-61. Which of the following statements about cleft lip and palate is correct?

a. It is one of the most frequent congenital anomalies.
b. Cleft lip and palate are always associated.
c. It is advisable to repair a cleft lip as soon as possible.
d. If a first child has a cleft lip, the risk of the next child in the family having the problem is the same as for the general population.
e. If two children in a family are affected, a third child has an increased probability of having cleft lip.
f. If a parent has a cleft lip, the incidence of the first child being affected is increased.

39-62. What is an omphalocele?

39-63. Which of the following statements about omphalocele is correct?

a. The defect occurs when the rectus muscles and their fascial sheaths do not cover the entire abdomen.
b. Rupture with evisceration and peritonitis are grave complications.
c. The defect is associated with elevated levels of α-fetoprotein in maternal serum and amnionic fliud.
d. The defect is associated with increased levels of bilirubin in amnionic fluid.
e. The appropriate management is surgical correction.

Instructions for Items 39-64 to 39-66: Match the type of hernia in the neonate with the appropriate statement.

a. Umbilical hernia
b. Inguinal hernia

39-64. May undergo incarceration, especially in premature infants
39-65. Strangulation of the bowel is extremely rare
39-66. May correct spontaneously in some cases

39-67. Atresia of the anus, where the rectum ends in a blind pouch, gives rise to the condition known as ______________.

39-68. Sacrococcygeal teratomas are never malignant.

a. True
b. False

39-69. Genetic counseling is the appropriate function of any licensed obstetrician-gynecologist.

a. True
b. False

39-70. List the elements that should be included in the complete evaluation of a malformed infant who dies in the perinatal period.

39-71. A mutant gene that can produce its effects when present on one chromosome of a given pair is

a. Dominant
b. Recessive

39-72. A dominant trait is always sex-linked.

a. True
b. False

39-73. The degree of penetrance of a given dominant gene is defined as ______________________________.

39-74. When a single gene manifests itself in a variety of ways in different people, the characteristic is called ______________________________.

39–75. Which of the following developmental abnormalities are examples of multifactorial or polygenic inheritance?

a. Cleft lip
b. Pyloric stenosis
c. Spina bifida
d. Anencephaly
e. Down's syndrome
f. Congenital heart defects

39–76. In general, as the number of malformed children in a family rises, the risk of subsequent children being malformed

a. Increases
b. Remains the same
c. Decreases

40. FAMILY PLANNING

40–1. When a fertile couple does not use any contraceptive method, what percent of the women will conceive within 1 year?

a. 20
b. 40
c. 60
d. 80
e. 98

40–2. Sexually active young women do not need to use contraceptives until they begin to menstruate.

a. True
b. False

40–3. Which of the following statements about fertility in older women is correct?

a. Women with regular menstrual cycles almost always ovulate normally.
b. Extremely irregular or absent menstrual cycles usually mean the absence of ovulation.
c. Pregnancy is rare over the age of 50.
d. Documented hypergonadotropic, hypoestrogenic amenorrhea eliminates the possibility of pregnancy.

40–4. Supply the failure rates of the following common methods of contraception during the first year of their use.

Method	Percent
Oral contraceptives	(1)
Intrauterine devices	(2)
Condom	(3)
Spermicides	(4)
Diaphragm	(5)
Rhythm	(6)

40–5. There is a strong negative correlation between the failure rate for a given method and both the age of the woman and the length of time she has been using the method.

a. True
b. False

40–6. Which of the following statements about estrogen-progestin contraceptives is correct?

a. Ethinyl estradiol, or estrogens that metabolize to it, are used in most estrogen-progestin pills in the United States.
b. Virtually all pills use norethindrone as the progestational agent.
c. The main effect of estrogen-progestin pills is the suppression of hypothalamic-releasing factors.
d. Oral estrogen-progestin contraceptives probably alter the receptiveness of the endometrium to implantation and also make cervical mucus less penetrable to sperm.
e. Once a patient begins to correctly use an estrogen-progestin contraceptive, she is immediately protected against conception.

40–7. Which of the following statements about the administration of estrogen-progestin oral contraceptives is correct?

a. It is generally recommended that oral contraceptive use be initiated on the 5th day of the menstrual cycle.
b. An additional method of birth control should be utilized during the first pill cycle by any woman who does not begin oral contraceptive use immediately after a normal menstrual cycle or within 3 weeks of delivery.
c. Women should be encouraged to establish a regular routine for pill ingestion.
d. If a woman misses one pill, she should use an additional method of birth control for the remainder of the cycle.
e. An oral contraceptive should not be restarted immediately after withdrawal bleeding.

40–8. The amount of estrogen in oral contraceptives has been steadily reduced in recent years because of the rising cost of synthetic hormones.

a. True
b. False

40–9. Most estrogen-progestin oral contraceptives used in the United States contain ________________ μg of either mestranol or ethinyl estradiol.

a. 10 to 15
b. 30 to 50
c. 70 to 90
d. 110 to 130

40–10. All estrogen-progestin oral contraceptives are formulated to deliver a constant daily dosage of progestin throughout the cycle.

a. True
b. False

40–11. When used correctly by appropriately selected patients, effects of estrogen-progestin oral contraceptives include a reduced incidence of

a. Functional ovarian cysts
b. Cervical cancer
c. Endometrial cancer
d. Ovarian cancer
e. Rheumatoid arthritis
f. Pelvic inflammatory disease

40–12. The major adverse reaction to the estrogen-progestin oral contraceptive may be the anxiety generated in the public and medical community by any reported side effects.

a. True
b. False

40–13. Which of the following statements about the metabolic effects of estrogen-progestin oral contraceptives is correct?

a. Some of the metabolic changes are qualitatively similar to those seen in pregnancy.
b. Plasma thyroxine, thyroid-binding globulin, and triiodothyronine uptake by resin are all elevated.
c. Plasma cortisol and transcortin levels are lowered.
d. Serum glucose levels are lowered.
e. High density lipoprotein cholesterol levels are lowered.

40–14. Estrogen-progestin oral contraceptives should be withheld from women with a history of viral hepatitis.

a. True
b. False

40–15. Which of the following statements about complications from the use of estrogen-progestin oral contraceptives is correct?

a. Contraceptive steroids may intensify existing diabetes.
b. Cholestasis and cholestatic jaundice are relatively common complications that do not usually clear when oral contraceptive use is discontinued.
c. Hepatic focal nodular hyperplasia and tumor formation have been linked to oral contraceptive use.
d. Oral estrogen-progestin contraceptives are a common cause of vitamin B_6 deficiency.
e. Oral estrogen-progestin contraceptives often result in iron deficiency.

40–16. Use of oral estrogen-progestin contraceptives results in ________________ (1) menstrual blood loss and ____________ (2) dysmenorrhea.

a. Increased
b. Decreased

40–17. Which of the following statements about the cardiovascular effects of oral estrogen-progestin contraceptives is correct?

a. The risk of deep vein thrombosis and pulmonary embolism is increased.
b. The risk of postoperative thromboembolic disease is unchanged.
c. The risk of stroke in all women taking oral contraceptives is increased about fourfold.
d. The risk of developing hypertension is increased, especially in older patients.
e. The frequency and intensity of migraine headache is increased.
f. The risk of myocardial infarction is increased.
g. Even in young, healthy women, the risk of death as a consequence of oral contraceptive use is greater than the risk from pregnancy and delivery.

40–18. List the important contraindications to the use of estrogen-progestin oral contraceptives.

40–19. Most women resume regular ovulation within 3 months after discontinuing the use of oral estrogen-progestin contraceptives.

a. True
b. False

40–20. Estrogen-progestin oral contraceptives

a. Are a common cause of cervical mucorrhea
b. Are associated with Candida vulvovaginitis
c. Can aggravate acne in some cases
d. May result in the increased growth of uterine myomas
e. Are a troublesome cause of weight gain in most women
f. Are a relatively common cause of congenital malformations in the children of women who become pregnant soon after taking them

40–21. Breast feeding should not be combined with the use of estrogen-progestin oral contraceptives because of the large amounts of hormones excreted in the milk.

a. True
b. False

40–22. Why have oral progestin-only contraceptives not achieved widespread popularity in the United States?

40–23. Which of the following statements about injectable hormonal contraceptives is correct?

a. The effectiveness of injected medroxyprogesterone acetate is comparable to that of combined oral contraceptives.
b. Lactation is not likely to be impaired.
c. Prolonged amenorrhea or uterine bleeding may occur during or after their use.
d. There may be prolonged anovulation after their use is discontinued.
e. The risk of venous thrombosis and thromboembolism is increased.

40–24. The "morning after pill" is composed of what compound?

40–25. The "ideal" intrauterine device would have what properties?

40–26. What are the two general types of intrauterine devices?

40–27. Which of the following meets the criteria of the "ideal" intrauterine device?

a. Lippes Loop
b. Copper T
c. Cu7
d. Progestasert

Instructions for Items 40–28 to 40–31: Match the type of intrauterine device with its chemically active substance.

a. Copper
b. Progesterone
c. No active substance

40–28. Lippes Loop
40–29. Cu7
40–30. Progestasert
40–31. Copper T

40–32. Which type of intrauterine device (IUD) may be effective where use of another type of IUD has caused bleeding or cramping?

a. Lippes Loop
b. Copper T
c. Cu7
d. Progestasert

40–33. How does the chemically inert type of intrauterine device prevent pregnancy?

40–34. Copper-containing intrauterine devices work through a long-range, systemic action.

a. True
b. False

40–35. In general, the serious side effects of intrauterine devices have not been common while the common side effects have not been serious.

a. True
b. False

40–36. Which of the following statements about the side effects of intrauterine devices (IUDs) is correct?

a. Most uterine perforations are due to migration of the IUD through the uterine wall over the period of several years.
b. Bleeding and cramping are more likely with a larger device.
c. Blood loss during menstruation may be twice normal when an IUD is in place.
d. An increased incidence of pelvic infections is associated with the use of an IUD.
e. Mortality due to the uses of an IUD is higher than either that due to pregnancy or to the use of oral contraceptives.

40–37. The use of an intrauterine device is usually discouraged in women

a. Of no parity
b. Of high parity
c. At increased risk of developing infections of the pelvic viscera
d. Who smoke

40–38. If actinomyces bodies are identified in Papanicolaou smears from an asymptomatic patient with an intrauterine device, it should be removed immediately and parenteral antibiotics should be administered.

a. True
b. False

40–39. Which of the following statements about locating and managing a lost intrauterine device (IUD) is correct?

a. When an IUD tail is not visible, it is best to insert another device immediately in order to ensure that pregnancy does not occur.
b. Ultrasound and/or hysteroscopy may be helpful in locating the device.
c. Extrauterine location of an IUD may be confirmed radiographically utilizing an opaque probe in the uterine cavity.
d. It is best not to remove any extrauterine IUD, particularly if it is adherent to bowel.

40–40. If pregnancy is recognized and the IUD tail is visible through the cervix, the device should be removed.

a. True
b. False

40–41. What additional risks are present if pregnancy occurs with an IUD still in place?

a. Abortion
b. Low birth weight
c. Prematurity
d. Ectopic pregnancy
e. Septic abortion
f. Congenital malformations
g. Future infertility

40–42. If an intrauterine device is promptly removed when a pregnancy is recognized the abortion rate is ________ (1) percent and if the device is left in place the rate is ________ (2) percent.

a. 12
b. 25
c. 54
d. 76

40–43. A woman at high risk for ectopic pregnancy is a ____________ candidate for an intrauterine contraceptive device.

a. Good
b. Poor

40–44. Which of the following statements about the insertion of an intrauterine device (IUD) is correct?

a. Prior to insertion, patients must be informed about the potential risks and side effects.
b. Insertion should be timed to coincide with ovulation.
c. Insertion at or soon after the time of delivery is associated with a high expulsion rate.
d. Postpartum insertion should be delayed 3 months.
e. In the absence of infection, an IUD may be inserted immediately after abortion.

40–45. Which of the following is a contraindication to the use of an intrauterine device?

a. Recent pelvic infection
b. Untreated gonorrhea
c. Cervical stenosis
d. Anemia
e. Severe dysmenorrhea
f. Abnormalities of blood coagulation
g. Abnormalities of the uterine cavity

40–46. Place the following steps involved in the insertion of an intrauterine device (IUD) in the proper sequence.

a. Grasp cervix with tentaculum
b. Perform a thorough pelvic examination
c. Sound the uterus
d. Apply traction to the uterus
e. Place the IUD inserter into the uterus
f. Cut the IUD marker tail
g. Remove the inserter

40–47. Which of the following statements about expulsion of an intrauterine device (IUD) is correct?

a. Loss of an IUD from the uterus is most common during the first month it is in place.
b. The IUD string is rarely palpable.
c. The woman should be examined 1 month after insertion to check for proper placement.
d. Ideally, barrier contraception should be used with an IUD during the fertile period of each month.

Instructions for Items 40–48 to 40–51: Match the type of intrauterine device with the correct replacement schedule.

a. Annually
b. Every 3 years
c. Every 6 years
d. Indefinite placement

40–48. Lippes Loop
40–49. Cu7
40–50. Copper T
40–51. Progestasert

40–52. Which of the following statements about the use of condoms is correct?

a. It is the only reversible "male method" of contraception.
b. The failure rate for condom use is usually higher during the first year than subsequently.
c. Condoms may provide protection against some sexually transmitted diseases.
d. Condoms have been implicated in the progression of premalignant changes in the cervix.

40–53. Which of the following statements about intravaginal contraceptives is correct?

a. A prescription is needed to purchase intravaginal contraceptives.
b. These contraceptives usually function as a physical barrier as well as a spermicide.
c. To be effective, the agents must be deposited high in the vagina in contact with the cervix.
d. One application is usually effective for 6 hours.
e. High pregnancy rates are due to inconsistency of use.
f. This type of contraception appears to provide protection from some sexually transmitted diseases.

40–54. The use of vaginal spermicides during the year before pregnancy has been associated with a well-defined syndrome of congenital malformations.

a. True
b. False

40–55. To what parts of the vaginal diaphragm is the spermicidal jelly or cream applied?

40–56. Which of the following statements about diaphragm use is correct?

a. The diaphragm should be placed in close relative position to the pubic symphysis.
b. A cystocele or prolapsed uterus may cause instability in diaphragm position.
c. The diaphragm should be inserted 6 hours prior to coitus.
d. The risk of toxic shock syndrome requires that the diaphragm be removed immediately after each coitus.
e. The diaphragm is now generally considered an outdated method of contraception.

40–57. The "Today" contraceptive sponge has proved to be more effective than other vaginal methods.

a. True
b. False

40–58. Which of the following statements about breast feeding and contraception is correct?

a. For nursing mothers, ovulation during the first 10 weeks after delivery is unlikely.
b. Breast feeding provides excellent contraception until the first menstrual period.
c. Oral contraceptives may impair milk production.
d. Intrauterine devices should not be used by a woman who is breast feeding.

40–59. List the rhythm methods of contraception.

40–60. Which of the following statements about tubal sterilization is correct?

a. It is about twice as common as vasectomy.
b. The procedure should only be performed in the puerperium.
c. The likelihood of postpartum hemorrhage in multiparous women decreases during the 10 hours after delivery.
d. There is no correlation between postoperative morbidity and the time between delivery and sterilization.
e. A high failure rate is associated with sterilization procedures that do not include some form of tubal resection.

Instructions for Items 40–61 to 40–67: Match the procedure used for tubal sterilization with the appropriate description.

a. Irving procedure
b. Pomeroy procedure
c. Parkland procedure
d. Madlener procedure
e. Fimbriectomy

40–61. The tube is divided and the end of the medial segment is buried in the myometrium and the proximal end of the lateral segment is buried within the mesosalpinx
40–62. Plain catgut is used to ligate a knuckle of tube
40–63. The oviduct is ligated twice with 0 chromic suture and the intervening segment excised
40–64. A knuckle of tube is crushed and ligated with nonabsorbable suture but not resected
40–65. The distal end of the tube is removed
40–66. The procedure that is least likely to fail
40–67. The simplest procedure

40–68. After puerperal sterilization, the patient should

a. Be kept in bed for 2 days
b. Remain hospitalized for 3 days
c. Eat a regular diet as tolerated
d. Not breast feed for 1 week

40–69. What general types of surgical procedures are available for nonpuerperal tubal sterilization?

40–70. Which of the following are the principal hazards associated with tubal sterilization?

a. Complications of anesthesia
b. Inadvertent coagulation of vital structures
c. Pulmonary embolism
d. Failure to produce sterility with a resulting ectopic pregnancy

40–71. What is the leading cause of death related to tubal sterilization?

40–72. What factors appear to increase morbidity in patients undergoing tubal sterilization?

a. Previous abdominal or pelvic surgery
b. Diabetes
c. General anesthesia
d. Obesity
e. History of previous pelvic infection

40–73. The "posttubal ligation syndrome," which includes pain, cyst formation, and abnormal bleeding, can be prevented by utilizing the Pomeroy procedure when performing a tubal sterilization.

a. True
b. False

40–74. The patient who is considering tubal sterilization should be informed that reversal of the procedure is possible and often successful.

a. True
b. False

40–75. Which of the following factors makes hysterectomy for the purpose of sterilization (in the absence of uterine and/or pelvic disease) difficult to justify?

a. Cost
b. Blood loss potentially leading to blood transfusion
c. Potential injury to the urinary tract
d. Risk of death

40–76. Which of the following is the most cost-effective method of female sterilization?

a. Hysterectomy
b. Tubal sterilization
c. Hysteroscopic tubal occlusion

40–77. Which of the following statements about vasectomy is correct?

a. The cost is approximately one-fifth that of tubal sterilization.
b. The failure rate is 1 in 100.
c. Sterility is immediate.
d. Restoration of fertility occurs in over 90 percent of all cases of surgical reversal.

40–78. What factors are important in the restoration of fertility after previous vasectomy?

40–79. Which of the following statements about male contraception is correct?

a. Storage of sperm prior to vasectomy has had excellent results.
b. Antibodies to sperm are rarely found after vasectomy in humans.
c. Vasectomy predisposes to atherosclerosis.
d. A safe and effective reversible male contraceptive is as yet to be developed.

41. FORCEPS DELIVERY AND RELATED TECHNIQUES

41–1. Obstetric forceps are designed for what basic purpose?

41–2. List the parts of each forceps branch.

41–3. The cephalic curve of the forceps blade conforms to the shape of the ________ (1), while the pelvic curve conforms to the shape of the ________________ (2).

a. Birth canal
b. Fetal head

41–4. Fenestrated forceps blades permit a firmer hold on the fetal head.

a. True
b. False

Instructions for Items 41–5 to 41–9: Match the type of forceps with the correct lock.

a. English lock
b. Sliding lock
c. French lock

41–5. Kielland forceps
41–6. Simpson forceps
41–7. Barton forceps
41–8. Tucker-McLane forceps
41–9. Tarnier forceps

41–10. In a low forceps (outlet forceps) operation, the instrument is applied after the fetal head has reached the ________ (1), the sagittal suture is in the ________ (2) diameter of the outlet, and the scalp is visible at ________________ (3).

41–11. Which of the following statements about midforceps operations is correct?

a. Forceps are applied before the criteria for low forceps are met but after the fetal head is engaged.
b. The fetal head is usually engaged when the lowermost part of the skull has descended to the level of the ischial spines.
c. All midforceps operations are of approximately equal difficulty.
d. A low midforceps delivery requires that the biparietal diameter be at or below the level of the ischial spines and the leading part be within a finger's breadth of the perineum between contractions.
e. In a low midforceps delivery, the head partially fills the hollow of the sacrum.

41–12. Which of the following types of midforceps deliveries has the greater potential for fetal and maternal trauma?

a. The fetal head has never reached the perineum and the sagittal suture has never achieved the anteroposterior diameter.
b. Due to uterine contraction and maternal expulsive efforts the fetal head lay firmly on the perineum, but receded slightly after anesthesia.

41–13. Under what circumstances is a high forceps delivery indicated?

41–14. Increased perinatal morbidity and mortality and maternal morbidity result from midforceps delivery as compared to spontaneous delivery.

a. True
b. False

41–15. Which of the following influences the decision to utilize low forceps delivery as opposed to spontaneous delivery?

a. Parity of the mother
b. Type of analgesia used in labor
c. Type of anesthesia used in labor
d. Attitudes of staff

41–16. What two physical forces can forceps apply?

41–17. Which of the following are possible treatments for deep transverse arrest?

a. Cesarean delivery
b. Forceps delivery
c. Oxytocin stimulation

41–18. Which of the following maternal or fetal conditions may be an indication for forceps delivery?

a. Maternal heart disease
b. Maternal pulmonary edema
c. Maternal intrapartum infection
d. Maternal exhaustion
e. Prolapse of the umbilical cord
f. Fetal distress
g. Placental abruption

41–19. Which of the following statements about the elective low forceps operation is correct?

a. It constitutes the vast majority of forceps operations in the United States.
b. It is commonly the most reasonable procedure when anesthesia interferes with the patient's voluntary expulsive efforts.
c. If enough time is allowed, the strict criteria for low forceps can usually be met despite the effects of analgesia and anesthesia.
d. Forceps should not be used electively until the criteria for low forceps are fulfilled.

41–20. When is "prophylactic" forceps delivery utilized?

41–21. Prophylactic low forceps delivery improves neonatal outcome in low birth weight infants.

a. True
b. False

41–22. List the prerequisites for the successful application of forceps.

41–23. Which of the following forms part of a low forceps delivery?

a. The bladder should be catheterized
b. The patient's buttocks should rest on the edge of the delivery table
c. The patient's legs should rest in stirrups
d. The patient should be scrubbed and draped
e. General anesthesia should be administered

41-24. Which of the following statements about the technique of forceps application is correct?

a. The biparietal diameter of the fetal head corresponds to the greatest distance between appropriately applied blades.
b. The long axis of appropriately applied blades corresponds to the occipitomental diameter.
c. The tips of the blades should be over the cheeks, while the concave blade margins should be directed toward either the sagittal suture or the face.
d. If one blade is applied over the brow and the other over the occiput, most forceps cannot be locked.
e. The position of the head can be determined by examination of the sagittal suture and fontanels.
f. The posterior ear of the fetus can be helpful in determining the exact position of the head.

41-25. The term pelvic application means that the left blade is applied to the ________ (1) side and the right blade to the ________ (2) side of the woman's pelvis, irrespective of the position of the fetal head.

a. Left
b. Right

41-26. Pelvic application of forceps should not be practiced because the procedure can potentially cause injury to the fetus.

a. True
b. False

41-27. What are the major obstacles to delivery with a low forceps operation?

41-28. Which of the following statements about a low forceps application is correct?

a. The left branch of the forceps is inserted with the left hand.
b. The palmar surface of the fingers of the right hand serve as a guide for the left branch.
c. The handle and branch are inserted directly horizontally.
d. An assistant must be utilized to stabilize one branch while the other is being applied.
e. Application should be checked prior to applying traction.

41-29. Describe the locations of appropriately applied blades for the occiput anterior and occiput posterior positions.

41-30. If cervical tissue has been grasped in a low forceps application, it is appropriate to apply gentle traction for three to five contractions in order to free the fetal head from the incompletely dilated cervix.

a. True
b. False

41-31. Which of the following statements about traction during a low forceps delivery is correct?

a. Gentle intermittent horizontal traction is applied until the perineum bulges.
b. After vulvar distention, the handles are gradually elevated.
c. Episiotomy usually precedes the application of forceps.
d. During the birth of the head, traction should be intermittent.
e. The modified Ritgen maneuver, when used in conjunction with forceps, predisposes to maternal lacerations.

41-32. Which of the following statements about midforceps operations is correct?

a. The first blade should always be applied over the posterior ear.
b. In the occiput transverse position, one blade lies in front of the sacrum and the other lies behind the symphysis.
c. If the occiput is obliquely anterior, it rotates spontaneously to the symphysis as traction is exerted.
d. In exerting traction and rotation, the operator's body weight must often be used.

41-33. The fetal head is often improperly flexed when it is in the right occiput posterior or left occiput posterior positions.

a. True
b. False

41-34. A vital part of manual rotation of the fetal head in posterior positions is the disengagement of the head from the pelvis.

a. True
b. False

41-35. If manual rotation of the head to the occiput anterior position is accomplished, the need for forceps delivery is eliminated.

a. True
b. False

41-36. Which of the following statements about forceps delivery from the occiput posterior position is correct?

a. If manual rotation cannot be accomplished easily, delivery from the persistent occiput posterior position may be the safest procedure.
b. Extraction is easier from the posterior position than from the anterior position.
c. Perineal laceration is less common in the posterior position than in the anterior position.
d. Forceps rotation should only be done with Kielland forceps.
e. Forceps rotation is less traumatic to the mother and the fetus than delivery of the head in the occiput posterior position.

41-37. Which of the following is characteristic of the Scanzoni-Smellie maneuver?

a. It is utilized for the obliquely posterior occipital position.
b. There is a double application of forceps.
c. The head must be disengaged from the pelvis.
d. An exaggerated arc is described by the forceps handles.

41-38. Which of the following statements about Kielland midforceps rotation operations is correct?

a. The Kielland forceps have virtually no cephalic curve.
b. The safer approach for applying the anterior blade is the "wandering" method.
c. Rotation is performed at the station at which it can be most easily accomplished.
d. The procedure should only be utilized for occiput transverse positions.
e. The same forceps may be used for both rotation and extraction.

41-39. What forceps with a hinged anterior blade and a sliding lock is especially useful when the sagittal suture occupies the transverse diameter of a platypelloid pelvis with a straight sacrum?

41-40. In which of the following situations could midforceps delivery be a substitute for cesarean section?

a. Fetal distress
b. Prolapse of the umbilical cord
c. Maternal exhaustion
d. Secondary arrest of labor due to conduction anesthesia

41-41. As compared to cesarean delivery, midforceps procedures generally carry ________ (1) risk of maternal morbidity and ________ (2) risk of short-term fetal morbidity.

a. Decreased
b. Increased

41-42. It has been well documented that midforceps rotation operations are associated with a higher incidence of cerebral palsy and lower intelligence that persists over time.

a. True
b. False

41-43. Forceps should not be applied in a face presentation when the chin is directed to the ________.

Instructions for Items 41-44 to 41-46: Match the procedure with the appropriate description.

a. Trial forceps
b. Failed forceps

41-44. Performed in an operating room ready for cesarean delivery

41-45. Vigorous but unsuccessful attempt to deliver with forceps

41-46. The possibility of fetopelvic disproportion is known to the operator in advance

41-47. What are the fundamental factors responsible for failed forceps?

41-48. Which of the following is a theoretic advantage associated with vacuum extraction?

a. It is a simpler operation than forceps delivery.
b. Rotation can be accomplished with less trauma to the mother.
c. Less intracranial pressure is applied during traction.

41-49. What are the reported complications of vacuum extraction?

41-50. Which of the following is a commonly used obstetric procedure in the United States?

a. Craniotomy
b. Pubiotomy
c. Symphysiotomy
d. Hysterostomatomy (Dührssen incision)
e. Manual dilation of the cervix

42. TECHNIQUES FOR BREECH DELIVERY AND VERSION

42-1. Which of the following statements about the mechanism of labor in the breech presentation is correct?

a. Descent usually takes place with the bitrochanteric diameter of the breech in one of the oblique diameters of the pelvis.
b. Internal rotation occurs as a response to resistance from the pelvic floor.
c. The anterior hip is born before the posterior hip.
d. The posterior portion of the neck is normally brought to a position just under the pubic symphysis.
e. The head is born in extension.

42-2. In the vaginal delivery of a breech presentation, attempts should be made to rotate the back of the fetus toward the maternal vertebral column.

a. True
b. False

Instructions for Items 42-3 to 42-5: Match the type of breech delivery with the correct description.

a. Spontaneous breech delivery
b. Partial breech extraction
c. Total breech extraction

42-3. The infant is delivered spontaneously as far as the umbilicus
42-4. No traction or manipulation is required except support of the infant
42-5. The entire body of the fetus is extracted by the obstetrician

42-6. List the members of the delivery team (and their functions) that must be present at a vaginal breech delivery.

42-7. Delivery is easier and perinatal mortality and morbidity are lower when the breech is allowed to deliver spontaneously.

a. True
b. False

42-8. What options are available if fetal distress develops during labor in a breech presentation?

42-9. Which of the following statements about extraction of the complete or incomplete breech is correct?

a. The obstetrician's hand is introduced through the vagina and the infant's ankles are grasped.
b. The anterior foot should be brought through the introitus first.
c. Episiotomy is required only in a preterm birth.
d. As the buttocks emerge, the operator's thumbs should be placed over the sacrum with the fingers over the hips and downward traction should be continued.
e. The legs are wrapped in a towel to allow a better grip as downward traction is exerted.
f. No attempt should be made to deliver the shoulders and arms until one axilla becomes visible.

42-10. In a successful breech extraction, gentle steady downward traction is applied until the lower halves of the scapulas are delivered outside the vulva.

a. True
b. False

42-11. What two methods are available to deliver the shoulders in a breech extraction?

42-12. In extraction of the complete or incomplete breech, attempts to deliver the arms immediately after the costal margins emerge should be avoided.

a. True
b. False

42-13. Which of the following statements apply when it is necessary to first free and deliver the arms in a breech extraction?

a. Free the posterior arm first.
b. Apply downward traction at all times.
c. Splint the infant's arm with two fingers.
d. Never manipulate the scapulas.

42–14. Which of the following statements about a nuchal arm is correct?

a. One or both fetal arms may be draped around the back of the neck.
b. The presence of a nuchal arm usually requires cesarean delivery.
c. In cases where the arm cannot be delivered, rotation of the fetus so as to force the elbow toward the face may be effective.
d. To free the nuchal arm, the fetus should be pulled downward.
e. Forcible extraction of a nuchal arm by hooking a finger over it often leads to fracture of the humerus or clavicle.
f. Fracture of a humerus or clavicle usually leads to permanent deformity.

42–15. The Mauriceau maneuver is utilized to help ______________ the fetal head.

a. Flex
b. Extend

42–16. What are important aspects of the Mauriceau maneuver?

a. Index and middle finger placed over infant's maxilla
b. Infant's body resting on operator's palm and forearm
c. Two fingers of operator's other hand hooked over fetal neck, grasping shoulders
d. Downward traction until suboccipital region appears under symphysis
e. Moderate suprapubic pressure by assistant
f. Body of fetus elevated toward maternal abdomen

42–17. Which of the following statements about the extraction of a frank breech is correct?

a. Moderate traction exerted by a finger in each groin may be adequate.
b. A generous episiotomy can facilitate delivery.
c. Breech decomposition converts the frank breech into a footling breech.
d. Breech decomposition can be more readily accomplished if there has been prolonged rupture of the membranes.
e. The Pinard maneuver should be used to aid in the delivery of the anterior shoulder.

42–18. Forceps should not be applied to the aftercoming head until it has been brought into the pelvis and is engaged.

a. True
b. False

42–19. Why is the fetal body suspended in a towel while forceps are applied to the aftercoming head?

42–20. When should Dührssen incisions be utilized in breech delivery?

42–21. Which of the following statements about anesthesia for breech delivery is correct?

a. Pudendal block and local infiltration are usually adequate.
b. Nitrous oxide should never be used in a breech delivery.
c. Halothane can be used to relax the uterus for decomposition and extraction.
d. Conduction anesthesia (spinal, epidural, caudal) should be reserved for vertex presentations.

42–22. List the increased maternal risks due to manipulation and anesthesia in cases of complicated breech delivery.

42–23. In general, the prognosis for the mother whose fetus is delivered by breech extraction is probably ______________ (1) as compared to cesarean delivery and the prognosis for the fetus is ______________ (2).

a. More favorable
b. Less favorable

42–24. Which of the following are potential risks to the fetus in breech extraction?

a. Intracranial hemorrhage
b. Tentorial tears
c. Umbilical cord prolapse
d. Fractures
e. Epiphyseal separations
f. Paralysis

42–25. What is a version operation?

Instructions for Items 42–26 to 42–29: Match the type of version with the appropriate description.

a. Cephalic version
b. Podalic version
c. External version
d. Internal version

42–26. Breech is made the presenting part
42–27. Head is made the presenting part
42–28. Manipulations are performed through the abdominal wall
42–29. Manipulations are performed by a hand introduced into the uterine cavity

42–30. Which of the following conditions is necessary before attempting external version?

a. Presenting part must be engaged
b. Abdominal wall must not be flaccid
c. Uterine wall must not be irritable
d. Uterus must contain enough amnionic fluid to permit easy movement of the fetus

42–31. Which of the following statements about external cephalic version is correct?

a. It should be attempted in the last few weeks of pregnancy in all cases of breech or shoulder presentation.
b. It should not be attempted in the presence of marked disproportion between the fetus and the pelvis.
c. General anesthesia is preferable to conduction anesthesia for the version procedure.
d. Version can be attempted early in labor.
e. Version can usually be accomplished most easily after the membranes have ruptured and the cervix has fully dilated.

42–32. Which of the following is necessary whenever an external cephalic version is attempted?

a. Fetal presentation and position must be determined.
b. Fetal heart rate should be continuously monitored.
c. Version should be performed in a labor and delivery unit.
d. Use of tocolytic agents is required.

42–33. Which of the following may be an indication for an internal podalic version?

a. Delivery of a first twin
b. Delivery of a second twin
c. Delivery of a dead fetus
d. Transverse lie
e. Lack of descent after full cervical dilation

43. CESAREAN SECTION AND CESAREAN HYSTERECTOMY

43–1. Cesarean section is defined as the delivery of the fetus through ______________________.

43–2. Removal of the fetus from the abdominal cavity in the case of uterine rupture or abdominal pregnancy is a special case of cesarean delivery.

a. True
b. False

43–3. In general, what temporal factors affect the decision to utilize cesarean delivery?

43–4. Specific indications for cesarean delivery may include

a. Previous cesarean delivery
b. Breech presentation
c. Fetal distress
d. Dystocia

43–5. Increased use of cesarean delivery is the major reason for the absolute decrease in perinatal mortality.

a. True
b. False

43–6. Based on data from other countries, neonatal morbidity and mortality would be minimized if the cesarean delivery rate was below 10 percent.

a. True
b. False

43–7. The lower the birth weight, the ______________ the risk for a vaginal breech delivery.

a. Lower
b. Higher

43–8. Which of the following statements about the morbidity and mortality associated with cesarean delivery is correct?

a. Maternal mortality is due primarily to blood loss.
b. The most frequent cause of maternal morbidity is associated with the use of anesthesia.
c. The incidence and severity of maternal morbidity is similar to that seen with vaginal delivery.
d. Cesarean delivery provides a guarantee against fetal injury.
e. Fetal morbidity is decreased if cesarean delivery is utilized in breech presentations and transverse lie.
f. Respiratory distress is more common following cesarean delivery.

43–9. Which of the following statements about the timing of repeat cesarean delivery is correct?

a. A preset delivery date allows better arrangements to be made by hospital personnel and by the family.
b. Uterine rupture is more likely if labor occurs in a woman with a previous vertical uterine incision than with a previous horizontal uterine incision.
c. All repeat cesarean sections should first undergo amniocentesis to determine fetal lung maturity.
d. Sonography can be used in place of amniocentesis to determine fetal lung maturity.

43–10. At Parkland Memorial Hospital, what information is used to determine fetal maturity so as to correctly time repeat cesarean section?

43-11. Which of the following is an absolute contraindication to cesarean delivery?

a. Presence of a dead fetus
b. Prematurity
c. Placenta previa
d. Neglected transverse lie
e. Maternal coagulation defect

43-12. Which of the following statements about the use of vaginal delivery in a woman with a previous cesarean delivery is correct?

a. Vaginal delivery should only be considered in a young patient.
b. The cesarean delivery must have utilized a low transverse uterine incision.
c. The cesarean delivery cannot have been performed because of cephalopelvic disproportion.
d. When attempting a trial of labor, an operating room and all relevant personnel and equipment must be available.

43-13. Describe a classical cesarean incision.

Instructions for Items 43-14 to 43-21: Match the type of incision utilized for cesarean delivery with the appropriate statement.

a. Lower segment transverse (Kerr technique)
b. Lower segment vertical (Kronig technique)

43-14. May be easily extended if more room is required
43-15. Requires less dissection of the bladder
43-16. More likely to tear through the cervix into the vagina
43-17. Laceration may include large branches of the uterine artery
43-18. More likely to rupture in a subsequent pregnancy
43-19. Results in less blood loss
43-20. Less likely to promote bowel adherence
43-21. Easier to repair

43-22. For a cephalic presentation, a transverse incision through the lower uterine segment is usually the procedure of choice.

a. True
b. False

43-23. Which of the following steps in preparation for cesarean delivery should be completed prior to the induction of general anesthesia?

a. Abdomen shaved
b. Bladder emptied through an indwelling catheter
c. Operative field scrubbed
d. Operating team fully prepared

43-24. Which of the following types of anesthesia used in cesarean delivery is administered before the abdomen is scrubbed and draped?

a. Epidural
b. General
c. Spinal

43-25. Which of the following statements about the abdominal infraumbilical midline vertical incision for cesarean delivery is correct?

a. It is the quickest to make.
b. For all deliveries, the length of the incision should be 10 cm.
c. There is greater risk of incising underlying structures if the fascia is opened with scissors.
d. The peritoneum should be opened at the inferior end of the incision.
e. Bleeding sites anywhere in the abdominal incision should be ligated as soon as encountered.

43-26. Which of the following is characteristic of the Pfannenstiel incision?

a. Transverse skin incision
b. Incision just below the umbilicus
c. Transverse muscle incision
d. Longitudinal muscle incision

43-27. Which of the following statements about abdominal incisions utilized for cesarean delivery is correct?

a. The transverse incision has a cosmetic advantage.
b. There is less likelihood of dehiscence with a transverse incision.
c. With a vertical incision, there is superior exposure of the uterus and its appendages.
d. The horizontal incision should be used with obese women.
e. The horizontal incision should be used by a less skilled operator.
f. At repeat cesarean section, reentry through the transverse incision is more time consuming.

43-28. The uterus is palpated upon entry into the abdominal cavity in order to identify________________.

43-29. During cesarean section, placement of laparotomy packs in the lateral peritoneal gutters minimizes the chance of uterine artery laceration.

a. True
b. False

43-30. Describe the process by which the upper margin of the bladder is pushed off the lower uterine segment during cesarean section.

43–31. Which of the following constitutes correct technique when incising the uterus for cesarean delivery?

a. The uterine incision is made 2 cm above the detached bladder.
b. The incision is begun transversely and made with a scalpel.
c. The incision is extended laterally and upward with a scalpel.
d. The incision should never exceed 8 cm in length.

43–32. What steps should be taken if the placenta is encountered in the line of the uterine incision?

43–33. Describe the method for delivery of the infant through the uterine incision.

43–34. In cesarean section, what can be done to aid the delivery of an infant whose head is tightly wedged into the pelvis?

43–35. After the body of the fetus is delivered,

a. 20 Units of oxytocin should be administered as an IV bolus
b. The nares and mouth should be aspirated with a bulb syringe
c. The cord should be clamped
d. The newborn should be given to a member of the resuscitation team
e. A sample of cord blood should be obtained
f. Fundal massage should be initiated

43–36. At the time of cesarean section, manual removal of the placenta should never be attempted.

a. True
b. False

43–37. A longitudinal incision through the lower uterine segment might be advantageous when

a. The fetus is not in a vertex presentation
b. The fetus is macrosomic
c. There are multiple fetuses
d. A placental abnormality is present

43–38. What are the advantages and disadvantages of extraabdominal exteriorization for repair of the uterus after cesarean delivery?

43–39. The principal reason that the uterus should not be exteriorized for repair is that the procedure markedly increases the risk of infection.

a. True
b. False

43–40. Which of the following steps is involved in repairing the uterus after cesarean delivery?

a. Inspect and wipe uterine cavity.
b. Probe endocervical canal to ensure patency.
c. Ligate large vessels individually with a suture ligature.
d. Incorporate posterior uterine wall into closure.

43–41. Describe the suturing technique that should be used for uterine repair after cesarean section.

43–42. After the uterine incision is closed, the peritoneal edge should be sutured above the bladder to strengthen the incision.

a. True
b. False

43–43. If tubal sterilization is to be performed along with cesarean section, it should be done after the repair of the uterus.

a. True
b. False

43–44. Outline the preferred method of tubal sterilization that is used at the time of cesarean section at Parkland Memorial Hospital.

43–45. Which of the following statements about closure of the abdomen after cesarean section is correct?

a. Blood and amnionic fluid are left in the abdomen to decrease the formation of adhesions.
b. If possible, the abdominal contents should be palpated.
c. The uterus is compressed to express blood.
d. As each layer is closed, identified bleeding sites are clamped and ligated.
e. A tight pressure dressing should always be applied.

Instructions for Items 43–46 to 43–49: Match the layer of the abdominal wall with the correct suture that is used to close it after cesarean delivery.

a. Interrupted 0 nonabsorbable sutures
b. Continuous 00 chromic catgut
c. Vertical 000 silk mattress sutures
d. Interrupted 000 plain catgut

43–46. Peritoneum
43–47. Rectus fascia
43–48. Subcutaneous adipose tissue
43–49. Skin

43–50. Which of the following is an indication for classical cesarean section?

a. Inability to expose the lower uterine segment
b. Presence of a myoma in the lower uterine segment
c. Invasive cervical carcinoma
d. Transverse lie of a large fetus
e. Placenta previa

43–51. Which of the following statements about classical cesarean section is correct?

a. The abdominal incision is the same as that utilized in a lower segment cesarean.
b. The uterine incision is begun in the fundus and carried caudad as far as necessary.
c. Bleeders in the uterine wall should be clamped and tied as soon as they are encountered.
d. One layer is usually sufficient for closure.
e. An assistant should compress the myometrium medially to aid in closure of the uterus.

43–52. Extraperitoneal cesarean section is particularly useful in patients with a bleeding disorder.

a. True
b. False

43–53. Fetal outcome from a postmortem cesarean section is dependent upon which of the following factors?

a. Anticipation of maternal death
b. Fetal gestational age
c. Adequate personnel and equipment
d. Postmortem support of the mother
e. Prompt delivery
f. Effective infant resuscitation

43–54. Which of the following may be indications for cesarean hysterectomy?

a. Intrauterine infection
b. Defective uterine scar
c. Uterine atony
d. Uterine vessel laceration
e. Invasive cervical carcinoma
f. History of abnormal menses
g. Placenta increta

43–55. What are the two major dangers/complications of cesarean hysterectomy?

Instructions for Items 43–56 to 43–57: Match the average blood loss with the procedure.

a. 500 ml
b. 1000 ml
c. 1500 ml
d. 2000 ml

43–56. Cesarean section
43–57. Cesarean hysterectomy

43–58. Which of the following statements about cesarean hysterectomy is correct?

a. The adnexa usually must be removed.
b. The tissue planes are usually easy to develop.
c. Administration of oxytocin is unnecessary.
d. The bladder and its peritoneal flap should be fully developed prior to ligating the round ligaments.
e. All pedicles should be doubly ligated.

43–59. In a cesarean hysterectomy, the ureters are most likely to be injured when the round ligament is incised.

a. True
b. False

43–60. In a supracervical hysterectomy, the body of the uterus is amputated after doubly clamping and ligating what structures?

43–61. Which of the following is an important step in performing a total cesarean hysterectomy?

a. Extensive mobilization of the bladder
b. Identification of the cervix
c. Ligation of the pedicles to include only a small volume of tissue in each clamp
d. Excision of the entire cervix

43–62. In a total cesarean hysterectomy, what is the advantage of using a running-lock stitch around the vaginal mucosal edge rather than a series of figure-of-eight sutures?

43–63. Which of the following should be routinely performed as part of a cesarean hysterectomy?

a. Appendectomy
b. Oophorectomy
c. Reperitonealization
d. The peritoneum and fascia closed as a single layer with permanent nonreactive sutures
e. The skin and subcutaneous tissue left open

43–64. Which of the following is a recommended preoperative step when elective repeat cesarean section is contemplated?

a. Type and cross-match so as to have at least 1000 ml of blood available.
b. Administer a sedative 1 hour prior to surgery.
c. Administer nothing by mouth for 8 hours prior to surgery.
d. Administer an antacid shortly before the induction of anesthesia.

43–65. Which of the following statements about the management of fluids at the time of cesarean section is correct?

a. Each milliliter of blood lost at surgery should be replaced by a milliliter of transfused blood.
b. The only intravenous fluid that should be utilized is 5 percent dextrose in water.
c. Oxytocin should be added to the IV infusion when the shoulders of the infant are delivered.
d. Throughout the procedure, blood pressure and urine flow should be monitored.
e. Urine flow need not be monitored in the recovery area.

43–66. What might contribute to the underestimation of blood loss from cesarean delivery?

43–67. Which of the following statements about recovery room care after cesarean delivery is correct?

a. The best method to assure that the uterus is well contracted is to watch for excessive vaginal bleeding.
b. Withholding analgesia in the recovery room allows for better monitoring of clinical signs.
c. A thick abdominal dressing should be applied if only a small one was applied in the operating room.
d. Deep breathing and coughing should be encouraged.

43–68. A woman may be returned to her room when she

a. Is fully awake
b. Has minimal bleeding
c. Has a satisfactory blood pressure
d. Has a urine output of at least 30 ml per hour

43–69. What type and dosage of analgesia is recommended for the postoperative cesarean section patient?

43–70. At what intervals should the vital signs of the patient be monitored during the first 24 hours after cesarean section?

43–71. Which of the following should routinely be monitored at the prescribed intervals during the first day after cesarean delivery?

a. Blood pressure
b. Pulse rate
c. Urine flow
d. Hematocrit
e. Temperature
f. Amount of bleeding
g. Status of the fundus
h. Degree of dilation of pupils

43–72. Due to the sequestration of large amounts of extracellular fluid, patients undergoing an uncomplicated cesarean section usually require approximately 6 liters of IV fluids in the first 24 hours.

a. True
b. False

43–73. After cesarean section, a urine output of less than 30 ml per hour should be evaluated only if it persists for at least 12 consecutive hours.

a. True
b. False

Instructions for Items 43–74 to 43–81: Match the time after cesarean section with the events that should normally occur.

a. Postoperative day 1
b. Postoperative day 2
c. Postoperative day 3
d. Postoperative day 4

43–74. Oral fluids tolerated
43–75. General diet tolerated
43–76. Bladder catheter removed
43–77. Active bowel sounds
43–78. Gas pains from incoordinate bowel action
43–79. Ambulation with assistance
43–80. Bathing by shower or tub
43–81. Skin sutures removed

43–82. Which of the following statements about the routine management of a patient after cesarean delivery is correct?

a. A complete blood count is preferred over a hematocrit.
b. Initial blood testing is performed 2 days after surgery.
c. Blood transfusion should be immediately instituted if the initial hematocrit is low.
d. If the patient is stable and no further blood loss is anticipated, iron therapy is preferable to transfusion.

43–83. Which of the following statements about postcesarean section breast feeding is correct?

a. Breast feeding should begin on the third postoperative day.
b. A breast binder may suppress lactation in a woman not wishing to breast feed.
c. Bromocriptine is effective for suppressing lactation.
d. Suppression of lactation removes a possible source of postpartum fever.

43–84. In the absence of complications, the mother can be safely released from the hospital after cesarean delivery on the ______________ postpartum day.

43–85. What instructions for home care and follow-up visits are advisable at the time of discharge after cesarean delivery?

43–86. Which of the following statements about the use of prophylactic antibiotics in cesarean delivery is correct?

a. Prophylactic antibiotics should be administered to all women having a cesarean delivery.
b. Febrile morbidity appears to be more common among indigent women.
c. Women undergoing cesarean delivery whose membranes have been ruptured for more than 6 hours are at greater risk of infection.
d. Antibiotics should be administered prior to clamping the cord.

ANSWERS

1–1. b
*p 1**
obstetrics, definition

1–2. c
p 2
fertility rate

1–3. a
p 2
birth rate

1–4. c
p 2
live birth

1–5. a
p 2
abortus

1–6. b
p 2
stillbirth

1–7. a,b,c
p 2
live birth, criteria

1–8. the number of fetal deaths (stillbirths) plus neonatal deaths per 1000 total births
p 2
perinatal mortality rate, definition

1–9. c
p 2
stillbirth rate; fetal death rate

1–10. d
p 2
postterm infant, definition

1–11. e
p 2
low birth weight infant, definition

1–12. b
p 2
preterm infant, definition

1–13. c
p 2
term infant, definition

1–14. b
p 2
maternal death, indirect

1–15. d
p 2
maternal death rate, definition

1–16. deaths resulting from the use of contraceptive techniques plus deaths that are the consequence of pregnancy per 100,000 women
p 2
reproductive mortality, definition

1–17. a,c,d
p 3
maternal mortality

1–18. a,c,d
p 3
maternal mortality

1–19. d
p 4
obstetric care, quality; perinatal mortality rate

1–20. a,c,d
p 4
neonatal death

1–21. a,b,c,d
p 5
birth certificate

2–1. c
p 7
vulva, anatomy

2–2. a,b,c,d
p 7
vulva, anatomy

2–3. a,d,e
p 7
vulva; labia majora; perineum

2–4. a,b,d
p 7
vulva, anatomy; labia majora

2–5. b,d,e
pp 7–8
vulva, anatomy; labia minora

2–6. b,c,d,e
pp 8–9
vulva, anatomy; clitoris

2–7. a
pp 7–9
vulva; clitoris

2–8. b,c,d
p 9
vestibule

2–9. a,b,d,e
p 9
vulva; Bartholin glands

* *All page numbers refer to Pritchard J, et al:* Williams Obstetrics, 17th Edition.

2–10. c
pp 8–10
vulva, innervation; hymen; innervation, genitals

2–11. b
pp 9–10
vulva; hymen

2–12. b
p 11
hymen; virginity

2–13. myrtiform caruncles
p 11
hymen; myrtiform caruncles

2–14. A
pp 8 (Fig. 2-1), 9
vulva; clitoris

2–15. K
pp 7, 8 (Fig. 2-1)
vulva; labia majora

2–16. D
p 8 (Fig. 2-1)
vulva; hymen

2–17. F
p 8 (Fig. 2-1)
vulva; perineal body

2–18. B,L
p 8 (Fig. 2-1)
vulva; frenulum; prepuce

2–19. a,b,d
p 11
vagina

2–20. a,b,c,e
pp 11–12
vagina, anatomy; vagina, embryology; parturition

2–21. pouch (cul-de-sac) of Douglas
p 12
vagina; cul-de-sac of Douglas

2–22. b
p 12
vagina, anatomy

2–23. b,c,d
p 12
vagina, anatomy

2–24. c,d
pp 12–13
vagina; exfoliative cytology, vagina

2–25. c
p 13
vagina, vasculature

2–26. a
p 13
vagina, vasculature

2–27. b,d
p 13
vagina, vasculature

2–28. a,b,d
pp 7,9,13
vulva; vaginal delivery; genitalia, venous system; hematoma, parturition

2–29. hypogastric (internal iliac)
p 13
vagina, vasculature

2–30. a
p 13
vagina, lymphatics; vulva, lymphatics; inguinal nodes

2–31. b
p 13
vagina, innervation

2–32. b,c
p 13
perineum; pelvic diaphragm

2–33. a,d
pp 13,15
perineum; urogenital diaphragm

2–34. a,b,c
p 15
perineum; perineal body

2–35. b
p 15
uterus, anatomy

2–36. d
p 15
uterus, anatomy; uterus, corpus

2–37. b
p 15
cervix

2–38. a
p 15
uterus, anatomy; uterus, cornu

2–39. c
p 15
uterus, anatomy; uterus, fundus

2–40. b
p 15
uterus

2–41. b
p 16
uterus, anatomy; uterus, isthmus; lower uterine segment

2-42. b,c
p 16
cervix, anatomy

2-43. a
p 16
cervix; external cervical os

2-44. a
p 17
cervix; incompetent cervix

2-45. c,d
p 17
cervix, anatomy; Nabothian cysts

2-46. just above the bladder and at the lateral margins
p 17
uterus, anatomy

2-47. a,c
p 17
endometrium

2-48. a,b
p 18
uterus, vasculature; uterine artery; ovarian artery

2-49. a,b,c
p 18
uterus, blood supply; endometrium; coiled arterioles; basal arteries

2-50. b
p 18
myometrium

2-51. a,b,c
p 19
broad ligament; uterus, ligaments; mesosalpinx; infundibulopelvic ligament; cardinal ligament

2-52. b
p 19
cardinal ligament; uterus, ligaments

2-53. a
p 19
infundibulopelvic ligament; uterus, ligaments; ovarian artery; ovarian vein

2-54. c
p 20
round ligaments; uterus, ligaments

2-55. d
p 20
uterosacral ligament; uterus, ligaments

2-56. D
p 19 (Fig. 2-14)
cervix

2-57. I
p 19 (Fig. 2-14)
round ligament

2-58. J
p 19 (Fig. 2-14)
ovarian artery; ovarian vein

2-59. G
p 19 (Fig. 2-14)
urethra

2-60. B
p 19 (Fig. 2-14)
utero-ovarian ligament

2-61. a,b,c
p 20
uterus, position

2-62. hypogastric (internal iliac) artery
p 20
uterus, vasculature; hypogastric artery; uterine artery

2-63. a,b,c,d
p 20
uterus, vasculature; uterine artery

2-64. c
p 20
uterine artery; ureter

2-65. There is the possibility of surgical injury to the ureter when clamping and ligating uterine vessels.
p 20
uterine artery; ureter

2-66. b,c,d
p 20
uterus, vasculature; ovarian artery; infundibulopelvic ligament; uterine artery

2-67. a,b,d
p 20
uterus, vasculature; uterus, veins; ovarian vein; pampiniform plexus

2-68. a
p 20
cervix, lymphatics; hypogastric nodes; pudendal nerve

2-69. a,b
p 20
uterus, lymphatics; hypogastric nodes; periaortic nodes

2-70. a,b,c,d
pp 20,23
reproductive tract, innervation

2-71. b
pp 23-24
oviduct

2–72. a,b,d
p 24
oviduct

2–73. a
p 24
oviduct

2–74. a
p 25
oviduct

2–75. Diverticula
p 25
oviduct; ectopic pregnancy

2–76. a,b,c,e
p 25
oviduct, embryonic development; uterus, embryonic development

2–77. a,b,e
pp 25-26
ovary, anatomy; ovary, vascular supply; infundibulopelvic ligament

2–78. a
p 26
ovary, cortex

2–79. a,b
p 26
ovary, cortex; ovary, medulla

2–80. a
p 26
ovary, cortex

2–81. a
p 26
ovary, cortex

2–82. b
p 26
ovary, medulla

2–83. b
p 26
ovary, medulla

2–84. b
p 26
ovary

2–85. The ventral surface of the embryonic kidney at 4 weeks.
p 26
ovary, embryonic development

2–86. b
p 26
ovary, embryonic development; primordial germ cells

2–87. a,b,c,d
p 26
testis, embryonic development; mesonephros

2–88. a,e
pp 26–27,30
ovary, embryonic development; oogenesis

2–89. mesovarium
p 29
ovary, embryonic development; mesovarium

2–90. a
pp 29–30
ovary, cortex; primordial follicles

2–91. a
p 30
mesonephric duct, embryonic remnants; Gartner duct

2–92. b
p 30
mesonephric tubules, embryonic remnants; paroophoron

2–93. a
p 30
mesonephric duct, embryonic remnants; parovarium

3–1. ovulation
p 31
ovulation; menses

3–2. a
pp 32–33
ovary, embryology

3–3. a
p 33
ovary, embryology

3–4. b
p 33
ovary, embryology; oogonia

3–5. b
p 33
oogonia

3–6. d
p 33
oogonia

3–7. c
p 33
oogonia

3–8. a
p 33
oogonia

3–9. b
p 36
graafian follicle, histology

3-10. E
p 36 (Fig. 3-9)
graafian follicle, histology

3-11. F
p 36 (Fig. 3-9)
graffian follicle, histology

3-12. D
p 36 (Fig. 3-9)
graafian follicle, histology

3-13. C
p 36 (Fig. 3-9)
graafian follicle, histology

3-14. A
p 36 (Fig. 3-9)
graafian follicle, histology

3-15. a
p 37
graafian follicle

3-16. b
p 34
graafian follicle

3-17. b
pp 33-34
graafian follicle

3-18. d
p 38
oocyte, maturation

3-19. a,b
p 38
oocyte, maturation

3-20. a,b,c,d
p 39
FSH

3-21. a,d
p 39
androstenedione; estrone; testosterone

3-22. a,b,c
p 39
androstenedione; virilization; feminization; masculinization

3-23. c
p 40
progesterone, synthesis; cholesterol

3-24. a,b,c
p 41
ovulation

3-25. a
p 43
ovulation, timing; luteal phase

3-26. c
p 43
ovulation, timing; menstrual cycle

3-27. c
p 44
ovulation; progesterone, actions

3-28. None
pp 43-44
ovulation; progesterone, actions

3-29. c
p 44
ovulation; LH

3-30. a,b,c
pp 44-45
corpus luteum

3-31. a,c,d
pp 45-46
corpus luteum

3-32. b
p 47
corpus luteum, pregnancy

3-33. d
p 47
corpus luteum, pregnancy

3-34. corpora albicantes (corpus albicans)
p 47
corpora albicantes; corpus luteum

3-35. a,b,c
p 48
follicle, atresia

3-36. a,b,c,d
p 48
ovary, hormones

3-37. a,c,d
p 48
estrogen; estradiol-17β; estriol; estrone

3-38. catechol estrogens
p 48
catechol estrogens; estrone, metabolism; estradiol-17β, metabolism

3-39. a
p 50
estrogen, synthesis; estrone; androstenedione

3-40. a,c,d
p 50
estrogen, synthesis; menopause, estrogen production

3-41. a,c
p 50
estrogen, synthesis; androstenedione

3-42. a
p 50
estrogen, synthesis; ovary, hormones

3-43. a,b
pp 50-51
estrogen, synthesis; ovary, hormones; estradiol-17β, synthesis

3-44. A
p 51
cholesterol; estrogen, synthesis

3-45. E
p 51
estradiol; estrogen, synthesis

3-46. H
p 51
androstenedione; estrogen, synthesis

3-47. J
p 51
progesterone; estrogen, synthesis

3-48. F
p 51
testosterone; estrogen, synthesis

3-49. b
p 51
estrogen, synthesis; estradiol-17β

3-50. 1 = a; 2 = b
p 51
estrogen, metabolism

3-51. b
pp 51-52
estrogen, metabolism

3-52. a,b,c,d,e
pp 52-53
estrogen, actions; estradiol-17β

3-53. b,c,d,f
pp 52-53
estrogen, actions

3-54. a
p 53
progesterone, synthesis; corpus luteum, hormone production

3-55. pregnanediol
p 53
progesterone. metabolism; pregnanediol

3-56. c
p 54
progesterone

3-57. a
p 53
estrogen, actions; bone growth

3-58. b
p 54
progesterone, actions; smooth muscle

3-59. b
p 54
progesterone, actions; respiration, rate

3-60. a
p 54
estrogen, actions; ovulation

3-61. b
p 54
progesterone, actions; implantation

3-62. a,b
p 55
placenta, hormone production; progesterone, pregnancy; corpus luteum

3-63. the electrochemical gradient
p 55
progesterone, actions; myometrium, contractions

3-64. a,b
p 55
progesterone, actions; oviduct

3-65. a
p 55
progesterone, actions; cervical mucus

3-66. b
p 55
progesterone, actions; breast, development

3-67. a
pp 53,55
estrogen, actions; breast, function

3-68. b
p 55
progesterone, actions; breast, function; prolactin

3-69. a,b
pp 55-56
androgens, synthesis; androstenedione

3-70. b
p 56
androgens, synthesis; dehydroisoandrosterone

3-71. b
p 56
androgens, synthesis; dehydroisoandrosterone sulfate

3-72. c, lesser amounts from a
p 56
androgens, synthesis; testosterone

3-73. a,b
p 56
estrogen, synthesis; testosterone, synthesis; androstenedione

3–74. a,b,c
p 56
relaxin

3–75. a,b,e
p 56
relaxin

3–76. a
p 57
hypothalamus; puberty

3–77. a,b,c
p 57
FSH, actions

3–78. 1 = b; 2 = a
p 57
estrogen, menopause; FSH

3–79. a
p 57
LH

3–80. c
p 58
LH; estrogen, action

3–81. b,c,d
p 58
prolactin

3–82. a,b,c,d
p 59
prolactin

3–83. folliculostatin
p 59
folliculostatin; FSH

3–84. b
p 60
folliculostatin; progesterone, actions

3–85. a
p 60
folliculostatin; androstenedione

3–86. a
p 60
folliculostatin; testosterone, actions

3–87. b
p 60
folliculostatin; estradiol-17β

3–88. a polypeptide biosynthesized, processed, and released by a cell that affects the function of another cell in the vicinity
p 60
cybernin

4–1. a,b,c,d
p 65
estrogen, action; estradiol-17β; progesterone, receptors

4–2. a,b,c
p 65
progesterone action; estradiol-17β

4–3. b
p 66
progesterone, receptors; breast, tumors

4–4. c
p 66
menstruation

4–5. a
pp 66, 71
menstrual cycle; ovarian cycle

4–6. b
p 67
ovarian cycle; endometrial cycle, follicular phase; follicular phase

4–7. a
p 67
ovarian cycle; endometrial cycle, follicular phase; follicular phase

4–8. c
p 67
ovarian cycle; endometrial cycle; luteal phase

4–9. a,c
p 66
menstrual cycle; ovarian cycle; follicular phase; proliferative phase

4–10. a,b,c
p 66
endometrial cycle, proliferative phase

4–11. a
p 68
endometrial cycle, secretory phase

4–12. a
p 68
endometrial cycle, secretory phase

4–13. b
p 68
endometrial cycle, proliferative phase

4–14. c
p 68
endometrial cycle, premenstrual phase

4–15. d
p 68
endometrium cyclical changes

4-16. a
p 67
endometrium, cyclical changes

4-17. c
p 68
endometrium, cyclical changes

4-18. e
p 68
endometrium, cyclical changes

4-19. b
pp 67-68
endometrium, cyclical changes

4-20. a,b
pp 68-69
menstrual cycle; menstruation

4-21. a,b,c
pp 66,69
decidua

4-22. a,b,c,d
p 69
prostaglandins

4-23. a,b,c
pp 71-72
menstrual cycle

4-24. b
p 71
ovulation; menstruation

4-25. a,c
p 72
cervical mucus; menstrual cycle

4-26. d
pp 73-74
menstrual cycle; cervical mucus

4-27. a
p 74
cervical mucus; estrogen, actions

4-28. b
p 74
cervical mucus; progesterone, actions

4-29. a
p 74
vagina, menstrual cycle

4-30. b
p 74
vagina, menstrual cycle

4-31. a
p 74
vagina, menstrual cycle

4-32. b
p 74
vagina, menstrual cycle

4-33. b,c
p 75
menarche; puberty

4-34. c
p 75
menopause

4-35. b
p 75
puberty

4-36. a
p 75
menarche

4-37. d
p 75
climacteric

4-38. a,b,c
p 75
menstrual cycle

4-39. b
p 75
menstrual cycle; fertility

4-40. b,d
pp 75-77
menstrual cycle

4-41. b
p 77
menstrual cycle

5-1. meiosis
p 79
meiosis

5-2. d
p 80
gametogenesis; germ cells; autosomes

5-3. b
p 80
gametogenesis; germ cells

5-4. b
p 81
meiosis; mitosis

5-5. b
p 81
meiosis, prophase

5-6. c
p 81
meiosis, prophase

5-7. a
p 81
meiosis, prophase

5-8. d
p 81
meiosis, prophase

5-9. zona pellucida
p 81
follicle; zona pellucida

5-10. b,c,d
p 81
oogenesis; meiosis

5-11. a
p 81
oogenesis

5-12. c
pp 81-82
gametogenesis, meiosis; meiosis

5-13. c
p 82
oogenesis

5-14. b
p 81
meiosis

5-15. b
p 82
cybernin; oocyte maturation inhibitor

5-16. b,c
p 82
oogenesis; meiosis

5-17. at the time of fertilization
p 82
oogenesis; fertilization; meiosis

5-18. b
p 82
fertilization

5-19. b
p 83
primordial germ cells; gametogenesis

5-20. d
p 83
spermatogenesis

5-21. a,b
p 83
oogenesis; spermatogenesis

5-22. b
pp 83-84
spermatogenesis

5-23. a
p 83
oogenesis

5-24. a,b
p 83
gametogenesis; oogenesis; spermatogenesis

5-25. a
p 80
spermatogenesis

5-26. a
p 83
spermatogenesis

5-27. b,c
p 83
spermatogenesis

5-28. b,c
p 83
spermatogenesis

5-29. b,c
p 83
spermatogenesis

5-30. e
p 85
fertilization; sperm migration

5-31. b
p 85
fertilization; sperm migration

5-32. a
pp 85-86
fertilization

5-33. 1 = 3 per 2000 live births; 2 = 1 per 100 live births
p 86
Down syndrome

5-34. a
p 87
chromosomal abnormality, incidence

5-35. a
pp 80-81
mitosis; oogenesis

5-36. b
p 81
oogenesis; meiosis

5-37. a
p 87
mitosis; cleavage of zygote

5-38. b
p 81
meiosis

5–39. b
p 87
embryo; embryonic period

5–40. a
p 88
implantation

5–41. e,c,b,f,d,a
pp 87–88
embryonic development

5–42. a,b,c,d
pp 87–88
embryonic development; implantation

5–43. a
p 87
inner cell mass; embryonic development

5–44. b,c
pp 89–90
syncytiotrophoblast

5–45. umbilical cord
p 92
embryonic development

5–46. G
p 93
embryonic period

5–47. E
p 93
embryonic period

5–48. C
p 93
embryonic period

5–49. H
p 93
embryonic period

5–50. I
p 93
embryonic period

5–51. D
p 93
embryonic period

5–52. A
p 93
embryonic period

5–53. F
p 93
embryonic period

5–54. a
p 92
germ layers, ectodermal derivatives

5–55. c
p 92
germ layers, endodermal derivatives

5–56. a
p 92
germ layers, ectodermal derivatives

5–57. b
p 92
germ layers, mesodermal derivatives

5–58. b
p 92
germ layers, mesodermal derivatives

5–59. c
p 92
germ layers, endodermal derivatives

5–60. b
p 92
germ layers, mesodermal derivatives

5–61. a,b,d
p 95
embryonic development; notochord

5–62. a
p 95
embryonic period

5–63. a,b
p 95
embryonic period, somite development

6–1. 1 = c; 2 = b
p 98
chorionic villi; angiogenesis

6–2. e
p 98
placenta, circulation

6–3. d
p 98
placenta, circulation

6–4. c
p 98
chorionic villi

6–5. b,c
p 98
chorionic villi; hydatidiform mole; trophoblast

6–6. a,b,c
p 98
chorionic villi; intervillous space

6–7. a,d
p 98
chorionic villi; intervillous space

6-8. e
p 98
embryonic development; placental development

6-9. a,b,c
p 98
placenta, cytotrophoblast; chorion

6-10. d,e
p 98
placenta, syncytiotrophoblast; chorion

6-11. 1 = b; 2 = a
p 98
chorion frondosum; chorion laeve; chorionic villi

6-12. c
pp 98-99
chorion frondosum; chorion laeve; chorion; prostaglandin, synthesis; labor

6-13. a
p 99
amniochorion

6-14. a stem villus and its branches
p 99
placenta, cotyledons

6-15. b
p 99
placenta, cotyledons

6-16. a,c,d
pp 100-101
placenta

6-17. a,e
pp 100-101
decidua; decidual reaction

6-18. d
p 101
decidua capsularis

6-19. E
p 102 (Fig. 6-6)
decidua vera

6-20. H
p 102 (Fig. 6-6)
decidua capsularis

6-21. B
p 102 (Fig. 6-6)
decidua basalis

6-22. C
p 102 (Fig. 6-6)
chorion frondosum

6-23. G
p 102 (Fig. 6-6)
chorion laeve

6-24. a
p 101
decidua; decidua vera; decidua basalis

6-25. d
p 101
decidua; zona basalis; endometrium, regeneration

6-26. b
p 102
decidua; zona spongiosa

6-27. a
p 101
decidua; zona compacta

6-28. b,c
pp 102-103
decidua basalis; decidua vera

6-29. Nitabuch layer
p 103
decidua; Nitabuch layer

6-30. a,b
p 103
decidua; placenta accreta; Nitabuch layer

6-31. a,b,c,d,e
p 103
decidua; abortion

6-32. a,e
p 104
decidua; prolactin; amnionic fluid, prolactin; arachidonic acid

6-33. a,b,d,e
p 104
decidua; relaxin; 1,25-dihydroxyvitamin D_3

6-34. b,c
pp 105,107
cytotrophoblast; syncytiotrophoblast

6-35. b
p 107
placenta

6-36. syncytiotrophoblast (syncytium)
p 107
placenta, hormones; syncytiotrophoblast

6-37. a,b,d
p 107
placenta

6-38. D
p 110 (Fig. 6-14)
myometrium

6-39. A
p 110 (Fig. 6-14)
chorionic plate

6–40. B
p 110 (Fig. 6-14)
placenta, villi

6–41. C
p 110 (Fig. 6-14)
decidua basalis

6–42. c
p 107
fetal circulation; umbilical vein

6–43. a,d,e,f
pp 107-108,110
placenta, circulation

6–44. b,c,d
pp 109-110
placenta, circulation; uterus, contractions; intervillous space

6–45. a,c,d
p 110
placenta, circulation; intervillous space

6–46. a,b,c,d,e
p 110
placenta; uteroplacental circulation; cytotrophoblasts

6–47. none of the explanations is *adequate*
p 110
placenta, immunology

6–48. a,e
pp 110-113
placenta, immunology; fetal circulation

6–49. e
pp 114-115
amnion; prostaglandins

6–50. a,b,d
p 115
umbilical cord; fetal circulation; umbilical artery; umbilical vein

6–51. Meckel's diverticulum
p 115
umbilical cord; Meckel's diverticulum

6–52. a
p 115
umbilical cord; congenital anomalies; umbilical artery

6–53. e
p 115
umbilical cord

6–54. a,b,c
pp 115-116
umbilical cord, false knots; fetal circulation; Wharton jelly

7–1. a,b,c
pp 119-120
hCG

7–2. a,d,e,f
p 120
hCG, alpha subunit; hCG, beta subunit

7–3. *None* of the glycoprotein hormones has an alpha subunit significantly different from the others.
p 120
hormones, glycoprotein; alpha subunit, glycoprotein hormones

7–4. a
p 120
hCG, beta subunit; hLH, beta subunit

7–5. a
p 120
hormones, glycoprotein; beta subunit, glycoprotein hormones

7–6. b,c
p 120
hCG, synthesis; hCG, pregnancy

7–7. b,c
p 120
hCG, secretion

7–8. maintenance of corpus luteum function in early pregnancy
p 120
hCG, actions; corpus luteum

7–9. a,b,c,d,f
pp 120-121
hCG, actions; hCG, metabolism

7–10. a,b
pp 121-122
pregnancy tests; hCG, beta subunit

7–11. a,b
p 122
hCG, metabolism

7–12. b,d
p 122
hCG, metabolism; hydatidiform mole, hCG levels; multifetal pregnancy, hCG levels; hCG, hydatidiform mole; hCG, multifetal pregnancy

7–13. b
p 122
hCG, metabolism; hCG, renal clearance

7–14. a
p 121
hCG, actions; testosterone, fetal

7-15. a,b,c,d,f
p 122
hPL, synthesis; hPL, secretion; syncytiotrophoblast; growth hormone

7-16. a,b,e
pp 122-123
hPL; fertilization

7-17. c
p 123
hPL

7-18. a,b,d
p. 123
hPL, actions; free fatty acids; glucose metabolism

7-19. b
p 123
hPL, actions

7-20. b
p 123
labor, ACTH; labor, associated hormones

7-21. a,b,c,d
pp 123-124
placenta, hormones; ACTH; LHRH; TRH; CRF

7-22. a,c
p 124
pregnancy specific proteins

7-23. b
p 124
estrogen, synthesis; pregnancy, estrogen metabolism

7-24. b,d
p 124
estrogen, pregnancy

7-25. b
p 125
estrogen, pregnancy; oophorectomy, effect on pregnancy

7-26. c
p 125
estriol, synthesis

7-27. The placenta lacks steroid 17α-hydroxylase activity and, therefore, cannot convert C_{21}-steroids to C_{19}-steroids which are the precursors of estrogen.
p 125
estrogen, synthesis

7-28. c
p 124
estriol, synthesis

7-29. b
p 125
estrone, synthesis

7-30. a
p 125
estradiol-17β

7-31. d
p 125
dehydroisoandrosterone sulfate (DS); adrenal cortex, fetal

7-32. a,b,c,d
p 125
estrogen, pregnancy; placenta

7-33. a
p 125
estrogen, pregnancy; placenta; dehydroisoandrosterone sulfate

7-34. a,b,d,e
pp 125-126
dehydroisoandrosterone sulfate; hypertension, pregnancy

7-35. b
p 126
estriol, pregnancy

7-36. a,b,d
p 127
estrogen, pregnancy; anencephaly

7-37. b
p 127
estrogen, pregnancy; Addison's disease

7-38. androgen is efficiently aromatized to estrogen by the placenta
p 127
virilization, fetus

7-39. a,b,c
pp 127-128
adrenal gland, fetal

7-40. a,b
p 127
adrenal gland, fetal; adrenal gland, maternal

7-41. a,b
p 128
adrenal gland, fetal

7-42. a
p 128
adrenal gland, fetal

7-43. a,b
p 129
adrenal gland, fetal

7-44. de novo synthesis from cholesterol
p 129
adrenal gland, fetal; cortisol

7-45. a,c,e
pp 127-130
adrenal gland, fetal

7-46. **a,c,d**
p 130
adrenal gland, fetal

7-47. **b**
p 130
dehydroisoandrosterone sulfate; hyperprolactinemia; bromocriptine

7-48. **1 = b; 2 = b**
p 130
adrenal gland; prolactin; puerperium, endocrine changes

7-49. **a,b,c**
pp 131-132
estriol; fetal well-being, estriol

7-50. **b**
p 131
estriol; fetal well-being, estriol

7-51. **c,d,e,f**
p 131
estriol; fetal well-being, estriol; multifetal pregnancy; placental sulfatase

7-52. **a**
p 131
estriol, urinary level; aspirin

7-53. **a**
p 131
estriol, urinary level; pyelonephritis

7-54. **a**
p 131
estriol, urinary level; anencephaly

7-55. **b**
p 131
estriol, urinary level; Rh isoimmunization

7-56. **a**
p 131
estriol, urinary level; glucocorticosteroids

7-57. ichthyosis
p 131
placental, sulfatase; ichthyosis

7-58. **a,b,c,d**
pp 132-133
estetrol; fetal well-being

7-59. **b**
p 133
estriol; fetal well-being, estriol

7-60. **b,c**
pp 133-134
progestrone, pregnancy; cholesterol

7-61. **d**
p 119
deoxycorticosterone

7-62. **a**
p 119
estradiol-17β

7-63. **b**
p 119
estriol

7-64. **c**
pp 119, 134
progesterone, levels

7-65. **e**
p 122
hPL, levels

7-66. **a,b,d**
p 135
placenta, hormones; adrenal gland, fetal

8-1. **c**
p 139
gestational age

8-2. **a and d; b and c**
p 139
fertilization age; ovulation age; gestational age; menstrual age

8-3. **c**
p 139
implantation

8-4. **a,d,c,b,e**
p 139
implantation; embryonic development

8-5. **d**
p 139
embryonic development

8-6. **a,b,c,d,e**
p 139
embryonic development; pregnancy testing

8-7. **a**
p 140
embryonic period; organogenesis

8-8. **b**
pp 142-143
fetal development

8-9. **a**
pp 142-143
fetal development

8-10. **e**
pp 142-143
fetal development

8-11. **d**
pp 142-143
fetal development

8–12. f
pp 142-143
fetal development

8–13. 1 = 36 cm; 2 = 3400 g
p 143
fetus, term; crown-rump length; fetal weight

8–14. a,c
pp 143-144
crown-rump length; gestational age determination

8–15. a,b,d
p 144
birth weight

8–16. e
pp 144-145
fetus, head

8–17. b,c
p 144 (*Fig. 8-7*)
fetus, head; sutures

8–18. e
p 144
fetus, head; sutures; labor, pelvic examination

8–19. b
p 144
fetus, head; fontanels

8–20. c
p 144
fetus, head; fontanels

8–21. a
p 144
fetus, head; fontanels

8–22. a,b
p 144
fetus, head; fontanels

8–23. b
p 145
fetus, head; biparietal diameter

8–24. d
p 145
fetus, head; occipitomental diameter

8–25. a
p 145
occipitofrontal diameter

8–26. 1 = occipitofrontal; 2 = suboccipitobregmatic
p 145
fetus, head; occipitofrontal diameter; suboccipitobregmatic diameter

8–27. b
p 145
molding, fetal head; accommodation

8–28. a
p 145
gestation age, determination

8–29. a,c
pp 145-146
placental transfer; intervillous space; Rh sensitization; maternal-fetal bleeding

8–30. a,b,c,d,e,f,g,h,i
p 146
placental transfer; intervillous space

8–31. a,c,d,e,f
pp 146-147
intervillous space; uteroplacental blood flow

8–32. b,c,d
p 147
placental transfer; intervillous space

8–33. b,c,d
p 147
placental transfer

8–34. c,d
p 147
placental transfer; simple diffusion; anesthesia, inhalation

8–35. b
p 147
placental transfer

8–36. a,b
pp 147-148
placental transfer; oxygen transfer

8–37. a,b,c
p 148
hemoglobin, fetal; oxygenation, fetal

8–38. a,c
pp 148-149
placental transfer; carbon dioxide, transfer

8–39. a,b,c,d,e
p 149
iron transport; placental transfer; selective transport; melanoma, malignant; intrauterine infection

8–40. a,c,e
p 149
circulation, fetal; inferior vena cava; superior vena cava

8–41. ductus arteriosus
p 149
ductus arteriosus; circulation, fetal

8–42. d,c,a,b
p 149-150
circulation, fetal; oxygenation, fetal

8–43. a,d
pp 150-151
circulation, fetal

8–44. b,c,e
p 151
circulation, fetal; ductus arteriosus; prostaglandins

8–45. a
p 151
circulation, fetal; ductus arteriosus; prostaglandins, actions; prostaglandin synthetase inhibitors; patent ductus arteriosus (PDA)

8–46. a,b
p 151
circulation, fetal; foramen ovale; circulation, neonatal; birth, circulatory changes

8–47. c
p 151
umbilical artery; umbilical ligament

8–48. a
p 151
ligamentum teres; umbilical vein

8–49. b
p 151
ligamentum venosum; ductus venosus

8–50. a,d,e
pp 151-152
blood, fetal; hematopoiesis, fetal; erythrocytes, fetal

8–51. e
p 152
hemoglobin, fetus; Gower-1

8–52. c
p 152
hemoglobin, fetus; Gower-2

8–53. d
p 152
hemoglobin, fetus; hemoglobin F

8–54. b
p 152
hemoglobin, fetus; hemoglobin A

8–55. a
p 152
hemoglobin, fetus; hemoglobin A_2

8–56. b
p 152
hemoglobin, fetus; hemoglobin A

8–57. at higher temperatures, the affinity of fetal blood for oxygen decreases
p 152
hypoxia, fetus; hemoglobin, fetus; oxygenation, fetal

8–58. a,b,c,d,f
pp 151-153
hematopoiesis, fetus; erythropoietin

8–59. a
p 153
erythropoietin

8–60. b
p 153
coagulation factors, neonate

8–61. b
p 153
coagulation factors, neonate

8–62. b
p 153
coagulation factors, neonate

8–63. b
p 153
coagulation factors, neonate

8–64. b
p 153
coagulation factors, neonate

8–65. a
p 153
platelets; blood, fetus

8–66. a
p 153
coagulation factors, neonate; thrombin time, neonate

8–67. VIII
p 153
coagulation factors, fetus; hemophilia; Factor VIII

8–68. a,c
p 153
immunoglobulins, fetus

8–69. fetal infection has provoked a fetal immune response
p 153
immunoglobulins, fetus; infection, fetal

8–70. c
p 153
urine, fetus

8–71. a,c,e
p 153
urinary system, fetus; intrauterine growth retardation; urinary tract, anomalies

8–72. b
p 153
urinary system, fetus

8–73. a,b,c,d,e
p 154
respiratory system, fetus; surfactant

8–74. d
p 154 (Fig. 8-14)
surfactant; phosphatidylcholine

8–75. phosphatidylglycerol
p 154
phosphatidylglycerol; surfactant; respiratory distress syndrome

8–76. 1 = lecithin; 2 = sphingomyelin
p 155
surfactant; L/S ratio; lung maturity, fetal

8–77. a,b,c,d
p 155
surfactant; phosphatidylglycerol

8–78. phosphatidate phosphohydrolase (PAPase)
p 156
surfactant

8–79. 1 = a; 2 = c
p 157
surfactant; lung maturation, fetus; phosphatidylglycerol; phosphatidylinositol

8–80. 1 = phosphatidylcholine and phosphatidylinositol; 2 = phosphatidylglycerol
p 159
respiratory distress syndrome; diabetes, maternal; surfactant; phosphatidylcholine; phosphatidylglycerol; phosphatidylinositol

8–81. b,d
pp 160-162
surfactant; corticosteriods, actions; prolactin, actions; respiratory distress syndrome

8–82. b
p 163
respiration, fetus; breathing, fetal

8–83. a,b,c,e
pp 163-164
respiratory system, fetus; fetal breathing

8–84. a,b,c
p 164
digestive system, fetus; fetal swallowing; amnionic fluid

8–85. a,b,c
p 165
digestive system, fetus; meconium; biliverdin; hypoxia, fetal

8–86. a,b,e
p 165
liver, fetus; bilirubin, fetal

8–87. b,c,d
p 165
pancreas, fetus; insulin, fetus

8–88. b
p 165
pancreas, fetus; glucagon, fetus

8–89. a,b,c,d,e
p 165
pituitary, fetus

8–90. b
p 165
pituitary, fetus; growth hormone

8–91. a,c,d,f
p 166
thyroid function, fetus

8–92. a
p 166
parathyroid, fetus

8–93. antidiuretic hormone
p 166
antidiuretic hormone, fetus; urine production, fetal

8–94. b
p 166
testosterone, fetus

8–95. c
pp 166-167
nervous system, fetus

8–96. e
pp 166-167
nervous system, fetus

8–97. f
pp 166-167
nervous system, fetus

8–98. b
pp 166-167
nervous system, fetus

8–99. f
pp 166-167
nervous system, fetus

8–100. b,c,d
p 167
immunology, fetus; immunoglobulins, fetus

8–101. c
p 168
nutrition, fetus; placental transfer

8–102. b
p 168
nutrition, fetus; glucose levels, fetal

8–103. b,c,d,f
pp 168-169
intrauterine growth retardation; placental transfer; vascular disease, maternal; uteroplacental blood flow; nutrition, maternal

8–104. a,b,c,d
p 169
amnionic fluid

8–105. b
p 169
amnionic fluid; hydramnios; postterm pregnancy; prolonged pregnancy

8–106. a,c,d
pp 169–170
amnionic fluid

8–107. urinary, gastrointestinal, respiratory
pp 169–170
amnionic fluid

8–108. b
p 170
hydramnios; esophageal atresia

8–109. a
p 170
oligohydramnios; renal agenesis

8–110. a
p 170
oligohydramnios; rupture of the membranes

8–111. a
p 170
oligohydramnios; pulmonary hypoplasia

8–112. b
p 170
sex ratios

8–113. b
p 170
sex differentiation

8–114. a,b,c,d,e
pp 170–172
sex differentiation

8–115. androgens
p 172
sex differentiation; ambiguous genitalia

8–116. a,c
pp 172–175
sex differentiation; female psuedohermaphroditism; dysgenetic gonads; true hermaphroditism

8–117. b
pp 172–175
sex differentiation; male pseudohermaphroditism

8–118. a
pp 172–175
sex differentiation; female pseudohermaphroditism

8–119. a,c
pp 172–175
female pseudohermaphroditism; dysgenetic gonads; true hermaphroditism

8–120. b
pp 172–175
sex differentiation; male pseudohermaphroditism

8–121. a
pp 172–175
sex differentiation; female pseudohermaphroditism

8–122. c
pp 172–175
sex differentiation; dysgenetic gonads; true hermaphroditism

8–123. adrenal gland
p 172
female pseudohermaphroditism; sex differentiation

8–124. capacity of trophoblast to convert aromatizable C_{19}-steroids to estrogens
p 172
female pseudohermaphroditism; virilization, fetal

8–125. a
p 172
sex differentiation; female pseudohermaphroditism

8–126. a,b
p 173
sex differentiation.

8–127. a,b,c,e
p 173
testicular feminization; sex differentiation.

8–128. familial male pseudohermaphroditism; a spectrum of abnormalities affecting genital virilization
p 173
sex differentiation; male pseudohermaphroditism

8–129. c
p 175
Turner syndrome; dysgenetic gonads; sex differentiation

8–130. a,b,d
p 175
sex differentiation

8–131. b
p 175
genital ambiguity; sex differentiation

9–1. b
p 181
uterus, pregnancy; myometrial cell hypertrophy

9–2. a,b,d,e
p 181
uterus, pregnancy; uterus, blood supply; uterus, nerve supply

9–3. b
p 181
uterus, pregnancy; uterine enlargement, pregnancy; uterine hypertrophy; pregnancy, first trimester

9-4. b
p 181
polyamine levels, pregnancy; pregnancy, first trimester

9-5. c
pp 181-182
uterus, pregnancy; uterine enlargement, pregnancy

9-6. a
p 182
uterine enlargement, pregnancy; placenta, implantation site

9-7. a,b,d
p 182
uterus, pregnancy

9-8. a,c,d,e
p 182
uterus, pregnancy; uterine contractions; Braxton Hicks contractions

9-9. c
p 183
uteroplacental blood flow; cardiovascular changes, pregnancy

9-10. a
p 183
uteroplacental blood flow; uterus, contractions

9-11. a,b,c,e
pp 183-184
uteroplacental blood flow; estrogen, actions; angiotensin II

9-12. cyanosis and softening
pp 184-185
cervix, pregnancy

9-13. a,b
pp 185-186
cervix, pregnancy; cervical mucus; erosions of the cervix

9-14. b,c
p 186
ovary, pregnancy; corpus luteum, pregnancy

9-15. a,c
p 186
relaxin, pregnancy; corpus luteum, pregnancy

9-16. b,c,d
pp 186-187
luteoma, pregnancy; virilization, maternal; virilization, fetal

9-17. a
p 187
ovary, pregnancy; decidual reaction, ovary

9-18. c
p 187
oviduct, pregnancy

9-19. a,c,d
p 187
vagina, pregnancy

9-20. Chadwick sign
p 187
vagina, pregnancy; Chadwick sign

9-21. a,c,d
p 187
vagina, pregnancy; vaginal secretions, pregnancy; vagina, pH; Lactobacillus; *cervix, pregnancy; cervical secretions, pregnancy*

9-22. b,c
p 187
striae gravidarum; cutaneous changes, pregnancy

9-23. diastasis recti
p 187
diastasis recti

9-24. a
p 188
linea nigra; cutaneous changes, pregnancy

9-25. b
p 188
chloasma; cutaneous changes, pregnancy

9-26. b
p 188
chloasma; oral contraceptives, side effects

9-27. a,b
p 188
vascular spiders; palmar erythema; cutaneous changes, pregnancy

9-28. a,b
p 188
vascular spiders; palmar erythema; hyperestrogenemia, pregnancy; cutaneous changes, pregnancy

9-29. a,b
p 188
vascular spiders; palmar erythema; cutaneous changes, pregnancy

9-30. a
p 188
vascular spiders; nevus; telangiectasis; cutaneous changes, pregnancy

9-31. a,b,c,d,e
p 188
breasts, pregnancy; colostrom; striae gravidarum

9-32. glands (follicles) of Montgomery
p 188
breasts, pregnancy; glands of Montgomery

9-33. 27 to 28 pounds (earlier reported values were about 24 pounds)
pp 188, 189 (Table 9-1)
pregnancy, weight gain

9-34. a,c,d
pp 188-189
water metabolism, pregnancy; pregnancy, weight gain; puerperium, weight loss; puerperium, diuresis

9-35. b
p 189
protein metabolism, pregnancy

9-36. b
p 189
carbohydrate metabolism, pregnancy; lipid metabolism, pregnancy; fatty acid metabolism, pregnancy

9-37. a,b,c
pp 189-190
carbohydrate metabolism, pregnancy; hPL; pancreas, pregnancy

9-38. c
p 190
carbohydrate metabolism, pregnancy; tolbutamide

9-39. a,b,d
p 190 (Table 9-2)
lipid metabolism, pregnancy; free fatty acids; cholesterol

9-40. a,d,e
pp 190-191
lipid metabolism, pregnancy; breast feeding; progesterone, actions

9-41. a,b,c,d
p 191
acid-base equilibrium, pregnancy; 2,3-diphosphoglycerate; respiratory function, pregnancy

9-42. a
p 191
minerals, pregnancy; copper

9-43. b
p 191
sodium levels, pregnancy

9-44. b
p 191
minerals, pregnancy; magnesium

9-45. c
p 191
minerals, pregnancy; phosphorus

9-46. b
p 191
potassium levels, pregnancy

9-47. b,d
p 191
blood volume, pregnancy; hematologic changes, pregnancy

9-48. c
p 191
blood volume, pregnancy; hematologic changes, pregnancy; erythrocyte volume, pregnancy

9-49. 33
p 192
hematologic changes; pregnancy; erythrocytes, pregnancy

9-50. b,c,d
p 192
hematologic changes, pregnancy; erythrocytes, pregnancy

9-51. b
p 192
hemoglobin, pregnancy; anemia, pregnancy

9-52. b
p 192
iron requirements, pregnancy

9-53. a
p 193
iron requirements, pregnancy; hematologic changes, pregnancy; erythrocytes, pregnancy

9-54. b,d
p 193
iron requirements, pregnancy; iron absorption, pregnancy

9-55. c
p 193
blood loss, vaginal delivery

9-56. b
p 193
blood loss, vaginal delivery; blood loss, cesarean section; multifetal pregnancy, blood loss

9-57. a,b
p 193
blood volume, labor; blood volume, delivery; blood volume, puerperium; erythrocytes, pregnancy

9-58. c
p 193
leukocyte count, pregnancy; leukocyte count, labor; puerperium

9-59. a
p 193
alkaline phosphatase levels, leukocytes

9-60. a
p 193
blood coagulation, pregnancy

9-61. a (slightly)
p 194
blood coagulation, pregnancy

9-62. a
p 194
blood coagulation, pregnancy

9-63. a
p 194
blood coagulation, pregnancy

9-64. a
p 194
blood coagulation, pregnancy

9-65. a
p 194
blood coagulation, pregnancy

9-66. b
p 194
blood coagulation, pregnancy

9-67. b
p 194
blood coagulation, pregnancy

9-68. a
p 194
sedimentation rate, pregnancy

9-69. b
p 194
blood coagulation, pregnancy; Quick one-stage prothrombin time

9-70. b
p 194
blood coagulation, pregnancy; partial thromboplastin time

9-71. c
p 194
blood coagulation, pregnancy; clot retraction test

9-72. a,b
p 194
blood coagulation, pregnancy; platelets, pregnancy; fibrinogen

9-73. a,b,d,e
p 194
blood coagulation, pregnancy; fibrinolysis, pregnancy; fibrin degradation products

9-74. b,c,d
p 194
cardiovascular system, pregnancy; heart displacement, pregnancy

9-75. b
p 194
cardiovascular system, pregnancy; cardiomegaly

9-76. a
p 194
cardiovascular system, pregnancy; cardiac volume

9-77. a
p 194
cardiovascular system, pregnancy; ventricular wall mass

9-78. a
pp 194-195
cardiovascular system, pregnancy; stroke volume

9-79. c
p 195
cardiovascular system, pregnancy; inotropic state of the myocardium

9-80. a
p 194
cardiovascular system, pregnancy; heart rate, pregnancy

9-81. a,c,d,e,f
p 195
cardiovascular system, pregnancy; heart sounds; heart murmurs

9-82. d
p 195
cardiovascular system pregnancy; electrocardiogram changes, pregnancy

9-83. a,c,d
p 195
cardiovascular system, pregnancy; cardiac output; labor, cardiovascular function

9-84. c
p 195
circulation, pregnancy; blood pressure, pregnancy

9-85. a
p 195
blood pressure, pregnancy

9-86. c,d
pp 195-196
venous pressure, pregnancy; supine hypotension, pregnancy; blood flow, pregnancy

9-87. b,c,d
p 196
venous pressure, pregnancy; hemorrhoids; varicose veins; edema, pregnancy; circulation, pregnancy

9-88. a,b,c,d
p 196
circulatory system, pregnancy; supine position, pregnancy; supine hypotension, pregnancy; cardiac output, pregnancy

9-89. b
p 196
circulatory system, pregnancy; blood pressure, pregnancy; uteroplacental function

9-90. b,c
pp 195-196
circulatory system, pregnancy; supine position, pregnancy; blood pressure; cardiac output, pregnancy; blood flow, pregnancy

9–91. a
p 196
circulatory system, pregnancy; cutaneous changes, pregnancy; blood flow, pregnancy

9–92. a,b,c
p 196
respiratory function, pregnancy; musculoskeletal system, pregnancy

9–93. b
p 196
respiratory tract pregnancy; pulmonary function, pregnancy; maternal arteriovenous oxygen difference

9–94. c
p 196
respiratory system, pregnancy; pulmonary function, pregnancy; maximum breathing capacity

9–95. b
p 196
respiratory system, pregnancy; pulmonary function, pregnancy; functional residual capacity

9–96. c
p 196
respiratory system, pregnancy; pulmonary function, pregnancy; lung compliance

9–97. a
p 196
respiratory system, pregnancy; pulmonary function, pregnancy; airway conductance

9–98. a
p 196
respiratory system, pregnancy; pulmonary function, pregnancy; tidal volume

9–99. b
p 196
respiratory system, pregnancy; pulmonary function, pregnancy; total pulmonary resistance

9–100. the effects of progesterone and to a lesser extent estrogen on the respiratory center
p 197
respiratory system, pregnancy; progesterone, actions; estrogen, actions

9–101. a,c,d
pp 197-198
urinary system, pregnancy; vitamins, pregnancy; renal function, pregnancy

9–102. c
p 198
renal function tests, pregnancy; creatinine clearance

9–103. water accumulated during the day as dependent edema is mobilized and excreted at night (therefore, concentrated urine may not be excreted even after withholding fluids for 18 hours)
p 198
renal function tests, pregnancy

9–104. a,b
pp 190, 198
urinary system, pregnancy; glucosuria, pregnancy

9–105. b
p 198
urinary system, pregnancy; proteinuria, pregnancy; preeclampsia

9–106. a,b,c,d
pp 198-200
urinary system, pregnancy; progesterone, actions; ureters, pregnancy

9–107. b,c
p 200
urinary system, pregnancy; bladder, pregnancy; urinary tract infection, pregnancy

9–108. a,b,c
p 200
gastrointestinal system, pregnancy; gastric-emptying time

9–109. upward and laterally
p 200
gastrointestinal system, pregnancy; appendix, pregnancy

9–110. b
p 201
liver, pregnancy

9–111. a
p 201
liver, pregnancy; alkaline phosphatase activity, serum

9–112. b
p 201
liver, pregnancy; albumin concentration, plasma

9–113. b
p 201
liver, pregnancy; cholinesterase activity, plasma

9–114. a
p 201
liver, pregnancy; leucine aminopeptidase activity, serum

9–115. a,c,d,e
pp 200-201
gastrointestinal system, pregnancy; gallbladder, pregnancy; hemorrhoids, pregnancy

9–116. b
p 201
pituitary gland, pregnancy

9–117. a,c,d
pp 201-202
pituitary gland, pregnancy; prolactin; microadenomas, pituitary; growth hormone

9–118. b
p 202
pituitary gland, pregnancy; prolactin

9-119. a,b,d
p 202
pituitary gland, pregnancy; β-endorphins

9-120. a,d
pp 202-203
thyroid gland, pregnancy; goiter, maternal; hydatidiform mole; hCG, actions

9-121. a = increased; b = not increased; c = increased; d = increased; e = increased; f = increased; g = increased; h = increased; i = not increased; j = not increased; k = not increased; l = increased; m = not increased; n = not increased; o = increased
p 203 (Table 9-5)
thyroid gland, pregnancy

9-122. 1 = a; 2 = c
p 203
thyroid gland, pregnancy

9-123. c,d
p 203
parathyroid gland, pregnancy; calcitonin; vitamin D

9-124. c,d,e
p 204
adrenal gland, pregnancy; aldosterone, pregnancy; renin; angiotensin

9-125. a,b,c
p 205
musculoskeletal system, pregnancy; lordosis, maternal

9-126. b
p 205
musculoskeletal system, pregnancy

9-127. b
p 205
precocious puberty; menarche

9-128. a
p 205
pregnancy, complications; maternal age, effect on pregnancy

10-1. c,d,e
p 211
pregnancy, positive evidence; pregnancy, diagnosis; fetal movement; fetal heart tones

10-2. 120 to 160 beats per minute
p 211
fetal heart rate

10-3. c,d
p 211
ultrasonography, real time; fetal heart activity; echocardiography

10-4. a,d,e,f
pp 211-212
fetal heart sounds

10-5. b
p 212
uterine souffle; auscultation of abdomen

10-6. a
p 211
funic souffle; auscultation of abdomen

10-7. d
p 211
auscultation of abdomen; intestinal peristalsis, maternal

10-8. c
p 212
auscultation of abdomen; fetal movement

10-9. a
p 211
funic souffle; auscultation of abdomen

10-10. b
p 212
uterine souffle; auscultation of abdomen

10-11. a
p 211
funic souffle; auscultation of abdomen

10-12. b
p 212
uterine souffle; auscultation of abdomen; leiomyoma uteri

10-13. b,c,d,e
p 212
fetal movement

10-14. a,c,d
p 212
diagnosis of pregnancy; ultrasonography

10-15. a,b,c
p 212
blighted ovum; abortion, spontaneous; ultrasonography

10-16. a,b,c,d,e,f
pp 212-213
ultrasonography

10-17. a
p 213
ultrasonography

10-18. 16
p 213
diagnosis of pregnancy; radiography; ossification, fetal bones

10-19. a
p 213
pregnancy, probable evidence

10-20. a,b
p 213
pregnancy, nulliparous; pregnancy, multiparous

10–21. b
p 213
pregnancy, multiparous

10–22. b
p 213
pregnancy, multiparous

10–23. a,b
p 213
pregnancy, nulliparous; pregnancy, multiparous

10–24. a,c,f
p 213
pregnancy, probable evidence; uterus, pregnancy; cervix, pregnancy

10–25. e
p 213
pregnancy, probable evidence; Braxton Hicks contractions

10–26. ballottement
p 214
pregnancy, probable evidence; ballottement

10–27. diagnostic errors may arise from the presence of anatomic abnormalities (such as leiomyomata) or variations in the size of the normal uterus
p 214
pregnancy, probable evidence.

10–28. b
p 214
pregnancy tests

10–29. hCG (human chorionic gonadotropin)
p 214
pregnancy tests; hCG

10–30. c,d
p 214
pregnancy tests; hCG; LH; radioimmunoassay

10–31. b
p 215
hCG, levels

10–32. a
pp 212, 215
pregnancy, diagnosis; pregnancy tests; hCG; ultrasonography

10–33. a,b,c
p 215
pregnancy tests, false results; pregnancy, diagnosis; menopause

10–34. c
p 215
pregnancy tests, home kits; pregnancy, diagnosis

10–35. b
p 216
pregnancy tests, progesterone withdrawal; amenorrhea; pregnancy, diagnosis

10–36. a,c
pp 216–217
pregnancy tests; hCG; ectopic pregnancy

10–37. d
p 217
hCG, postabortion monitoring

10–38. a,b,c,d,e,f,g,i,j
p 217
pregnancy, presumptive evidence; pregnancy, diagnosis

10–39. c,e
p 217
pregnancy, presumptive evidence; amenorrhea

10–40. a,b,c,d
pp 216–217
pregnancy, presumptive evidence; breasts

10–41. c
p 218
pregnancy, presumptive evidence; Chadwick sign

10–42. a
p 218
pregnancy, presumptive evidence; skin pigmentation; oral contraceptives, side effects

10–43. b,c,e
p 218
pregnancy, presumptive evidence

10–44. b
p 218
pregnancy, differential diagnosis; hematometra

10–45. a,b,c,e,f
p 218
pseudocyesis

10–46. a,b
p 219
pregnancy, multiparous; pregnancy, nulliparous; striae gravidarium

10–47. a
p 219
pregnancy, nulliparous; labia majora

10–48. b
p 219
pregnancy, multiparous

10–49. b
p 219
pregnancy, multiparous; myrtiform caruncles

10–50. a
p 219
pregnancy, nulliparous

10–51. b,d
p 219
fetal death; ultrasonography, real time

10–52. a,e
p 219
fetal death

11–1. accommodation
p 221
labor; pelvis; accommodation

11–2. linea terminalis
p 221
pelvis, anatomy; linea terminalis

11–3. c
p 221
pelvis, anatomy; false pelvis

11–4. b
p 221
pelvis, anatomy; false pelvis

11–5. a
p 221
pelvis, anatomy; false pelvis

11–6. d
p 221
pelvis, anatomy; false pelvis

11–7. a = pubic bones, the ascending superior rami of the ischial bones; b = anterior surface of sacrum; c = inner surface of the ischial bones, sacrosciatic notches, and sacrosciatic ligaments; d = promontory and alae of sacrum, linea terminalis, and the upper margins of the pubic bones; e = pelvic outlet
p 221
pelvis, anatomy; true pelvis

11–8. a,c,e,f,g
p 221
pelvis, anatomy; true pelvis

11–9. a,b
p 221
pelvis, anatomy; sacrum; clinical pelvimetry

11–10. b
pp 222-223
clinical pelvimetry; pelvic inlet; obstetric conjugate

11–11. b
p 223
clinical pelvimetry; obstetric conjugate

11–12. subtract 1.5 to 2.0 cm from the measured length of the diagonal conjugate (which is the distance from the lower margin of the symphysis to the promontory of the sacrum)
p 223
clinical pelvimetry; obstetric conjugate

11–13. b
p 223
pelvis, anatomy; clinical pelvimetry

11–14. a = horizontal rami of the pubic bones and symphysis pubis; b = pubic arch; c = linea terminalis; d = sacrosciatic ligaments and the ischial tuberosities; e = promontory and alae of the sacrum; f = tip of sacrum; g = obstetric conjugate; h = lower margin of the symphysis pubis to the top of the sacrum; i = greatest distance between the linea terminalis; j = from the tip of the sacrum to a right angled intersection with a line between the ischial tuberosities
pp 222-223
pelvis, anatomy; planes of the pelvis

11–15. D
p 223 (Fig. 11-5)
pelvis, anatomy; midpelvis

11–16. B
p 223 (Fig. 11-5)
obstetric conjugate; pelvis, anatomy

11–17. A
p 223 (Fig. 11-5)
true conjugate; pelvis, anatomy

11–18. C
p 223 (Fig. 11-5)
diagonal conjugate; pelvis, anatomy

11–19. d
p 223
midpelvis; pelvis, anatomy

11–20. a,e
p 223
pelvis, anatomy

11–21. e
p 224
pelvis, anatomy; pelvic joints

11–22. a,f
p 224
pelvis, mobility; pelvic joints, pregnancy

11–23. b
pp 224-225
pelvis, mobility

11–24. a,b
p 225
pelvic types; Caldwell-Moloy classification

11–25. a
p 225 (Fig. 11-9)
pelvic shape; gynecoid pelvis

11–26. d
p 226 (Fig. 11-9)
pelvic shape; platypelloid pelvis

11–27. b
p 226 (Fig. 11-9)
pelvic shape; android pelvis

11-28. c
p 226 (Fig. 11-9)
pelvic shape; anthropoid pelvis

11-29. c
p 226
pelvic shape, frequency; anthropoid pelvis

11-30. a
p 226
pelvic shape, frequency; gynecoid pelvis

11-31. b
p 226
pelvic shape, frequency; android pelvis

11-32. d
p 226
pelvic shape, frequency; platypelloid pelvis

11-33. a,c
p 226
pelvic shape, frequency; gynecoid pelvis; anthropoid pelvis

11-34. b
p 226
pelvic shape; Caldwell-Moloy classification

11-35. b
p 226
pelvic shape; android pelvis

11-36. b,c,d
pp 226-227
pelvis, anatomy; pelvic size

11-37. a
pp 226-227
pelvis, anatomy; diagonal conjugate; clinical pelvimetry

11-38. descent of the biparietal plane of the fetal head to a level below that of the pelvic inlet
p 227
engagement

11-39. a,b,c
p 227
engagement

11-40. b
p 228
engagement

11-41. a,c,d
pp 227-228
engagement

11-42. a,b,c
p 228
pelvis, anatomy; pelvic outlet

11-43. c
p 228
pelvis, anatomy; pelvic outlet

11-44. d
p 229
midpelvis; pelvimetry, x-ray; clinical pelvimetry

11-45. a
p 229
pelvimetry, x-ray

11-46. a,d,e
p 229
pelvis, anatomy; pelvimetry, x-ray

11-47. a,b
p 230
pelvimetry, x-ray

11-48. a,b,c,d
p 231
pelvis, anatomy

11-49. b,c
p 231
pelvis, anatomy

11-50. a,b,c
p 231
pelvis, anatomy

12-1. habitus/attitude
p 235
fetus, attitude; habitus

12-2. a,c,d,e
p 235
fetus, attitude

12-3. b
p 235
fetus, posture; accommodation

12-4. relation of the long axis of the fetus to that of the mother
p 235
fetus, lie

12-5. b
p 235
fetus, lie; oblique lie

12-6. c
p 235
fetus, lie

12-7. a,b
p 235
fetus, presentation; fetus, lie; longitudinal lie

12-8. A
p 236
cephalic presentation, vertex; fetus, presentation

12-9. D
p 236
cephalic presentation, face; fetus, presentation

12–10. B
p 236
cephalic presentation, sinciput; fetus, presentation

12–11. C
p 236
cephalic presentation, brow; fetus, presentation

12–12. b
p 235
cephalic presentation, vertex; fetus, presentation

12–13. a
p 235
cephalic presentation, face; fetus, presentation

12–14. c
p 235
cephalic presentation, brow; fetus, presentation

12–15. d
p 235
cephalic presentation, sinciput; fetus, presentation

12–16. a
p 235
cephalic presentation, sinciput; cephalic presentation, brow; fetus, presentation

12–17. b
p 235
breech presentation, complete; fetus, presentation

12–18. a
p 235
breech presentation, frank; fetus presentation

12–19. c
p 235
breech presentation, incomplete; breech presentation, footling; fetus, presentation

12–20. the right or left side of the maternal birth canal
p 235
fetus, position

12–21. a = 96 percent; b = 3.5 percent; c = 0.3 percent; d = 0.4 percent
p 237
fetus, vertex presentation

12–22. c
p 237
breech presentation; prematurity, presentation

12–23. a,c,d,e
pp 237–238
fetus, presentation; hydrocephalus

12–24. a,b,c,d,e
p 238
fetus presentation, diagnostic methods; fetus position, diagnostic methods; ultrasonography; x-ray

12–25. c
pp 239–240
Leopold maneuvers; fetus presentation, diagnostic methods; fetus position, diagnostic methods

12–26. b
pp 238–239
fetus presentation, diagnostic methods; fetus position, diagnostic methods

12–27. a
pp 238–239
Leopold maneuvers; fetus presentation, diagnostic methods; fetus position, diagnostic methods

12–28. d
p 240
Leopold maneuvers; fetus presentation, diagnostic methods; fetus position, diagnostic methods

12–29. a,b,c,d
p 240
Leopold maneuvers; fetus presentation, diganostic methods; fetus position, diagnostic methods

12–30. sagittal
p 242
presentation; position; sagittal suture

12–31. b,c
p 242
presentation; position; auscultation

12–32. b
pp 242–243
ultrasonography; x-ray; fetus presentation, diagnostic methods; fetus position, diagnostic methods

13–1. a,b,c
p 245
prenatal care

13–2. b; ideally, prenatal care should be a continuation of a regimen of physician-supervised health care already established for the woman
p 245
prenatal care

13–3. d
p 246
primipara

13–4. b
p 245
gravida

13–5. c
p 246
nullipara

13–6. g
p 246
puerpera

13–7. f
p 246
parturient

13–8. e
p 246
multipara

13–9. a
p 245
nulligravida

13–10. primipara
p 246
primipara

13–11. d
p 246
obstetric history

13–12. d
p 246
pregnancy, duration

13–13. March 10
p 246
Naegele's rule; gestational age, determination; EDC (estimated date of confinement)

13–14. b
p 246
gestational age; menstrual age

13–15. c
p 246
gestational age

13–16. a,b,c,d
p 247
prenatal care, initial comprehensive obstetric evaluation; gestational age, determination

13–17. a,b,c
p 247
gestational age; prenatal care, initial comprehensive obstetric evaluation; oral contraceptives, effects

13–18. a,d
pp 247, 248
prenatal care, initial comprehensive obstetric evaluation; cervical cytology; gonorrhea, culture

13–19. c
p 248
vaginal secretions, pregnancy; prenatal care, initial comprehensive obstetric evaluation

13–20. b
p 248
prenatal care, initial comprehensive obstetric evaluation; clinical pelvimetry

13–21. the height of the fundus in cm equals the gestational age in weeks in most normal singleton pregnancies
p 248
gestational age; prenatal care; fundal height

13–22. b
p 248
dental care, pregnancy; caries, pregnancy

13–23. (1) vaginal bleeding; (2) swelling of the face or fingers; (3) severe or continuous headache; (4) dimness or blurring of vision; (5) abdominal pain; (6) persistent vomiting; (7) chills or fever; (8) dysuria; (9) escape of fluid from the vagina; (10) marked change in frequency or intensity of fetal movements
p 248
pregnancy, danger signals; prenatal care

13–24. a,b,c,d
p 248
high-risk pregnancy

13–25. c
p 248
prenatal care, return visits

13–26. b
p 248
prenatal care, return visits

13–27. a
p 248
prenatal care, return visits

13–28. a,b,e
p 249
prenatal care, return visits; fundal height; fetal heart sounds; gestational age, determination

13–29. a,b,c,d,e
p 249
prenatal care, routine monitoring; fetal heart rate; fetal movement

13–30. a,b,c
p 249
prenatal care, routine monitoring; fundal height

13–31. none of the tests *must* be repeated at *every* prenatal visit
p 249
prenatal care, routine monitoring; prenatal care, laboratory testing

13–32. b
p 250
nutrition pregnancy; preeclampsia

13–33. seven
p 250
low birth weight; neonatal mortality rate; weight gain, pregnancy

13-34. a,b,c,d,e,f
p 251
nutrition, pregnancy; high-risk pregnancy; weight gain, pregnancy

13-35. a,b,c,d
pp 250-251
weight gain, pregnancy; birth weight; low birth weight; diet, pregnancy

13-36. 300
p 251 (*Table 13-1*)
nutrition, pregnancy; caloric requirements, pregnancy

13-37. a,b
pp 251-252
nutrition, pregnancy; protein requirements, pregnancy; caloric requirements, pregnancy

13-38. iron; iodized salt should be utilized
p 252
nutrition, pregnancy; minerals, pregnancy; iron, pregnancy; iodine, pregnancy

13-39. a,d,e
pp 252-253
iron, pregnancy; nutrition, pregnancy

13-40. a,c,d
pp 252-253
iron, pregnancy; nutrition, pregnancy; nausea, pregnancy

13-41. b,c
p 253
calcium, pregnancy; nutrition, pregnancy

13-42. a,b,d
pp 253-254
zinc, pregnancy; nutrition, pregnancy; wound healing; acrodermatitis enteropathica

13-43. b,c,e
pp 253-254
minerals, pregnancy; nutrition, pregnancy; cretinism; goiter, fetal; potassium, pregnancy

13-44. b
p 254
sodium, pregnancy; nutrition, pregnancy; preeclampsia, etiology

13-45. c
p 254
fluoride, pregnancy

13-46. b
p 254
vitamins, pregnancy

13-47. a,c
p 255
folic acid, pregnancy; vitamins, pregnancy

13-48. a,b,c,d
p 255
vitamin B_{12}, *pregnancy; vitamins, pregnancy; breast milk, composition*

13-49. a,c
pp 255-256
vitamin B_6, *pregnancy; vitamins, pregnancy*

13-50. b
p 256
vitamin C, pregnancy; vitamins, pregnancy

13-51. b
p 254
iodine, pregnancy; minerals, pregnancy; cretinism, fetal

13-52. d
p 255
folic acid, pregnancy; vitamins, pregnancy

13-53. e
p 253
zinc, pregnancy; minerals, pregnancy; acrodermatitis enteropathica

13-54. c
p 254
iodine, pregnancy; vitamins, pregnancy; goiter, fetal

13-55. a
p 256
vitamin C, pregnancy; vitamins, pregnancy; scurvy

13-56. d
p 255
folic acid, pregnancy; vitamins, pregnancy; megaloblastic anemia

13-57. h
p 256
vitamin B_6, *pregnancy; vitamins, pregnancy; progressive sensory ataxia*

13-58. b,c
p 256
nutrition, pregnancy; weight gain, pregnancy; iron, pregnancy

13-59. a
p 256
exercise, pregnancy

13-60. a,b,c
p 256
exercise, pregnancy; multifetal pregnancy; hypertension, pregnancy; intrauterine growth retardation

13-61. a,b,c,d
pp 256-257
prenatal care; high-risk pregnancy, activity

13-62. b,c
p 257
prenatal care; travel, pregnancy

13-63. b
p 257
prenatal care

13-64. b
p 257
prenatal care; gastrointestinal system, pregnancy; laxatives, pregnancy

13-65. a
pp 257-258
prenatal care; coitus, pregnancy

13-66. b,c
p 258
prenatal care; douching, pregnancy; air embolism, pregnancy

13-67. b
p 258
striae gravidarum

13-68. a,c
p 258
smoking, pregnancy; perinatal death; low birth weight

13-69. a,b,c,d
p 258
smoking, pregnancy

13-70. a,b,c,d,e,f
p 259
fetal alcohol syndrome; alcohol, pregnancy; birth defects; intrauterine growth retardation

13-71. b,c,d
p 259
drug abuse, pregnancy; low birth weight

13-72. b,c,e
pp 259-260
prenatal care; immunization, pregnancy

13-73. a
p 260
medications, pregnancy; vitamin K, pregnancy; fetal coagulopathy

13-74. b
p 260
medications, pregnancy; platelet dysfunction

13-75. c
p 260
medications, pregnancy; ductus arteriosus

13-76. a
p 260
medications, pregnancy; fetal malformation

13-77. b
p 260
medications, pregnancy; placental function

13-78. b,e
pp 260-261
pregnancy, common complaints; nausea, pregnancy

13-79. a,c
p 261
pregnancy, common complaints; back pain, pregnancy; musculoskeletal system, pregnancy

13-80. b
pp 261-262
pregnancy, common complaints; varicosities, pregnancy

13-81. a,b,c,d
p 262
pregnancy, common complaints; hemorrhoids, pregnancy

13-82. b
p 262
pregnancy, common complaints; gastrointestinal system, pregnancy

13-83. b
p 262
nutrition, pregnancy; pica

13-84. b,d
pp 261-263
pregnancy, common complaints

13-85. a,b,c,d
p 263
vagina, pregnancy; vaginitis, pregnancy; Trichomonas; Candida

14-1. a,b,c,d,e,f,g,h
pp 267-268
antepartum care; fetal well-being; perinatal death rate

14-2. a,b,c,d,e,f
p 268
amniocentesis, risks; abortion; premature labor; Rh isoimmunization; umbilical cord trauma; intrauterine infection

14-3. a,b,c,d,e,f
pp 269-271
amniocentesis; amnionic fluid; congenital abnormalities; birth defects

14-4. a,b,c,d
pp 268, 272
amniocentesis; Rh isoimmunization; ultrasonography

14-5. a,b,c,d,e
pp 268, 272
amniocentesis, risks; postterm pregnancy; oligohydramnios

14-6. when the fetus is mature enough to have a reasonable chance of survival if delivery becomes necessary. This is especially the case after a suspected traumatic tap.
p 272
amniocentesis, risks; electronic fetal monitoring

14-7. e
p 272
amniocentesis; prenatal diagnosis

14-8. a,c
pp 272-273
amniocentesis, bloody tap; L/S ratio

14-9. type II pneumocytes
p 273
surfactant; fetal lung maturity

14-10. d
p 273
respiratory distress syndrome; L/S ratio; fetal lung maturity

14-11. a,b,
pp 273-274
L/S ratio; respiratory distress syndrome

14-12. 14
p 273
L/S ratio; respiratory distress syndrome; perinatal mortality; neonatal mortality

14-13. a,b,d
p 274
respiratory distress syndrome; L/S ratio; diabetes; erythroblastosis fetalis

14-14. a
p 274
respiratory distress syndrome; phosphatidylglycerol, amnionic fluid

14-15. a,b,c,d,e,f
p 274
surfactant; L/S ratio; foam stability test; phosphatidylglycerol

14-16. b
p 274
surfactant; foam stability test

14-17. a,c
pp 274-275
bilirubin, amnionic fluid

14-18. a,b,c
p 275
bilirubin, amnionic fluid; sickle cell anemia

14-19. a,b,c,d,e
p 275
amniocentesis, cytogenetic studies; spontaneous abortion; Down syndrome; neural tube defects; birth defects

14-20. f
p 276 (Table 14-2)
Trisomy 13; chromosomal abnormalities

14-21. d
p 276 (Table 14-2)
Trisomy 18; chromosomal abnormalities

14-22. a
p 276 (Table 14-2)
chromosomal abnormalities; Trisomy 21 (Down syndrome)

14-23. c
p 276 (Table 14-2)
chromosomal abnormalities

14-24. b
p 276 (Table 14-2)
chromosomal abnormalities

14-25. e
p 276 (Table 14-2)
chromosomal abnormalities

14-26. a,c,d
pp 275-276
amniocentesis

14-27. b
p 276
chromosomal abnormalities; amniocentesis, cytogenetic studies

14-28. b
p 276
amniocentesis; fetal sex determination; sex-linked inherited diseases

14-29. a,b
p 276
fetal sex determination; amniocentesis, cytogenetic studies

14-30. c
p 276
chromosomal abnormalities; inborn errors of metabolism; sex-linked inherited diseases

14-31. b,c
pp 276-277
β-thalsassemia; fetal hemoglobinopathy

14-32. b,c,d,e
p 277
α-fetoprotein, amnionic fluid; α-fetoprotein, fetal serum

14-33. a,b,c,d,e,f,g,h
p 277
α-fetoprotein, amnionic fluid

14-34. a,b,d
pp 277-278
α-fetoprotein, maternal serum; neural tube defects; congenital nephrosis

14-35. b
p 276
amniocentesis, cell fraction; fetal sex determination

14-36. a
p 273
amniocentesis, supernatant fraction; fetal lung maturity

14–37. a
pp 274-275
amniocentesis, supernatant fraction; bilirubin; hemolytic disease of the newborn

14–38. a
pp 277-278
amniocentesis, supernatant fraction; α-fetoprotein; neural tube defects

14–39. fetal neural tissue
p 278
acetylcholinesterase, amnionic fluid

14–40. the diagnosis is made earlier. Therefore, pregnancy terminations can be performed with more ease and safety.
p 278
chorionic villus biopsy; amniocentesis

14–41. a,b,c,d,e,f
pp 278-279
ultrasonography; multifetal pregnancy; oligohydramnios; hydramnios; placentation; gestational age, determination

14–42. a,b,c,d
p 279
ultrasonography; fetal movement; fetal heart activity

14–43. a,b,c,d
pp 278-279
ultrasonography; radiography; hydatidiform mole; gestational age

14–44. b
p 280
fetoscopy

14–45. a
p 280
amnioscopy

14–46. d
p 280
fetography

14–47. c
p 280
amniography

14–48. a,b,c,d
p 280
amnioscopy

14–49. none of the tools has been *proved* to be consistently clinically useful for assessing fetal well-being
pp 280, 281
fetal well-being

14–50. c,e
p 281
fetal movement; fetal well-being

14–51. b,e
p 281
fetal well-being; contraction stress test

14–52. a,b,c,e,f,g,h,i
p 282
contraction stress test; oxytocin

14–53. b
p 282
contraction stress test

14–54. b
p 282
contraction stress test, interpretation; contraction stress test, negative

14–55. d
p 282
contraction stress test, interpretation

14–56. c
p 282
contraction stress test, interpretation; contraction stress test, suspicious

14–57. e
p 282
contraction stress test, interpretation; contraction stress test, unsatisfactory

14–58. a
p 282
contraction stress test, interpretation; contraction stress test, positive

14–59. c
p 282
contraction stress test; fetal well-being; contraction stress test, negative

14–60. a
p 282
contraction stress test; fetal well-being; contraction stress test, negative

14–61. 1 percent or less
p 282
contraction stress test; contraction stress test, false negative

14–62. b
pp 282-283
contraction stress test; fetal well-being; contraction stress test, positive

14–63. a
p 282
fetal heart rate, acceleration; nonstress test; electronic fetal monitoring

14–64. three or more fetal movements are accompanied by acceleration of the fetal heart rate of 15 beats/minute or more
p 284
nonstress test

14–65. a
p 284
fetal well-being

14–66. b
p 284
fetal well-being; nonstress test

14–67. a,b,c,d,e
p 284
fetal well-being; fetal monitoring; anesthesia, obstetric; analgesia, obstetric

14–68. a,c,d
p 285
fetal monitoring, internal; spiral electrode

14–69. b
pp 285-286
fetal monitoring; fetal heart rate; spiral electrode

14–70. b,c,d
pp 284-286
fetal monitoring, internal; fetal monitoring, external

14–71. b
p 286
fetal monitoring

14–72. c
p 286
fetal heart rate, baseline

14–73. a
p 286
fetal heart rate, baseline; bradycardia, fetal

14–74. d
p 286
fetal heart rate, baseline; tachycardia, fetal

14–75. deviations from baseline that are related to uterine contractions
p 286
fetal heart rate, periodic

14–76. c
p 287
fetal heart rate, deceleration; variable deceleration; cord compression

14–77. b
p 287
fetal heart rate, deceleration; Type II deceleration; uteroplacental insufficiency

14–78. a
p 287
fetal heart rate, deceleration; Type I deceleration; fetal head compression

14–79. a
p 287
fetal heart rate, deceleration; Type I deceleration; vagus nerve, effect of stimulation

14–80. a
p 287
fetal heart rate, deceleration; Type I deceleration; atropine, maternal stimulation

14–81. a,b,c
p 287
fetal heart rate, deceleration; Type I deceleration; Type II deceleration; variable deceleration; maternal position, labor

14–82. a,b,c
p 287
fetal heart rate, deceleration; Type I deceleration; Type II deceleration; variable deceleration; fetal distress

14–83. a
p 287
fetal heart rate, deceleration; Type I deceleration

14–84. b
p 287
fetal heart rate, deceleration; Type II deceleration

14–85. a,b,c,d,e
p 287
fetal heart rate; beat-to-beat variability

14–86. a,c,d,e
pp 287-288
fetal heart rate; sinusoidal pattern; tachycardia, persistent; bradycardia, persistent; hypoxia, fetal; hypothermia, maternal

14–87. a
pp 287-288
fetal heart rate; sinusoidal pattern; anemia, fetal

14–88. d
pp 287-288
persistent fetal bradycardia, severe; heart block, fetal

14–89. b
pp 287-288
persistent fetal tachycardia; fever, maternal

14–90. a,b,c,d
p 288
fetal well-being; fetal blood sampling

14–91. c
p 288
fetal blood sampling; fetal distress; fetal blood, pH; cesarean delivery, indications

14–92. b
p 288
fetal blood sampling; fetal distress; fetal blood, pH

14–93. a
p 288
fetal blood sampling; fetal distress; fetal blood, pH

14-94. **b,c**
pp 288-289
fetal blood sampling; fetal blood, pH

14-95. **b,c,d**
p 289
amniotomy; fetal monitoring, internal; umbilical cord, prolapse

14-96. **a,b,c,d**
pp 289-290
fetal monitoring, internal

14-97. **b**
p 290
fetal monitoring, external

14-98. **c,d,e**
p 290
fetal blood sampling; vacuum extraction; hemophilia; coagulation defect, fetal

14-99. **b**
p 290
fetal monitoring; fetal well-being

15-1. **b,c,d,e**
p 296
oxytocin, pregnancy; labor, third stage; blood loss, postpartum; lactation

15-2. **b,c,e**
pp 295-296
oxytocin, labor

15-3. **b**
p 296
oxytocin, pregnancy; placental transfer

15-4. **a**
p 296
oxytocin, neonatal levels

15-5. **b**
p 296
progesterone, labor

15-6. **a,b,c,d**
p 297
prostaglandins, myometrial contractions

15-7. **a,b,d,e**
pp 297-298
cortisol, labor; labor, initiation

15-8. **a,c**
p 299
anencephaly; postmaturity; adrenal gland, fetal

15-9. **b**
p 299
cortisol, labor

15-10. **a,b,c,d**
p 299
prostaglandins, labor; labor, induction

15-11. prostaglandins
p 300
prostaglandins, labor; organ communication system

15-12. **a,b**
p 300
organ communication system; fetal membranes; prostaglandins

15-13. **1 = a; 2 = b**
p 300
prostaglandins; fetal membranes

15-14. arachidonic acid
p 300
prostaglandins, synthesis; arachidonic acid

15-15. **a**
p 300
prostaglandins, metabolism; 15-hydroxyprostaglandin dehydrogenase (PGDH)

15-16. Ca^{2+}
pp 301-302
arachidonic acid; prostaglandins, synthesis; calcium

15-17. **a**
p 303
labor, initiation; kidney, fetal

15-18. **a**
p 303
uterus, contractions; uterus, smooth muscle; calcium

15-19. **b**
p 302
uterus, contractions; uterus, smooth muscle; calcium

15-20. it functions to facilitate and integrate transmission of forces generated by the contraction of myometrial cells
p 304
myometrium, extracellular matrix; uterus, contractions; labor

15-21. facilitate intercellular communication by the passage of current (electrical or ionic coupling) or metabolites (metabolic coupling) between cells
p 304
gap junctions; uterus, contractions

15-22. **b,e,g**
pp 304-305
gap junctions; uterus, contractions; progesterone, actions; estrogen, actions

15-23. **a,b,c,e**
pp 305-306
smooth muscle contraction; calcium, muscle contraction; myosin

15-24. calmodulin
p 306
cervix, ripening; calmodulin

15-25. a,c,e
pp 17, 306
cervix, ripening; collagen, cervix; glycosamoglycans

15-26. a,b
p 306
cervix, ripening; prostaglandins, actions

15-27. a
p 306
prostaglandins, synthesis; estrogen, actions

15-28. a = uterine contractions reach sufficient frequency, intensity, and duration to bring about readily demonstrable effacement and dilation of the cervix; b = the cervix is sufficiently dilated to allow passage of the fetal head; c = dilation of the cervix is complete; d = the fetus is expelled; e = delivery of the infant; f = delivery of the placenta and fetal membranes
pp 306-307
labor, stages

15-29. b
p 307
labor, latent phase

15-30. a
p 307
prelabor

15-31. fourth stage of labor
p 307
labor, fourth stage

15-32. a
p 307
cervix, ripening; labor, prelabor

15-33. a,b,c,d
p 307
lightening, labor; lower uterine segment; fundal height

15-34. b
p 307
labor, false

15-35. a
p 307
labor, true

15-36. b,c
p 307
labor, false

15-37. "show" or "bloody show"
p 307
cervix, mucus; bloody show

15-38. a,b,d
pp 307-308
uterus, contractions; labor; paraplegia; epidural block; pain, labor

15-39. Ferguson reflex
p 308
Ferguson reflex; labor

15-40. a,b,c,d
p 308
labor; uterus, contractions; Ferguson reflex

15-41. a
p 308
labor; uterus, contractions; fetal distress; fetal hypoxia

15-42. 1 = b; 2 = a
p 308
upper uterine segment; lower uterine segment; labor

15-43. b
p 308
lower uterine segment

15-44. a
pp 308-309
upper uterine segment

15-45. a
pp 308-309
upper uterine segment

15-46. b
p 309
lower uterine segment

15-47. a
p 309
upper uterine segment

15-48. b
p 310
lower uterine segment

15-49. a
p 308 (Fig. 15-10)
upper uterine segment; uterus, corpus

15-50. b
p 308 (Fig. 15-10)
lower uterine segment; uterus, isthmus

15-51. pathologic retraction ring (the ring of Bandl)
p 310
pathologic retraction ring; labor, obstructed; Bandl's ring

15-52. a
p 310
labor; upper uterine segment; lower uterine segment; labor, contractions

15–53. 1 = b; 2 = a
pp 310-311
labor; uterus, contractions; uterus, shape

15–54. b,c
p 311
labor, stages; "pushing"

15–55. b
p 311
labor

15–56. cervical effacement
p 311
labor; cervix, effacement; lower uterine segment

15–57. a,d
pp 313-314
cervix, dilation; labor

15–58. cervical dilation and fetal descent
p 314
labor; Friedman's curve; fetal descent; cervical dilation

15–59. a
p 314
labor, latent phase

15–60. b
p 314
labor, active phase

15–61. a
p 314
labor, latent phase

15–62. b
p 314
labor, active phase

15–63. 1 = b; 2 = c; 3 = a
p 314
labor, acceleration phase; labor, maximum slope; labor, deceleration phase; cervix, dilation; Friedman's curve

15–64. b
p 314
labor; engagement

15–65. a
p 315
labor, preparatory phase; cervix, ripening

15–66. b
p 315
labor, dilational phase; cervix, dilation

15–67. a
pp 314-315
labor, preparatory phase

15–68. c
p 315
labor, pelvic phase

15–69. c
p 315
labor, pelvic phase; labor, cardinal movements

15–70. caul
p 315
fetal membranes; caul

15–71. f,e,a,d,h,g,b,c
pp 13-14; 316-317
pelvic floor, anatomy

15–72. b,c,e
pp 13-14; 316-317
pelvic floor, anatomy

15–73. a,b,e,f
pp 13-15; 317
urogenital diaphragm; perineum, anatomy

15–74. stretching of fibers of the levator ani muscles and the thinning of the central portion of the perineum
p 317
perineum, anatomy; labor

15–75. a disproportion between the relatively unchanged size of the placenta and the reduced size of the uterus
p 318
labor, third stage

15–76. c,d
pp 319-320
labor, third stage

15–77. a
p 320
placenta, extrusion; mechanism of Schultze

15–78. b
p 320
placenta, extrusion; mechanism of Duncan

15–79. a
p 320
placenta, extrusion; mechanism of Schultze

15–80. a
p 320
placenta, extrusion; mechanism of Schultze

16–1. 95
p 323
occiput (vertex) presentation

16–2. a,c,d
p 323
occiput (vertex) presentation; labor

16–3. a
p 323
occiput (vertex) presentation; labor

16–4. b,c,d
p 323
occiput posterior presentation; labor

16–5. e,d,c,b,a,f,g
p 324
labor, cardinal movements

16–6. a,d,e,f
pp 324-325
labor, cardinal movements

16–7. b
p 325
labor, engagement; labor, cardinal movements

16–8. asynclitism
p 325
asynclitism; labor; sagittal suture

16–9. a
p 325
asynclitism; labor; sagittal suture

16–10. a
p 325
asynclitism; labor

16–11. a,b,c,d
p 326
labor, cardinal movements

16–12. occipitofrontal
p 326
labor, flexion; labor, cardinal movements; accommodation

16–13. ischial spines
pp 326, 328
labor, internal rotation; labor, cardinal movements; engagement

16–14. a,b,c,d
p 328
labor, extension; labor, external rotation; labor, cardinal movements

16–15. a
p 329
persistent occiput posterior presentation; labor, transverse arrest

16–16. a,b,c,d
pp 329-330
caput succedaneum; fetal head, molding

17–1. a,c,d
p 331
labor; antepartum care; psychoprophylaxis

17–2. b
p 331
labor, false

17–3. a
p 331
labor, true

17–4. a
p 331
labor, true

17–5. b
p 331
labor, false

17–6. b
p 331
labor, false

17–7. b
p 331
labor, initial presentation; antepartum care

17–8. a,b,c,d,e,f
pp 331-332
labor; bloody show; admissions procedures; membranes, rupture

17–9. b
p 332
admissions procedures; bloody show; third trimester bleeding; labor

17–10. c,d,f
p 332
labor; vaginal examination; clinical pelvimetry

17–11. c
p 332
labor; vaginal examination; cervical effacement

17–12. c
p 332
labor; vaginal examination; cervical dilation

17–13. c
p 332
cervix, position; premature labor

17–14. a,b,c
p 332
labor, station; vaginal examination; cervix; engagement

17–15. c
p 332
labor, station

17–16. a,b,c,
p 333
labor, membranes, rupture; labor, infection; unbilical cord prolapse

17–17. 1 = 4.5 to 5.5; 2 = 7.0 to 7.5
p 333
amnionic fluid; membranes, rupture; vagina, pH

17–18. a,c,d
p 333
membranes, rupture; bloody show; rupture of membranes, detection; amnionic fluid, pH

17-19. d
p 333
vaginal examination; labor, management

17-20. b
pp 334-335
labor, first stage

17-21. c,d
p 335
labor, management; fetal monitoring; fetal heart rate; fetal distress, diagnosis

17-22. a,b,e
pp 335, 337
labor, management; uterus, contractions; fetal monitoring

17-23. a,b,c,d
pp 335, 337
labor, management; analgesia

17-24. c,d
p 337
labor, management; amniotomy; umbilical cord prolapse

17-25. d
p 337
labor, management

17-26. a,d
p 337
labor, management; bladder function; urinary tract infection

17-27. a,b,c,d
p 337
labor, second stage

17-28. b
p 337
labor, second stage

17-29. a,c,d,e
pp 337-338
labor, second stage; fetal heart rate; placental abruption; fetal distress; nuchal cord; electronic fetal monitoring

17-30. a,d
p 338
labor, second stage; maternal explusive efforts (pushing)

17-31. dorsal lithotomy position
p 338
delivery, dorsal lithotomy position

17-32. b
p 338
labor, second stage; leg cramps, labor

17-33. none of these *absolutely assures* a noninfected outcome
p 339
labor, infection; perineal preparation, labor

17-34. crowning
p 339
labor, second stage; crowning

17-35. a,b,c
p 339
delivery, head; episiotomy; pelvic relaxation

17-36. Ritgen maneuver (modified)
pp 339-340
Ritgen maneuver; labor, second stage

17-37. a,b,c,d
p 340
delivery, head; umbilical cord; nuchal cord

17-38. a,b
p 340
delivery, shoulders; second stage, management

17-39. a,b
p 340
fetus, injury; delivery, shoulders; second stage, management

17-40. b,d,f
pp 340, 342
umbilical cord; labor, second stage; hyperbilirubinemia; nuchal cord; infant transfusion syndrome

17-41. a,b,d,e
p 342
labor, third stage; placenta, separation; third stage management

17-42. a,b,c,e
pp 342-343
labor, third stage; postpartum hemorrhage; placental separation

17-43. inversion of the uterus
pp 342-343
uterine inversion; placenta, delivery

17-44. a
p 343
placenta, manual removal; postpartum hemorrhage

17-45. a,c,d,e
pp 343, 345
placenta, manual removal; third stage, management

17-46. a,b,c,d
p 345
labor, fourth stage; hemorrhage, obstetric; uterus, atony

17-47. vasoconstriction produced by a well-contracted myometrium
p 345
postpartum hemorrhage

17-48. a,b,d
p 345
oxytocic agents; labor, third stage; labor, fourth stage; oxytocin; ergonovine maleate; methylergonovine maleate

17-49. b,e,f
pp 345-346
oxytocin

17-50. a,b,c,d,e
p 346
ergonovine; methylergonovine

17-51. entrapment of a second, undiagnosed twin
p 347
oxytocics; multifetal pregnancy

17-52. b
p 347
birth canal, lacerations

17-53. c
p 347
birth canal, lacerations

17-54. a
p 347
birth canal, lacerations

17-55. d
p 347
birth canal, lacerations

17-56. a,b,c,d,e
pp 347, 349-350
episiotomy; birth canal, lacerations

17-57. a
p 348
episiotomy, midline

17-58. b
p 348
episiotomy, mediolateral

17-59. b
p 348
episiotomy, mediolateral

17-60. a
p 348
episiotomy, midline

17-61. a
p 348
episiotomy, midline

17-62. b
p 348
episiotomy, mediolateral

17-63. a
p 348
episiotomy, midline

17-64. hemostasis; anatomic restoration without excessive suturing
p 350
episiotomy, repair

17-65. d,e,f
p 350
episiotomy

17-66. vulvar, paravaginal, or ischiorectal hematoma or abscess
p 350
episiotomy

18-1. a,b,c,d
p 353
anesthesia, surgical; anesthesia, obstetric

18-2. a,b,c,d,e
pp 353-354
anesthesia, obstetric; analgesia, obstetric; labor, management

18-3. a,b
p 354
analgesia, obstetric; meperidine

18-4. none; all narcotics and tranquilizers used for analgesia during labor can reach the fetus
p 354
analgesia, obstetric; analgesia, fetal effects; placental transfer

18-5. a
p 355
narcotic antagonists; fetal respiratory depression; naloxone (Narcan)

18-6. a,d,e
p 355
narcotic antagonists; fetal respiratory depression; naloxone (Narcan)

18-7. c,d
pp 196, 355
anesthesia, obstetric; anesthesia, general; placental barrier.

18-8. a,c,d,e
p 355
anesthesia, obstetric; nitrous oxide; anesthetics, volatile

18-9. none; all are capable of crossing the placenta and producing fetal narcosis
p 355
anesthesia, obstetric; anesthetics, volatile; placental barrier; ether; halothane (Fluothane); methoxyflurane (Penthrane); enflurane (Ethrane)

18-10. a,b,c,d
pp 355-356
anesthesia, obstetric; anesthetics, volatile; ether; halothane (Fluothane); methoxyflurane (Penthrane); enflurane (Ethrane)

18-11. c
p 356
anesthesia, obstetric; anesthetics, volatile; methoxyflurane (Penthrane)

18–12. b
p 356
anesthesia, obstetric; anesthetics, volatile; halothane

18–13. a,b,c,d,e
p 356
anesthesia, obstetric; anesthetics, intravenous; thiopental

18–14. c,d
p 356
anesthesia, obstetric; anesthetics, intravenous; thiopental

18–15. b
p 356
anesthesia, obstetric; anesthetics, intravenous; fetal respiratory depression

18–16. a,b,c,d
p 356
anesthesia, obstetric; anesthetics, intravenous; ketamine; hypertension, maternal; respiratory depression of the newborn

18–17. aspiration and consequent chemical pneumonitis from the inhalation of acidic gastric contents
p 356
anesthesia, obstetric; aspiration, pneumonia; maternal death, causes

18–18. b,d,e
p 357
anesthesia, obstetric; aspiration, prevention

18–19. a
p 357
anesthesia, obstetric; aspiration

18–20. a,b,e
pp 357-358
anesthesia, obstetric; aspiration; aspiration pneumonitis

18–21. a,d
p 358
anesthesia, obstetric; aspiration, treatment; aspiration pneumonitis

18–22. a
p 358
anesthesia, obstetric; anesthesia, risks of exposure

18–23. a,b,c,d
pp 20, 23, 358
uterus, innervation; Frankenhaüser's ganglion; analgesia, labor

18–24. a,b,c
pp 23, 359
genital tract, innervation; pudendal nerve

18–25. second, third, and fourth sacral
p 359
genital tract, innervation; pudendal nerve

18–26. b,c,d,e,f
pp 359-360
anesthesia, obstetric; anesthesia, CNS toxicity; regional anesthesia; ephedrine; succinylcholine; thiopental; diazepam; convulsions, maternal

18–27. b,c,e
p 360
anesthesia, obstetric; anesthesia, local

18–28. a,b,c,d,e
p 360
anesthesia, obstetric; pudendal block; local infiltration

18–29. d
p 360
anesthesia, obstetric; pudendal block; vaginal delivery

18–30. a,b,c
p 360
anesthesia, obstetric; pudendal block; convulsions, maternal

18–31. a,b,d
p 360
anesthesia, obstetric; paracervical block; bradycardia, fetal; postparacervical bradycardia

18–32. a,c,d
p 361
anesthesia, obstetric; spinal block

18–33. a,b,c,d,e,f
pp 361-362
anesthesia, obstetric; spinal block, complications; spinal headache

18–34. a,b,c
p 361
anesthesia, obstetric; spinal block, complications; ephedrine; maternal hypotension

18–35. too large a dose of anesthetic
p 361
anesthesia, obstetric; spinal block, complications; total spinal block

18–36. a,b,c,d
p 362
anesthesia, obstetric; spinal block, complications; nitrous oxide; morphine; meperidine; fentanyl

18–37. leakage of cerebrospinal fluid from the site where the meninges have been punctured
p 362
anesthesia, obstetric; spinal block, complications; spinal headache

18–38. a,b,e,f,g
p 362
anesthesia, obstetric; spinal block, complications; spinal headache

18-39. a
p 362
anesthesia, obstetric; spinal block, complications; epidural block; hypertension, regional anesthesia; ergotamine

18-40. maternal hypovolemia; maternal hypotension or hypertension; maternal coagulation disorders; skin infection at the possible puncture site; maternal neurologic disorders
pp 362-363
anesthesia, obstetric; spinal block, contraindications

18-41. a,b,c
p 363
anesthesia, obstetric; epidural/peridural block; analgesia, obstetric

18-42. a,b,c,d,e
pp 363-364
anesthesia, obstetric; epidural block, complications; hypotension, maternal; labor, inhibition; spinal block

18-43. a
p 364
anesthesia, obstetric; epidural block; delivery, midforceps

18-44. maternal hemorrhage; overt hypertension; skin infection at or near the possible puncture site; neurologic disease
p 364
anesthesia, obstetric; epidural block, contraindications

18-45. b
pp 364-365
anesthesia, obstetric; analgesia, obstetric; psychoprophylaxis; Lamaze childbirth preparation

19-1. b
p 367
puerperium, definition

19-2. a
p 367
uterus, involution; puerperium

19-3. f
p 367
uterus, involution; puerperium

19-4. h
p 367
uterus, involution; puerperium

19-5. a
p 367
uterus, involution; puerperium

19-6. e
p 367
uterus, involution; puerperium

19-7. f
p 367
uterus, involution; puerperium

19-8. c,d
p 367
uterus, involution; puerperium

19-9. 1 = b; 2 = c
p 367
myometrium, involution

19-10. c
p 367
endometrium, postpartum regeneration

19-11. late puerperal hemorrhage
pp 367-368
placental site, involution; hemorrhage, postpartum

19-12. a,b
pp 367-368
placental site, involution

19-13. b
pp 368-369
uterus, vasculature; puerperium

19-14. b
p 369
cervix, puerperium; lower uterine segment, puerperium; vagina, puerperium; hymen, puerperium

19-15. a,d
p 369
abdominal wall, puerperium; striae gravidarum; diastasis recti

19-16. a,b,d
p 369
urinary system, puerperium; bladder, pregnancy

19-17. a,b,e
pp 369-370
breast development; lactation

19-18. a,d
p 370
colostrum; lactation

19-19. b,d
pp 370-372
colostrum; breast feeding, immunology

19-20. a,b,c,e
p 372
lactation; vitamins, breast milk; minerals, breast milk; breast milk; iodine

19-21. a,b,c,d,e,f
p 372
lactation, hormonal control

19-22. progesterone and estrogen
p 372
lactation, hormonal control; estrogen, actions; progesterone, actions

19-23. a,b,c,d,e
p 372
lactation; oxytocin, actions; prolactin, actions; suckling; milk letdown

19-24. a,b,c
pp 372-373
breast feeding, immunology; breast milk, IgA; colostrum

19-25. a,b
p 373
breast feeding

19-26. b,c,e
p 373
afterpains; puerperium

19-27. a,b,c,d
p 373
lochia

19-28. a,d,e
pp 373-374
lochia; oxytocics, puerperium; methylergonovine maleate

19-29. a,b
p 374
preeclampsia; puerperal diuresis

19-30. b,c,d
pp 373-374
puerperium; puerperal diuresis; urinary tract infection, puerperium; afterpains; leukocytosis, postpartum

19-31. a,b,d
p 374
puerperium; leukocytosis; lymphopenia; sedimentation rate (ESR)

19-32. a
p 374
puerperium, weight loss

19-33. b,c,d,e
pp 374-375
puerperium; postpartum hemorrhage; episiotomy

19-34. none; it is fairly common for the mother to experience some degree of depression a few days after delivery
p 375
postpartum depression

19-35. a,b,c
p 375
puerperium, early ambulation; puerperium, constipation; thromboembolism

19-36. a,c
p 375
puerperium, abdominal wall

19-37. d
p 375
puerperium, diet; lactation

19-38. a,b,c,d
p 375
puerperium, bladder function; puerperium, oxytocics

19-39. b
p 375
puerperium, bladder

19-40. a,b
p 376
puerperium, breast care; puerperium, constipation

19-41. c
p 376
puerperium

19-42. a,d,e
p 376
puerperium; postpartum, menstruation; postpartum, ovulation

19-43. none of these
p 377
puerperium

20-1. b
p 379
respiration, newborn; respiration, fetal; fetal breathing movements

20-2. a,c,d,e
p 379
respiration, newborn; transcient tachypnea of the newborn

20-3. fifth
p 379
respiration, newborn

20-4. a
p 379
ductus arteriosus; circulation, fetal

20-5. respiratory distress syndrome (hyaline membrane disease)
p 379
respiratory distress syndrome; surfactant; hyaline membrane disease

20-6. a,b,c,d
pp 379-380
respiration, newborn

20-7. a
p 380
respiration, newborn; cesarean section

20-8. a,b,c
p 380
neonate, immediate care; umbilical cord, management

20-9. a,b,c,d,e,f,g
p 380
neonate, immediate care; fetal well-being

20-10. auscultation over the chest; palpation of the base of the umbilical cord
p 380
neonate, heart rate; newborn, initial evaluation

20-11. c
p 380
neonate, heart rate

20-12. a
p 380
neonate, heart rate; neonate, respiration; neonate, resuscitation; suctioning, newborn nasopharynx

20-13. c,d
pp 380-381
neonate, respiration; neonate, resuscitation

20-14. a,b,c,d,e,f,g,h
p 381
respiration, initiation

20-15. heart rate; respiratory effort; muscle tone; reflex irritability; color
p 381
Apgar score; fetal well-being

20-16. a,b,d
p 381
Apgar score

20-17. 7
p 381
Apgar score

20-18. 4-7
p 381
Apgar score

20-19. failure to check equipment; use of a cold resuscitation table; unsuccessful intubation; inadequate ventilation; failure to manage bradycardia or poor chest movement; failure to manage hypovolemia; failure to perform cardiac massage
pp 381-382
resuscitation, neonate

20-20. skilled personnel immediately available; large, well-heated and lighted work area; equipment to deliver oxygen, positive pressure and suction; drugs and appropriate accompanying equipment
p 382
resuscitation, neonate

20-21. b
p 382
resuscitation, neonate

20-22. a
p 382
resuscitation, neonate; mask ventilation

20-23. a,c,d
p 382
resuscitation, neonate; endotracheal intubation

20-24. intermittent positive pressure ventilation with oxygen delivered from a bag; resuscitator puffing oxygen-rich air into the endotracheal tube
p 382
resuscitation, neonate; endotracheal intubation

20-25. a
p 382
endotracheal intubation, complications; pneumothorax

20-26. b
p 382
endotracheal intubation, complications

20-27. a
p 382
endotracheal intubation, complications; pneumomediastinum

20-28. a,b,c,d,e
p 382
resuscitation, neonate; acidosis; sodium bicarbonate

20-29. naloxone (Narcane)
p 382
resuscitation, neonate; respiratory depression; naloxone (Narcan); narcotics, respiratory depression

20-30. a,b,c,d,e
p 382
resuscitation, neonate; hypovolemia, newborn; sepsis, neonatal; twin-to-twin transfusion; hemorrhage; fetal to maternal

20-31. a
p 383
cardiac massage; resuscitation, neonate

20-32. a,b,e
p 383
cardiac massage; resuscitation, neonate

20-33. b
p 383
resuscitation, neonate; epinephrine; intracardiac injection

20-34. b
p 383
gestational age, determination

20-35. c,d
pp 383-384
gonorrheal ophthalmia; silver nitrate; penicillin; tetracycline

20-36. a,d
p 384
newborn, identification

20-37. a,b
p 384
newborn, temperature

20-38. a
p 384
vitamin K administration; coagulation defects

20-39. a,b,d,e
pp 384-385
umbilical cord, management

20-40. a
p 385
skin care, neonate; vernix caseosa

20-41. a,b,c,d
p 385
meconium

20-42. a,c
p 385
stool production, neonate

20-43. a,d,e
p 385
hyperbilirubinemia; icterus neonatorum; physiologic jaundice of the newborn

20-44. a,b,c,d
p 385
physiologic jaundice of the newborn; prematurity, effects; bilirubin; hemolysis, newborn

20-45. a,b,c,d
p 385
weight loss, newborn

20-46. a,c,d
p 385
weight loss, newborn; weight gain, infant; prematurity, effects

20-47. a,d
p 385
feeding, newborn; breast feeding

20-48. b
p 387
circumcision

20-49. a,b,d
p 387
circumcision, contraindications

21-1. Whole blood components are not immediately available.
p 389
obstetric hemorrhage; maternal mortality

21-2. a
p 389
obstetric hemorrhage; perinatal mortality; premature delivery; antepartum bleeding

21-3. a,d
p 389
blood loss, delivery; postpartum hemorrhage

21-4. 1000 to 2000 ml
p 389
pregnancy-induced hypervolemia; blood volume, pregnancy

21-5. b
p 389
obstetric hemorrhage

21-6. placenta previa; placental abruption; placenta accreta; ectopic pregnancy; midtrimester abortion; hydatidiform mole
p 389
obstetric hemorrhage, etiology; abnormal placental implantation

21-7. vaginal delivery other than spontaneous or outlet forceps; cesarean section or cesarean hysterectomy; uterine rupture
pp 389-390
obstetric hemorrhage, etiology; delivery, trauma

21-8. overdistended uterus; exhausted myometrium; anesthesia; previous atony
p 390
obstetric hemorrhage, etiology; uterine atony

21-9. small woman; pregnancy hypervolemia not yet maximal; pregnancy hypervolemia obtunded
p 390
obstetric hemorrhage, etiology; small blood volume

21-10. placental abruption; prolonged retention of dead fetus; amnionic fluid embolism; induced abortion; sepsis; gross intravascular hemolysis; massive hemorrhage treated with packed red cells plus electrolyte solution or old whole blood; eclampsia or severe preeclampsia; abnormalities of coagulation coincidental to pregnancy
p 390
obstetric hemorrhage, etiology; coagulation defects

21-11. b
p 390
obstetric hemorrhage; third trimester bleeding

21-12. b,c,d
p 391
obstetric hemorrhage, etiology; placental site; uterine atony

21-13. a
p 391
obstetric hemorrhage, etiology; genital tract lacerations

21-14. a
p 391
obstetric hemorrhage, management; oxytocics; uterine massage

21-15. uterine atony; retained placental fragments; trauma to genital tract
p 391
obstetric hemorrhage, etiology; uterine atony; placental fragments; genital tract, trauma

21-16. a,b,c,d
p 391
obstetric hemorrhage, management

21-17. None; all of the techniques are imprecise when used alone.
pp 391-392
obstetric hemorrhage, diagnosis; tilt test

21-18. a
pp 391-392
obstetric hemorrhage; tilt test; blood loss

21-19. venodilatation (reducing venous return); renal diarrhea (loss of fluids and electrolytes)
p 392
obstetric hemorrhage; diuretics, side effects

21-20. b
p 392
obstetric hemorrhage; oxytocics

21-21. a,b,c
pp 392-393
obstetric hemorrhage; blood volume measurements

21-22. a,c,d
p 393
obstetric hemorrhage; fluid replacement

21-23. Platelets in stored blood soon lose their functional capacity.
p 393
blood replacement; hypovolemia, management

21-24. b,c,d
pp 393-394
blood replacement; obstetric hemorrhage; coagulation defects; thrombocytopenia

21-25. a
pp 393-394
thrombocytopenia; blood replacement

21-26. b
pp 393-394
blood replacement; Factor V; Factor VIII

21-27. a,c,d,e,f
p 394
coagulation factors, pregnancy

21-28. d
p 394
coagulation, activation

21-29. b
p 394
coagulation, activation

21-30. a
p 394
coagulation, activation

21-31. c
p 394
coagulation, activation

21-32. delaying fibrin polymerization (prolonged thrombin time); causing defective fibrin clot structure (impaired clot retraction and stability)
p 394
coagulation, mechanism; fibrin degradation products

21-33. b
p 394
consumptive coagulopathy; DIC; heparin; fibrinogen; E-*amino caproic acid*

21-34. a,b,c
p 394
consumptive coagulopathy; DIC

21-35. b
p 395
hemostasis, defective

21-36. b,c,e,f
p 395
hemostasis, defective; petechiae; eclampsia

21-37. a,b,c,e
p 395
placental abruption; placenta previa; vasa previa; uterine bleeding; antepartum bleeding

21-38. a,b,c,d
pp 395-396
placental abruption

21-39. a
p 396
placental abruption; external hemorrhage

21-40. b
p 396
placental abruption; concealed hemorrhage

21-41. b
p 396
placental abruption; concealed hemorrhage

21-42. a,b,f
pp 396-397
placental abruption, frequency; neonatal mortality; maternal mortality

21-43. a,b,c,d,e,f,g,h,i
p 397
placental abruption; hypertension, pregnancy associated; multifetal pregnancy; preeclampsia; eclampsia; uterine decompression; short cord syndrome

21-44. a
p 397
placental abruption; hypertension

21-45. a
p 398
placental abruption, recurrent

21-46. None of these serves to reliably identify imminent placental abruption.
pp 398-399
placental abruption

21-47. a,c
p 398
placental abruption, pathology; spiral artery (arteriole) rupture

21-48. a,b,c,d
p 398
placental abruption; concealed hemorrhage

21-49. hemorrhage with retroplacental hematoma formation that is arrested without delivery occurring
p 398
placental abruption, chronic

21-50. b
p 398
placental abruption; fetal to maternal hemorrhage

21-51. d
p 398
placental abruption

21-52. b
pp 398-400
placental abruption; ultrasonography

21-53. b,d,f
p 399 (Table 21-3)
placental abruption, signs; placental abruption, symptoms; premature labor; fetal distress; vaginal bleeding, third trimester

21-54. a
p 400
placental abruption; placenta previa

21-55. b
p 400
placental abruption

21-56. placental abruption
p 400
placental abruption; consumptive coagulopathy

21-57. a,b
pp 400-401
consumptive coagulopathy; placental abruption

21-58. b,c,d
p 401
renal failure; placental abruption

21-59. There is widespread extravasations of blood into the uterine musculature and beneath the uterine serosa.
pp 401-402
Couvelaire uterus

21-60. b
pp 401-402
Couvelaire uterus

21-61. a,c
p 402
placental abruption, management; third trimester bleeding, management

21-62. b
p 402
placental abruption, management; third trimester bleeding, management

21-63. c, perhaps also (a) depending on the cause of the distress
p 402
placental abruption, management; third trimester bleeding, management

21-64. b
p 402
ultrasonography; placental abruption, diagnosis

21-65. placental separation; maternal hemorrhage; fetal hemorrhage; uterine hypertonus
p 402
fetal distress; placental abruption

21-66. None of these is recommended for the treatment of uterine hypertonicity associated with fetal distress and placental abruption.
p 402
placental abruption, management; fetal distress; tocolysis

21-67. a
p 403
placental abruption; cesarean delivery

21-68. a,b,c,d
p 403
vaginal delivery; placental abruption; fetal death; cesarean delivery; postpartum hemorrhage

21-69. b
p 403
placental abruption; amniotomy

21-70. a,b,d
pp 403-404
placental abruption, labor

21-71. b
p 404
placental abruption, delivery

21-72. None; the basic techniques for the management of obstetric hemorrhage apply in the case of placental abruption.
p 404
placental abruption; obstetric hemorrhage; hypovolemia

21-73. a,d,e,f
pp 404-407
coagulation defects, pregnancy; thrombocytopenia; consumptive coagulopathy; obstetric hemorrhage; placental abruption

21-74. hepatitis
p 405
hypofibrinogenemia, management

21-75. b
pp 406-407
placental abruption; coagulation defects, management

21-76. a,b,c,d,e
p 407
consumptive coagulopathy, newborn

21-77. The placenta is over or very near the internal os instead of being implanted in the body of the uterus.
p 407
placenta previa

21-78. c
p 407
placenta previa, marginal

21-79. b
p 407
placenta previa, partial

21-80. d
p 407
placenta previa, low-lying

21-81. a
p 407
placenta previa, total

21-82. b
p 407
placenta previa, degree; cervix, dilation

21-83. c
pp 407-408
placenta previa; placental abruption

21-84. a,b,c
p 407
abortion; placenta previa; implantation

21-85. c
pp 396, 408
placenta previa, incidence; placental abruption, incidence

21-86. a,b,c,d,e,f,g
p 408
placenta previa, associated factors; multifetal pregnancy; erythroblastosis; placenta accreta

21-87. Painless hemorrhage that does not usually appear until the end of the second trimester or after
pp 408-409
placenta previa

21-88. c,d
p 409
placenta previa; coagulation defects; obstetric hemorrhage

21-89. a,b,c,d,e
pp 408-410
placenta previa; ultrasonography; vaginal examination, placenta previa

21-90. b
p 410
placenta previa, management

21-91. The placenta may migrate away from the cervix.
p 410
placenta previa, management

21-92. a
p 411
placenta previa, management; cesarean delivery, placenta previa

21-93. b
p 411
placenta previa, management; vaginal delivery, placenta previa

21-94. a
p 411
placenta previa, management; vaginal delivery, placenta previa

21-95. a,b
p 411
placenta previa; cesarean delivery, placenta previa; placenta accreta

21-96. simple rupture of the membranes
p 411
vaginal delivery, placenta previa; tamponade

21-97. a,b,c,d,e
p 411
placenta previa, prognosis; perinatal mortality; cesarean delivery

21-98. b
p 412
intrauterine fetal demise, management

21-99. a,b,c
p 412
intrauterine fetal demise; coagulation defects; labor, induction

21-100. d
p 412
intrauterine fetal demise

21-101. a,b
p 412
consumptive coagulopathy; intrauterine fetal demise

21-102. a
pp 412-413
intrauterine fetal demise; consumptive coagulopathy; heparin

21-103. b
p 414
intrauterine fetal demise; intrauterine pregnancy; consumptive coagulopathy; multifetal pregnancy

21-104. d,e
p 414
intrauterine fetal demise; consumptive coagulopathy

21-105. a,b,d
p 414
intrauterine fetal demise; pregnancy termination; consumptive coagulopathy; laminaria; prostaglandin E_2; oxytocin

21-106. c
pp 414-415
pregnancy termination; prostaglandin E_2

21-107. a
pp 414-415
pregnancy termination; oxytocin

21-108. b
pp 414-415
pregnancy termination; laminaria

21-109. d
pp 414-415
pregnancy termination; hypertonic saline

21-110. A rent through the amnion and chorion; opened uterine or endocervical veins; a pressure gradient sufficient to force the amnionic fluid into the venous circulation
p 415
amnionic fluid embolism

21-111. a,b,c,d
p 415
amnionic fluid embolism

21-112. a,b,c
pp 416-417
amnionic fluid embolism, diagnosis; amnionic fluid embolism, management

21-113. a,b,c,d,e
p 418
consumptive coagulopathy; abortion

21-114. a,b,c
p 418
consumptive coagulopathy; thromboplastin

21-115. b
p 418
septic abortion; consumptive coagulopathy

21-116. a
p 419
consumptive coagulopathy, etiology; obstetric hemorrhage

21-117. a,d
p 429
preeclampsia; eclampsia; consumptive coagulopathy

22-1. b
p 423
ectopic pregnancy

22-2. a,b,c,d,e,f,g,h
p 423
ectopic pregnancy, etiology; pelvic inflammatory disease; endometriosis; infertility

22-3. a
p 423
ectopic pregnancy; hysterectomy

22-4. a
p 423
ectopic pregnancy, incidence

22-5. increased prevalence of sexually transmitted diseases; popularity of intrauterine devices; unsuccessful previous tubal sterilization; induced abortion followed by infection; fertility induced by ovulatory agents; previous pelvic surgery, specifically tubal surgery; in utero exposure to stilbestrol; better and earlier diagnostic techniques for ectopic pregnancy
pp 423-424
ectopic pregnancy, etiology

22-6. b
p 424
ectopic pregnancy, management

22-7. a,b,c,d
p 424
ectopic pregnancy, locations; tubal pregnancy

22-8. b,c,d
p 424
ectopic pregnancy; tubal pregnancy, implantation

22-9. a,b,c
p 424
ectopic pregnancy, uterine changes

22-10. a,c,d
p 424
ectopic pregnancy, endometrial changes; Arias-Stella reaction

22-11. a
p 424
ectopic pregnancy, endometrial changes; Arias-Stella reaction

22-12. a,b,c,d
pp 424-425
ectopic pregnancy, endometrial changes

22-13. separation of the products of conception from the implantation site and extrusion of the abortus through the fimbriated end of the oviduct
p 425
tubal abortion; tubal pregnancy

22-14. a,b,d,e
p 425
tubal abortion; ectopic pregnancy

22-15. a,e
p 425
ectopic pregnancy; tubal rupture; lithopedion; abdominal pregnancy

22-16. a,b,c
pp 425-426
ectopic pregnancy; broad ligament pregnancy; intraligamentous pregnancy

22-17. implants within the segment of the tube that penetrates the uterine wall
p 426
ectopic pregnancy; interstitial pregnancy

22-18. a,c,d,e
p 426
interstitial pregnancy; ectopic pregnancy; cornual pregnancy

22-19. a
p 426
ectopic pregnancy; cornual pregnancy; interstitial pregnancy; hysterectomy

22-20. a combined pregnancy
p 426
ectopic pregnancy; multifetal pregnancy; combined pregnancy

22-21. a,d
pp 426-427
combined pregnancy; ectopic pregnancy; multifetal pregnancy

22-22. b
p 427
tuboabdominal pregnancy; ectopic pregnancy

22-23. a
p 427
tubouterine pregnancy; ectopic pregnancy

22-24. c
p 427
tuboovarian pregnancy; ectopic pregnancy

22-25. a,b,c,d,e,f
p 428
ruptured tubal pregnancy, signs; ruptured tubal pregnancy, symptoms; tubal pregnancy

22-26. blood irritating the cervical sensory nerves on the inferior surface of the diaphragm
p 428
tubal pregnancy; ruptured tubal pregnancy, symptoms; hemoperitoneum; shoulder pain

22-27. b
p 428
ruptured tubal pregnancy, symptoms; pain, tubal pregnancy; hemoperitoneum

22-28. *None* of these rules out the presence of a ruptured tubal pregnancy.
pp 428-429
ruptured tubal pregnancy, diagnosis; amenorrhea; vaginal bleeding; pregnancy test

22-29. a,b,c
p 429
hypovolemia, detection; ruptured tubal pregnancy; hemorrhage

22-30. normocytic
p 429
ruptured tubal pregnancy; anemia

22-31. a,c,d
pp 429-430
ruptured tubal pregnancy, signs; hemoperitoneum; fever, hemoperitoneum

22-32. acute or chronic salpingitis; threatened or incomplete abortion of an intrauterine pregnancy; torsion of an ovarian cyst; appendicitis; gastroenteritis; pain from an intrauterine device; rupture of a corpus luteum or other ovarian cyst with intraperitoneal bleeding
p 430
ruptured tubal pregnancy, differential diagnosis; abortion; appendicitis; ovarian cyst; corpus luteum cyst; intrauterine device

22-33. b,d
p 430
ruptured tubal pregnancy, differential diagnosis; salpingitis

22-34. c,e
p 430
ruptured tubal pregnancy, differential diagnosis; abortion, intrauterine pregnancy; decidual cast; decidual reaction, ectopic pregnancy

22-35. b
p 430
ectopic pregnancy, diagnosis; multifetal pregnancy, ectopic

22-36. a
p 430
ruptured tubal pregnancy, differential diagnosis; amenorrhea

22-37. c
p 430
ruptured tubal pregnancy, differential diagnosis; twisted ovarian cyst

22-38. a
p 430
ruptured tubal pregnancy, differential diagnosis

22-39. b
p 430
ruptured tubal pregnancy, differential diagnosis; appendicitis

22-40. a,b,c
p 430
ruptured tubal pregnancy, management

22-41. a
p 430
ruptured tubal pregnancy, differential diagnosis; follicular cyst; corpus luteum cyst

22-42. a,c
p 430
ruptured tubal pregnancy, differential diagnosis; intrauterine device; tubal sterilization

22-43. b,c,d,e
pp 430-431
tubal pregnancy, diagnosis; ultrasonography; corpus luteum cyst; gestational sac

22-44. d
p 431
tubal pregnancy, diagnosis; culdocentesis

22-45. b
p 431
tubal pregnancy, diagnosis; curettage

22-46. a
p 431
tubal pregnancy, diagnosis; curettage

22-47. a
p 431
tubal pregnancy, diagnosis; curettage

22-48. b
p 431
tubal pregnancy, diagnosis; colpotomy

22-49. a,b,d
p 431
tubal pregnancy, diagnosis; laparoscopy

22-50. b
p 431
tubal pregnancy, diagnosis; culdoscopy; laparoscopy

22-51. d
p 431
tubal pregnancy, diagnosis; laparotomy

22-52. d
p 431
tubal pregnancy, maternal mortality

22-53. a
p 431
tubal pregnancy, maternal mortality; maternal mortality

22-54. b,c
p 432
tubal pregnancy, management; salpingectomy; cornual resection; infertility rate; oophorectomy

22-55. b
p 432
tubal pregnancy, management; methotrexate

22-56. a
p 433
autotransfusion; ruptured tubal pregnancy, management

22-57. b
p 433
autotransfusion; ruptured tubal pregnancy, management

22-58. b
p 433
autotransfusion; ruptured tubal pregnancy, management

22-59. b,c,d
p 433
Rh isoimmunization; ruptured tubal pregnancy, management

22-60. b
p 433
abdominal pregnancy

22-61. b,c,d,e
pp 434-435
abdominal pregnancy; lithopedion; adipocere; congenital malformations, abdominal pregnancy

22-62. a,b,c,d,e
p 435
abdominal pregnancy, diagnosis; abdominal pregnancy, symptoms

22-63. a,c,d,e
p 435
abdominal pregnancy, diagnosis; abdominal pregnancy, physical findings

22-64. b
p 435
abdominal pregnancy, diagnosis

22-65. b
p 435
abdominal pregnancy, diagnosis; oxytocin

22-66. b
pp 435-436
abdominal pregnancy, diagnosis; ultrasonography; isotope localization; x-ray

22-67. a,b,c
pp 436-437
abdominal pregnancy, management; hemorrhage

22-68. infection; abscess; intestinal obstruction; adhesions; wound dehiscence
p 436
abdominal pregnancy, complications of management

22-69. detect and manage ectopic pregnancy in the first trimester
pp 436-437
abdominal pregnancy, management; tubal pregnancy, management

22-70. the fallopian tube on the affected side is intact; the fetal sac occupies the position of the ovary; the ovary is connected to the uterus by the ovarian ligament; definite ovarian tissue is found in the wall of the sac
p 437
ovarian pregnancy, Spiegelberg criteria

22-71. a,b
p 437
ovarian pregnancy

22-72. within the cervix below the internal os
p 438
cervical pregnancy

22-73. a,c,d
p 438
cervical pregnancy, symptoms; cervical pregnancy, management

23-1. d
p 441
placenta succenturiata; placental abnormalities

23-2. a
p 441
placenta bipartita; placental abnormalities

23-3. b
p 441
placenta duplex; placental abnormalities

23-4. succenturiate lobe (accessory lobe)
p 441
succenturiate lobe; placenta succenturiata

23-5. b
p 441
succenturiate lobe; placenta succenturiata

23-6. c
p 441
succenturiate lobe; postpartum hemorrhage

23-7. a,c,d
p 441
ring-shaped placenta; fetal growth retardation; antepartum bleeding; postpartum bleeding

23-8. a,b,e
p 441
membranaceous placenta; placenta diffusa, retained placenta

23-9. a placenta in which the central portion is missing
p 441
fenestrated placenta

23-10. a
p 441
extrachorial placenta

23-11. a
pp 441-443
circumvallate placenta

23-12. b
pp 441-443
marginate placenta

23-13. a
pp 441-443
circumvallate placenta

23-14. b
pp 441-443
marginate placenta

23-15. a
pp 441-443
circumvallate placenta; fetal malformations; antepartum hemorrhage

23-16. b
p 443
placenta, weight

23-17. a,d
p 443
placental enlargement; syphilis; Rh sensitization; erythroblastosis fetalis

23-18. parts of a normal placenta or a succenturiate lobe that is retained after delivery
p 443
placental polyp; succenturiate lobe; retained placenta

23-19. changes associated with trophoblastic aging; impairment of the uteroplacental circulation causing infarction
p 443
placental infarcts; placenta, degeneration

23-20. a,b,c
p 443
placental infarcts; placenta, degeneration

23-21. a,e
pp 443-444
placental infarcts; placenta, degeneration

23-22. c
p 443
placental calcification; ultrasonography

23-23. a
p 444
villous arterial thrombosis

23-24. a,b,d
p 444
chorionic villi, hypertrophy; diabetes, placental effect; erythroblastosis (hydropic type); fetal congestive heart failure

23-25. a
pp 444-445
placental infection; infection, fetal; intrauterine infection

23-26. abnormalities of chorionic villi consisting of varying degrees of trophoblast proliferation and edema of the villous stroma
p 445
hydatidiform mole; neoplastic trophoblast

23-27. a,b
p 445
invasive mole; neoplastic trophoblast

23-28. b
p 445
choriocarcinoma; neoplastic trophoblast

23-29. A neoplastic trophoblast without stroma spreads locally or disseminates beyond the original site of zygote implantation and proliferates rapidly.
p 445
choriocarcinoma

23-30. a
p 445
invasive mole; chorioadenoma destruens

23-31. b
p 445
choriocarcinoma; chorionepithelioma

23-32. a,b,c
p 446
hydatidiform mole

23-33. Chorionic villi are converted to a mass of clear vesicles that often hang in clusters from thin pedicles. The mass may grow to the size of an advanced pregnancy. (Or, a small hairy creature with beady eyes and long whiskers.)
p 446
hydatidiform mole, complete; mole, small hairy

23-34. a
pp 446-447
hydatidiform mole, complete

23-35. b
pp 446-447
hydatidiform mole, partial

23-36. a
pp 446-447
hydatidiform mole, complete

23-37. b
pp 446-447
hydatidiform mole, partial

23-38. a
pp 446-447
hydatidiform mole, complete

23-39. b
pp 446-447
hydatidiform mole, partial

23-40. a,b
pp 446-447
hydatidiform mole, complete; hydatidiform mole, partial

23-41. moderate hydropic swelling of some villi without significant trophoblastic proliferation
p 447
molar degeneration

23-42. b
p 447
hydatidiform mole; choriocarcinoma

23-43. b,c,e
p 447
theca lutein cysts; hydatidiform mole

23-44. 1 per 1500 to 2000 pregnancies
p 447
hydatidiform mole

23-45. c
p 447
hydatidiform mole

23-46. a
p 448
hydatidiform mole

23-47. a,b,c,d,e
pp 448-449
hydatidiform mole, diagnosis

23-48. uterine bleeding
p 448
hydatidiform mole; uterine bleeding

23-49. c,d
p 448
hydatidiform mole; uterine bleeding; concealed hemorrhage

23-50. a
p 448
hydatidiform mole; gestational age

23-51. multiple lutein cysts
p 448
hydatidiform mole; theca lutein cysts

23-52. b
p 448
hydatidiform mole; hypertension

23-53. b,c
p 449
hydatidiform mole; hyperthyroidism, hydatidiform mole; TSH, hydatidiform mole

23-54. b
p 449
hydatidiform mole

23-55. a,b,c,d
p 449
hydatidiform mole; myomata; multifetal pregnancy; hydramnios; gestational age, determination

23-56. b
pp 449-451
hydatidiform mole; ultrasonography

23-57. a,d
p 451
hydatidiform mole; hCG, hydatidiform mole

23-58. a,b,c,d,e,f
p 451
hydatidiform mole, complete; hCG, hydatidiform mole; fetal heart sounds; vaginal bleeding, pregnancy; hydatidiform mole, ultrasonography; preeclampsia, hydatidiform mole

23-59. 0 percent
p 451
hydatidiform mole

23-60. a
p 451
hydatidiform mole; choriocarcinoma

23-61. c,d
p 452
hydatidiform mole, treatment

23-62. It allows a better assessment of malignant predisposition and prediction of subsequent biologic behavior of tissue that is left in the uterus.
p 452
hydatidiform mole

23-63. laparotomy
p 452
hydatidiform mole; obstetric hemorrhage, hydatidiform mole

23-64. a,b
p 452
hydatidiform mole; oxytocin

23-65. a,b
p 452
hydatidiform mole; prostaglandin

23-66. a
p 453
hydatidiform mole; hysterectomy

23-67. detection of any change suggestive of trophoblastic malignancy
p 453
hydatidiform mole; hydatidiform mole, follow-up

23-68. hCG levels
pp 453-454
hydatidiform mole, follow-up; hCG, hydatidiform mole

23-69. a,b,c,d
p 454
hydatidiform mole; actinomycin D; methotrexate; trophoblastic disease, treatment; hydatidiform mole, follow-up; persistent trophoblastic disease

23-70. b,c
p 454
persistent trophoblastic disease; curettage

23-71. a
p 454
persistent trophoblastic disease; hysterectomy

23-72. c
p 454
persistent trophoblastic disease; chemotherapy

23-73. a,d,e
p 454
persistent trophoblastic disease; hCG

23-74. b
p 454
hydatidiform mole; choriocarcinoma

23-75. d
pp 454-456
choriocarcinoma

23-76. b
p 456
choriocarcinoma; theca lutein cysts

23-77. a,b,c,d
p 456
choriocarcinoma

23-78. b
p 456
choriocarcinoma

23-79. a,c,d
p 456
choriocarcinoma; hydatidiform mole; hCG, hydatidiform mole

23-80. e
p 456
persistent trophoblastic disease

23-81. a,b,c,d
pp 456-457
choriocarcinoma; methotrexate; radiation therapy; actinomycin D

23-82. 24-hour urine hCG level less than 100,000 IU; duration of disease less than 4 months; no brain or liver metastases
p 457
choriocarcinoma, low risk

23–83. b
p 457
choriocarcinoma, treatment

23–84. b,c,d
p 457
invasive mole; methotrexate; choriocarcinoma

23–85. a,b,e
p 457
hemangioma, placenta; chorioangioma, placenta

23–86. malignant melanoma
p 457
placenta, metastatic tumors; melanoma

23–87. b
p 458
umbilical cord, abnormalities; long cord; knot, umbilical cord

23–88. b
p 458
umbilical cord, abnormalities; long cord; umbilical cord prolapse

23–89. a
p 458
umbilical cord, abnormalities; short cord; placental abruption

23–90. a
p 458
umbilical cord, abnormalities; short cord; intrafunicular hemorrhage

23–91. a,b,c,d,f
pp 458-459
umbilical cord, abnormalities; velamentous insertion; vasa previa; battledore placenta

23–92. c,d
pp 460-461
umbilical cord, abnormalities

23–93. b,c,d
pp 461-462
amnion; amnionic caruncles; amnion nodosum

23–94. excess amnionic fluid (>2000 ml)
p 462
hydramnios

23–95. a,b,c,d
pp 462-463
hydramnios

23–96. a,b,c,d,e,i
p 462
hydramnios; esophageal atresia; multifetal pregnancy; anencephaly; diabetes, maternal; erythroblastosis fetalis, hydropic; spina bifida

23–97. a,b,c,d,e
p 463
hydramnios

23–98. dyspnea; difficulty in palpating fetal small parts; difficulty in hearing fetal heart tones; pain with rapidly increasing uterine size; edema of the lower extremities, the vulva, and the abdominal wall
p 463
hydramnios

23–99. a,b,c,d
p 464
hydramnios

23–100. d
p 464
hydramnios; amniocentesis, therapeutic

23–101. b
p 464
hydramnios; amniocentesis; infection, fetal; intrauterine infection

23–102. a
p 464
hydramnios; amniocentesis; umbilical cord prolapse

23–103. a
p 464
hydramnios; amniocentesis; placental abruption

23–104. b
p 464
hydramnios; amniocentesis; hemorrhage, fetal

23–105. a,b,d,e
p 465
oligohydramnios; pulmonary hypoplasia, fetal; amnionic band amputation; postmaturity

23–106. a
p 465
oligohydramnios; fetal malformations

24–1. b; abortion is the termination of pregnancy by any means before the fetus is sufficiently developed to survive.
p 467
abortion

24–2. a
p 477
abortion, elective

24–3. b
pp 467, 477
abortion, therapeutic

24–4. c
p 467
abortion, elective

24-5. a
p 467
abortion

24-6. Viability may be defined as a reasonable potential for subsequent survival if the fetus is removed from the uterus.
p 467
viability, definition; abortion, viability

24-7. termination of pregnancy before 38 weeks of gestation but after the fetus has achieved some potential for survival
p 467
prematurity; preterm

24-8. 1 = 20 completed weeks; 2 = 500 grams
p 467
abortion, definition

24-9. c
p 467
immaturity; prematurity; gestational age

24-10. failure to include (or recognize) early spontaneous abortions; inclusion of actual induced abortions as early spontaneous abortions
pp 467-468
abortion, incidence; spontaneous abortion

24-11. a,b,c,d
p 468
abortion, spontaneous

24-12. a,b,e
p 468
abortion, spontaneous; chromosomal anomalies, abortion; fetal development, abnormal

24-13. 1 = b; 2 = a
p 468
abortion, spontaneous; chromosomal anomalies, abortion; trisomy; monosomy

24-14. a
p 469
abortion, spontaneous; gamete aging

24-15. a,b,c,d
p 469
abortion, spontaneous; uterine environment, abortion

24-16. b; (c) is still not certain but possible
pp 469-470
abortion, spontaneous; infection, abortion; toxoplasmosis; Listeria monocytogenes

24-17. b
p 470
abortion, spontaneous

24-18. None of these hormones is of great clinical utility in predicting the outcome of a particular pregnancy.
p 470
abortion, spontaneous; fetal well-being; hormone levels, spontaneous abortion

24-19. a,b,c
p 470
abortion, spontaneous; alcohol, abortion; smoking, abortion; nutrition, pregnancy

24-20. a
p 470
abortion, spontaneous; immunologic factors, abortion

24-21. b,c,d
p 470
abortion, spontaneous; laparotomy, spontaneous abortion; peritonitis, abortion; myomas, abortion

24-22. c,e,f
pp 470-471
abortion, spontaneous; reproductive tract abnormalities, spontaneous abortion; myomas, abortion

24-23. a
p 471
abortion, spontaneous; reproductive tract abnormalities, spontaneous abortion; uterine incarceration

24-24. Fertilization results in a zygote with too little or too much chromosomal material.
pp 471, 468
abortion, spontaneous; paternal factors, spontaneous abortion

24-25. b
p 471
abortion, spontaneous; carneous mole

24-26. a
p 471
abortion, spontaneous; blighted ovum

24-27. e
p 471
abortion, spontaneous; fetus papyraceus

24-28. c
p 471
abortion, spontaneous; tuberous mole

24-29. d
p 471
abortion, spontaneous; macerated fetus

24-30. a,b,c,d
pp 471-472
abortion, pathology; blighted ovum; fetus papyraceus; fetus compressus; multifetal pregnancy, fetal demise; twin pregnancy, fetal demise

24–31. a
pp 472–473
abortion, threatened

24–32. c
pp 472–473
abortion, incomplete

24–33. b
pp 472–473
abortion, inevitable

24–34. e
pp 472–473
abortion, habitual

24–35. d
pp 472–473
abortion, missed

24–36. a,c,d
p 472
abortion, threatened; antepartum bleeding

24–37. b,c,d
p 472
abortion, threatened; prematurity; low birth weight; perinatal death, abortion

24–38. b
p 472
abortion, inevitable; rupture of the membranes, preterm

24–39. a,b
p 472
abortion, incomplete

24–40. c
p 472
abortion, missed; fetal death

24–41. a
p 473
abortion, threatened; antepartum bleeding

24–42. 1 = a; 2 = b
p 473
abortion, threatened

24–43. a,b,c
p 473
abortion, threatened; pain, threatened abortion

24–44. b,c,e,f
pp 473–474
abortion, threatened; threatened abortion, management; hCG, serial determinations; progesterone

24–45. a
p 473
abortion, threatened; ultrasonography, abortion

24–46. b
p 474
abortion, threatened; antepartum bleeding; pain, threatened abortion

24–47. a,b,d
p 474
abortion, inevitable; rupture of the membranes; abortion, septic

24–48. a,d
p 474
abortion, incomplete; hemorrhage, abortion; suction curettage

24–49. b
p 474
abortion, missed

24–50. three or more consecutive spontaneous abortions
p 474
abortion, habitual

24–51. a
p 474
cytogenetic abnormalities, spontaneous abortion; abortion, spontaneous

24–52. b
p 474
maternal factors, spontaneous abortion; abortion, spontaneous

24–53. c
pp 474–475
abortion, habitual

24–54. a,b,c,d
p 475
incompetent cervix; abortion, habitual

24–55. a
p 475
incompetent cervix; abortion, habitual

24–56. a,b
p 475
incompetent cervix; abortion, habitual; stilbestrol, in utero exposure; cervix, trauma

24–57. b
p 475
incompetent cervix; abortion, habitual

24–58. bleeding; uterine contractions
p 475
cerclage, contraindications; incompetent cervix; abortion, habitual

24–59. a,b,c,e
p 475
incompetent cervix; cerclage; Shirodkar procedure; McDonald procedure; abortion, habitual

24–60. rupture of the uterus or cervix
p 475
incompetent cervix; uterus, rupture; cerclage, complications; abortion, habitual

24-61. b
p 475
incompetent cervix; cerclage; Shirodkar procedure; McDonald procedure; abortion, habitual

24-62. when the pregnancy may threaten the life of the woman or seriously impair her health; when the pregnancy has resulted from rape or incest; when continuation of the pregnancy is likely to result in the birth of a child with severe physical deformities or mental retardation
p 477
abortion, therapeutic

24-63. b
p 478
abortion, elective

24-64. a,b,c,d,e
curettage, complications; suction curettage; abortion, transvaginal

24-65. a
p 479
suction curettage; dilation and curettage

24-66. b
p 479
suction curettage; dilation and curettage

24-67. a,b,c,d
pp 479-480
abortion, transvaginal; laminaria, cervical dilation; prostaglandins, cervical softening; paracervical block anesthesia

24-68. Any instrument introduced into the uterine cavity may cause perforation.
p 480
uterine perforation; abortion, transvaginal

24-69. adequate dilation of the cervix; uterine evacuation without perforation; removal of all the products of conception but not the decidua basalis
p 481
abortion, transvaginal; morbidity, abortion

24-70. a,b,c
p 481
abortion, transvaginal; uterine perforation

24-71. a,d
p 481
abortion, transvaginal; uterine perforation

24-72. a,b,c
p 481
abortion, transvaginal; uterine synechiae; incompetent cervix; consumptive coagulopathy

24-73. a,b,c,d,e
p 481
menstrual aspiration

24-74. performing the procedure on a woman who is not pregnant; missing the implanted zygote with the small Karman curet; failure to recognize an ectopic pregnancy; uterine perforation
p 481
menstrual aspiration; uterine perforation; incomplete abortion

24-75. a
p 481
Rh isoimmunization, abortion; Rho (D) immune globulin, prophylaxis

24-76. b
p 481
menstrual aspiration

24-77. a,b,c,d
pp 481-482
hysterotomy; hysterectomy; second trimester abortion

24-78. b,c,e
p 482
oxytocin; abortion, induction

24-79. b,d,e
p 482
prostaglandins; abortion, induction

24-80. b,c,d
p 483
hyperosmotic solutions, abortion; abortion, induction

24-81. a,b,c,d,e,f,g,h,i,j,k
p 483
hyperosmotic solutions, abortion; hypertonic saline, side effects; abortion, induction

24-82. b,c,d
pp 483-484
abortion, sequelae; maternal mortality, abortion; Asherman's syndrome; incompetent cervix

24-83. a
p 484
abortion, sequelae; ovulation, abortion

24-84. uterine evacuation; administration of antibiotics
p 484
septic abortion

24-85. a,b,c,d,e
pp 484-485
septic shock

24-86. a,b,d
p 485
septic shock

24-87. perfusion of vital organs
p 485
septic shock

24-88. a,b,c,d
pp 485, 487
septic shock

24-89. a,b,d
p 487
septic shock

24-90. b,c,d
p 488
septic shock; renal failure

25-1. a
p 491
Bartholin glands; Bartholin glands, infection

25-2. b
p 491
Bartholin duct cyst

25-3. None of these should be surgically excised during pregnancy.
p 491
urethral diverticula; periurethral abscess; periurethral cyst

25-4. b,c,d
p 491
condyloma; cesarean delivery; podophyllin

25-5. a
pp 491-492
vulvar varices

25-6. vaginal delivery of a large infant without episiotomy and with tearing of the lower genital tract
p 492
cystocele; rectocele

25-7. b,c
p 492
cystocele; rectocele

25-8. b
p 492
stress incontinence, pregnancy

25-9. Gartner or Müllerian duct remnants
p 492
vaginal cysts, origin; Gartner duct; Müllerian duct

25-10. b
p 492
vaginal cysts, management

25-11. b,d
pp 492-493
cervical neoplasia, pregnancy; colposcopy

25-12. a,b,c,d
p 493
cervical dysplasia; conization

25-13. b
p 493
cervical dysplasia; endocervical curettage

25-14. c
p 493
cervical dysplasia

25-15. a
p 493
cervical carcinoma, pregnancy; staging, cervical carcinoma

25-16. a,b,c,d
pp 493-494
cervical carcinoma, invasive; staging, cervical carcinoma

25-17. a
p 493
cervical dysplasia, management

25-18. a
p 493
carcinoma in situ, management

25-19. e
pp 493-494
cervical carcinoma, management

25-20. c
pp 493-494
cervical carcinoma, management

25-21. b
p 494
uterine myoma, pregnancy; tumors, pregnancy

25-22. lack of or faulty fusion of the Müllerian ducts; unilateral maturation of the Müllerian duct with incomplete or absent development on the opposite side; defective canalization of the vagina
p 494
reproductive tract, developmental abnormalities; Müllerian duct

25-23. d
p 494
reproductive tract, developmental abnormalities; double uterus

25-24. c
p 494
reproductive tract, developmental abnormalities; bicornuate uterus

25-25. b
p 494
reproductive tract, developmental abnormalities; septate uterus

25-26. a
p 494
reproductive tract, developmental abnormalities; single uterus

25-27. single (normal cervix); septate (single muscular ring partitioned by a septum); double (two distinct cervices); single hemicervix
pp 494-495
cervix, developmental abnormalities

25-28. 1 = there is faulty longitudinal fusion of the Müllerian anlage; 2 = the united Müllerian anlage does not canalize normally
p 495
vagina, longitudinally septate; vagina, transversely septate; reproductive tract, developmental abnormalities

25-29. c
p 495
reproductive tract, developmental abnormalities

25-30. a,b,c,d,e
p 495
reproductive tract, developmental abnormalities; hemiuterus, obstetric significance; uterine abnormalities, obstetric significance

25-31. a
p 495
uterine abnormalities, obstetric significance

25-32. b
p 495
anatomic abnormalities, diagnosis

25-33. urinary tract
p 497
reproductive tract, developmental abnormalities; urinary tract, developmental abnormalities

25-34. a,b,c,d
p 497
uterine abnormalities, obstetric significance; cesarean delivery; abortion

25-35. c
p 497
anatomic abnormalities, treatment; metroplasty

25-36. a synthetic, nonsteroidal estrogen
p 497
stilbestrol

25-37. b,c
p 498
stilbestrol, reproductive tract abnormalities; clear cell adenocarcinoma

25-38. b,c,d,e
pp 499-500
uterus, retroversion; uterus, anteflexion; sacculation; uterine incarceration

25-39. extensive dilation of the lower portion of the body of the uterus
p 499
uterus, sacculation

25-40. a,b,c,d
p 500
uterus, prolapse; prolapsed uterus, management

25-41. a
p 500
cystocele; rectocele

25-42. Early in the second trimester, the chorion fuses with the decidua to completely obliterate the uterine cavity.
p 501
salpingitis, pregnancy

25-43. hydrorrhea gravidarum
p 501
hydrorrhea gravidarum; rupture of the membranes

25-44. none of these
p 501
endometriosis

26-1. abortion; increased perinatal mortality; low birth weight; fetal malformation; fetal-fetal hemorrhage; pregnancy induced or aggravated hypertension; maternal anemia; placental accidents; maternal hemorrhage; cord accidents; hydramnios; complicated labor
p 503
multifetal pregnancy, complications

26-2. a
p 503
twins, monozygotic

26-3. b
p 503
twins, monozygotic

26-4. c
pp 503-504
twins, monozygotic; monoamnionic, monochorionic twins

26-5. a
pp 503-504
twins, monozygotic; diamnionic, dichorionic twins

26-6. b
pp 503-504
twins, monozygotic; diamnionic, monochorionic twins

26-7. d
pp 503-504
twins, monozygotic; conjoined twins

26-8. c
pp 503-504
twins, monozygotic; monoamnionic, monochorionic twins

26-9. a
pp 503-504
twins, monozygotic; monoamnionic, monochorionic twins

26-10. b
pp 503-504
twins, monozygotic; diamnionic, monochorionic twins

26–11. a
p 503
twins, monozygotic; diamnionic, dichorionic twins

26–12. 1 set/250 births
p 504
twins, monozygotic

26–13. None of the factors seems to influence the incidence of monozygotic twins.
p 504
twins, monozygotic

26–14. a,b,c,d,e
p 504
twins, dizygotic

26–15. d,e
p 504-506
multifetal pregnancy; ovulation induction, multifetal pregnancy

26–16. a
p 506
twins, monozygotic

26–17. b
p 506
twins, dizygotic; twins, monozygotic

26–18. b,c
pp 506-507
zygosity

26–19. a
p 508
twins, conjoined; thoracopagus

26–20. d
p 508
twins, conjoined; ischiopagus

26–21. c
p 508
twins, conjoined; craniopagus

26–22. b
p 508
twins conjoined; pyopagus

26–23. thoracopagus
p 508
twins, conjoined; thoracopagus

26–24. a
p 508
twins, conjoined

26–25. a
p 509
twins, monozygotic; arteriovenous anastomoses, twins; twin-to-twin transfusion

26–26. b
p 509
twins, monozygotic; arteriovenous anastomoses, twins; twin-to-twin transfusion

26–27. b
p 509
twins, monzygotic; arteriovenous anastomoses, twins; twin-to-twin transfusion; cardiac hypertrophy, neonatal

26–28. a
p 509
twins, monozygotic; arteriovenous anastomoses, twins; twin-to-twin transfusion; microcardia, neonatal

26–29. b
p 509
twins, monozygotic; arteriovenous anastomoses, twins; twin-to-twin transfusion

26–30. b
p 509
twins, monozygotic; arteriovenous anastomoses, twins; twin-to-twin transfusion; polycythemia, neonatal

26–31. a
p 509
twins, monozygotic; arteriovenous anastomoses, twins; twin-to-twin transfusion; anemia, neonatal

26–32. a,b,c,d
p 510
twins, monozygotic; arteriovenous anastomoses, twins; twin-to-twin transfusion; hyperbilirubinemia

26–33. 1 = b; 2 = a
p 510
mosaicism; chimerism

26–34. b
p 510
chimerism; twin-to-twin transfusion; twins, monozygotic

26–35. multifetal pregnancy; bladder distention; inaccurate menstrual history; hydramnios; hydatidiform mole; uterine myomas or adenomyosis; closely attached adnexal mass; fetal macrosomia
p 510
multifetal pregnancy, diagnosis; uterine enlargement, differential diagnosis

26–36. a,b,c,f
pp 510-511
multifetal pregnancy, diagnosis; ultrasonography; x-ray

26–37. None of these biochemical tests clearly differentiates a multifetal pregnancy from a singleton pregnancy or from other possibilities such as hydatidiform mole.
pp 511-512
multifetal pregnancy, diagnosis; hCG; α-fetoprotein; estriol, urinary

26-38. a,d
pp 512-513
perinatal mortality rate, multifetal pregnancy; intrauterine fetal demise

26-39. 1 = 39; 2 = 35; 3 = 33; 4 = 29
p 514
multifetal pregnancy, duration

26-40. a
p 514
multifetal pregnancy, growth retardation; fetal growth retardation; intrauterine growth retardation

26-41. a
p 514
multifetal pregnancy, growth retardation; fetal growth retardation; intrauterine growth retardation

26-42. b
p 516
multifetal pregnancy, growth retardation

26-43. a
p 516
superfetation

26-44. b
p 516
superfecundation

26-45. a,b,c,d,e
p 517
multifetal pregnancy, maternal adaptation; hypervolemia, pregnancy; anemia, pregnancy; blood loss, vaginal delivery; hydramnios

26-46. prevention of delivery of markedly premature infants; identification and treatment of failure to thrive in one or both fetuses; prevention of birth trauma; provision for expert neonatal care
p 517
mortality, multifetal pregnancy; morbidity, multifetal pregnancy; multifetal pregnancy, management

26-47. a,b,c,d,f
pp 517-519
multifetal pregnancy, management; β-mimetics; bed rest, multifetal pregnancy; tocolysis

26-48. b
p 519
L/S ratio, multifetal pregnancy; fetal lung maturity, multifetal pregnancy

26-49. premature labor; uterine dysfunction in labor; abnormal fetal presentation; umbilical cord prolapse; premature separation of a normally implanted placenta; immediate postpartum hemorrhage
p 519
multifetal pregnancy, complications; umbilical cord prolapse; postpartum hemorrhage; abnormal presentation

26-50. a,b,c,d,e
p 520
anesthesia, multifetal pregnancy; analgesia, multifetal pregnancy

26-51. a,b,c,d,e
pp 520-522
ultrasonography; vaginal delivery, multifetal pregnancy; cesarean delivery, multifetal pregnancy

27-1. b,c,d,e
p 525
hypertension, pregnancy

27-2. a diastolic blood pressure of 90 mm Hg or more or a rise in diastolic pressure of 15 mm Hg; a systolic blood pressure of 140 mm Hg or more or a rise in systolic pressure of 30 mm Hg; these blood pressures measured on two or more occasions at least 6 hours apart
p 525
hypertension, pregnancy; diastolic blood pressure, hypertension; systolic blood pressure, hypertension

27-3. d
p 525
chronic hypertensive disease, pregnancy

27-4. a
p 525
preeclampsia

27-5. c
p 525
superimposed preeclampsia

27-6. the occurrence of convulsions not caused by neurologic disease in women with preeclampsia
p 525
eclampsia; preeclampsia

27-7. b
p 525
preeclampsia; gestational hypertension

27-8. a,b,c,d,e,f,g,h
pp 526, 541
pregnancy-induced hypertension; preeclampsia

27-9. the presence of 300 mg or more of protein in a 24-hour urine collection or a protein concentration of at least 1 g/L in two random urine specimens collected 6 hours apart
p 526
proteinuria

27-10. e
p 526
preeclampsia; pregnancy-induced hypertension; edema, preeclampsia; proteinuria, preeclampsia

27–11. placental infarction; small placental size; placental abruption
p 527
placental infarction; placental abruption; uteroplacental insufficiency; perinatal mortality, pregnancy-induced hypertension; intrauterine growth retardation; fetal growth retardation

27–12. b
p 527
proteinuria; eclampsia

27–13. a
pp 526–527
perinatal mortality, pregnancy-induced hypertension; pregnancy-induced hypertension

27–14. 1 = absent; 2 = present; 3 = absent; 4 = present; 5 = absent; 6 = present; 7 = absent; 8 = present; 9 = absent; 10 = present; 11 = absent; 12 = present; 13 = absent; 14 = present
p 527 (Table 27–2)
pregnancy-induced hypertension; abdominal pain, pregnancy; headache, pregnancy; thrombocytopenia, pregnancy; visual disturbance, pregnancy

27–15. b
p 528
intrauterine growth retardation, pregnancy-induced hypertension; intrauterine growth retardation, superimposed preeclampsia; fetal growth retardation

27–16. b
pp 527–528
eclampsia

27–17. a history of hypertension (>140/90) prior to pregnancy; the discovery of hypertension (>140/90) in a pregnant woman before the 20th week of gestation in the absence of hydatidiform mole or multifetal pregnancy
p 528
coincidental hypertension; chronic hypertension

27–18. a,c,d
p 528
chronic hypertension; intrauterine growth retardation; superimposed preeclampsia; fetal growth retardation

27–19. a,b,c,d
p 528
chronic hypertension; placental abruption; cerebrovascular accident

27–20. documentation of chronic hypertension; presence of a superimposed acute process: increase of systolic pressure of 30 mm Hg; increase of diastolic pressure of 15 mm Hg; development of edema and/or proteinuria
p 529
superimposed preeclampsia; pregnancy-aggravated hypertension

27–21. a,b,d
p 529
vasospasm; pregnancy-induced hypertension

27–22. a,b,e
pp 529–530
preeclampsia; eclampsia; angiotensin II, pregnancy-induced hypertension

27–23. a
pp 530–531
supine pressor response, pregnancy-induced hypertension

27–24. a,d
p 531
cardiac output, pregnancy; peripheral resistance, pregnancy

27–25. a,c
p 531
cardiac output, pregnancy-induced hypertension; peripheral resistance, pregnancy-induced hypertension

27–26. a,b,c,d
p 531
cardiac function, assessment; preload, cardiac function; afterload, cardiac function; inotropic state of the myocardium; heart rate

27–27. c
pp 531–532
afterload, cardiac function; α-adrenergic system

27–28. a
pp 531–532
preload, cardiac function

27–29. hydralazine
p 532
hydralazine; preeclampsia, treatment; eclampsia, treatment; antihypertensive medication, pregnancy

27–30. a
p 532
afterload, cardiac function

27–31. b
p 532
cardiac output, pregnancy-induced hypertension; peripheral resistance, pregnancy-induced hypertension

27–32. a,c,d
pp 533–534
preeclampsia, hematologic changes; eclampsia, hematologic changes; pregnancy hypervolemia, pregnancy-induced hypertension

27–33. intravascular permeability causing excess accumulation of extracellular fluid (probably the most important cause); generalized vasoconstriction
pp 533–535
hemoconcentration; blood volume; preeclampsia, vascular changes

27–34. b
p 534
eclampsia, blood volume; intravascular volume, pregnancy-induced hypertension

27–35. a
p 534
eclampsia, blood volume; intravascular volume, pregnancy-induced hypertension

27–36. b,d
p 534
preeclampsia, coagulation changes; eclampsia, coagulation changes

27–37. a
pp 534–535
preeclampsia, coagulation changes; eclampsia, coagulation changes

27–38. b
p 535
preeclampsia, endocrine changes; renin

27–39. b
p 535
preeclampsia, endocrine changes; angiotensin II

27–40. b
p 535
preeclampsia, endocrine changes; aldosterone

27–41. c; sometimes a
p 535
preeclampsia, endocrine changes; deoxycorticosterone

27–42. b
p 536
preeclampsia, endocrine changes; edema, preeclampsia; deoxycorticosterone

27–43. a,b
pp 536–537
pregnancy-induced hypertension, maternal effects; preeclampsia, renal changes

27–44. There is swelling of glomerular capillary endothelial cells and subendothelial deposition of proteinaceous material.
p 536
preeclampsia, renal changes; pregnancy-induced hypertension, renal changes

27–45. tubular necrosis; renal cortical necrosis
p 537
pregnancy-induced hypertension, renal changes

27–46. b,c,d
pp 537–538
pregnancy-induced hypertension, hepatic effects

27–47. a
p 538
pregnancy-induced hypertension, hepatic effects; subcapsular liver hemorrhage

27–48. None of these is abnormal in the brains of women with pregnancy-induced hypertension.
p 538
pregnancy-induced hypertension, brain

27–49. a
p 538
pregnancy-induced hypertension, brain; eclampsia, genetic determinant

27–50. a,b,c,d,e
p 538
pregnancy-induced hypertension, brain

27–51. c
p 538
placental perfusion; uteroplacental circulation

27–52. b
p 538
uteroplacental circulation, pregnancy-induced hypertension; intrauterine growth retardation; fetal growth retardation

27–53. a,b,c,e
pp 538–539
uteroplacental circulation, pregnancy-induced hypertension; hydralazine; thiazide diuretics; dehydroisoandrostrone sulfate

27–54. 1 = 5/100; 2 = 1/1000 to 1500 deliveries
p 539
preeclampsia, incidence; eclampsia, incidence

27–55. None of these has been clearly linked to the development of pregnancy-induced hypertension.
p 540
pregnancy-induced hypertension, etiology

27–56. a
pp 539–540
pregnancy-induced hypertension, genetic determinant

27–57. b
p 540
preeclampsia; headache, pregnancy; visual disturbance, pregnancy; hypertension, pregnancy; proteinuria, pregnancy

27–58. a,c
p 540
preeclampsia, clinical aspects; diastolic blood pressure, preeclampsia

27–59. a,d
pp 540–541
preeclampsia; proteinuria, pregnancy; headache, pregnancy; visual disturbance, pregnancy; epigastric pain, pregnancy; weight gain, preeclampsia

27–60. b
p 541
pregnancy-induced hypertension, prognosis

27-61. nulliparity; family history of preeclampsia-eclampsia; diabetes; chronic vascular or renal disease; hydatidiform mole; fetal hydrops; multifetal pregnancy
pp 526, 541
preeclampsia, predisposing factors; nulliparity; multifetal pregnancy; diabetes; hydatidiform mole; fetal hydrops

27-62. a,b,c,d
p 541
pregnancy-induced hypertension, detection

27-63. b
p 541
pregnancy-induced hypertension, weight gain

27-64. b,c,d
pp 541-542
pregnancy-induced hypertension, diuretics; thiazide diuretics

27-65. a
p 542
pregnancy-induced hypertension, sodium restriction

27-66. None of these statements about the treatment of pregnancy-induced hypertension is correct.
p 542
pregnancy-induced hypertension, treatment

27-67. a,b,c,e,f,g,h
pp 541-543
antepartum care, pregnancy-induced hypertension; preeclampsia, mild

27-68. severity of the preeclampsia; gestational age of the fetus; condition of the cervix
p 542
preeclampsia, management

27-69. mild cases that are near term
p 542
preeclampsia, management

27-70. a,b,c,d,e
pp 542-544
preeclampsia, management; hydralazine; magnesium sulfate; oliguria

27-71. a,b,c
p 543
preeclampsia, management; eclampsia, management; glucocorticosteroids, pregnancy-induced hypertension

27-72. None of these provides information that is otherwise unavailable.
p 543
pregnancy-induced hypertension, management

27-73. a
p 543
intrauterine growth retardation, pregnancy-induced hypertension; fetal growth retardation

27-74. a,b
p 544
pregnancy-induced hypertension, postpartum period

27-75. a
p 544
eclampsia

27-76. b,d,e
p 544
eclampsia, convulsions; eclampsia

27-77. a,c
pp 544-545
eclampsia, prognosis; pulmonary edema, eclampsia; fever, eclampsia

27-78. Intercurrent eclampsia is the uncommon situation where the woman returns to a completely oriented state after an eclamptic seizure and coma, occasionally with the disappearance of all evidence of the preeclampsia-eclampsia.
p 545
eclampsia, intercurrent

27-79. The likelihood of chronic vascular or renal disease increases as the duration of postpartum hypertension increases.
p 545
chronic hypertension; postpartum hypertension

27-80. a,b,c,d,e,f,g
p 545
eclampsia, differential diagnosis

27-81. a
p 547
eclampsia, differential diagnosis

27-82. control of convulsions; correction of hypoxia and acidosis; lowering of blood pressure as needed; delivery once the mother is free of convulsions
p 547
eclampsia, treatment

27-83. None of these changes tends to be permanent.
p 547
eclampsia

27-84. control convulsions with magnesium sulfate; intermittent intravenous administration of hydralazine whenever diastolic pressure is >110 mm Hg; avoid diuretics and hyperosmotic agents; limit fluid intake except when fluid loss is excessive; effect delivery
p 547
eclampsia, treatment

27-85. a,b,c,d,e
pp 547-548, 552
magnesium sulfate; eclampsia, treatment

27-86. c
p 548
magnesium sulfate, respiratory depression

27-87. b
p 548
magnesium sulfate

27-88. a
p 548
magnesium sulfate

27-89. calcium gluconate
p 548
magnesium sulfate, respiratory depression; calcium gluconate

27-90. a
p 549
hydralazine; hemorrhage, intracranial; preeclampsia, treatment; eclampsia, treatment

27-91. b
p 548
sodium nitroprusside, side effects

27-92. a
p 548
diazoxide, side effects

27-93. a
p 548
diazoxide, side effects

27-94. b
p 548
sodium nitroprusside, side effects

27-95. a,b,c,d,e
pp 549-550
eclampsia, diuretics

27-96. b,d,e
p 550
eclampsia, fluid; hematocrit, eclampsia

27-97. b
p 551
delivery, eclampsia; magnesium sulfate; induction of labor

27-98. e
p 551
delivery, eclampsia; anesthesia, eclampsia

27-99. a,b,c,d
p 551
anesthesia, eclampsia; delivery, eclampsia

27-100. a,c
pp 552-554
magnesium sulfate; myometrial contractility

27-101. c
p 553
eclampsia, treatment

27-102. a
pp 553-554
eclampsia, recurrence

27-103. b
p 553
eclampsia, multifetal pregnancy

27-104. a
p 554
preeclampsia, residual hypertension

27-105. a,b,c,d
p 554
chronic hypertension

27-106. e
pp 554-556
chronic hypertension; superimposed preeclampsia; antihypertensive medication

27-107. There is a sudden rise in blood pressure which is almost always complicated by substantial proteinuria; in neglected cases oliguria, convulsions, and coma are likely. The frequencies of fetal growth retardation and prematurity are increased.
p 556
pregnancy-aggravated hypertension

28-1. a,b,c,d
p 561
medical disease, pregnancy

28-2. a,b,c,d
p 561
anemia

28-3. a,b,c
p 561
anemia; anemia, pregnancy; anemia, puerperium

28-4. a
p 562
anemia; plasma expansion, pregnancy; red cell volume, pregnancy

28-5. a,b,d
pp 562-563
anemia, pregnancy; iron supplementation, pregnancy; red cell volume, pregnancy

28-6. iron deficiency and blood loss
p 563
anemia, pregnancy; iron deficiency, pregnancy; blood loss, vaginal delivery

28-7. d
p 563
iron, pregnancy

28-8. b
p 563
iron, pregnancy

28-9. c
p 563
iron, pregnancy

28-10. a
p 563
iron, pregnancy

28-11. a
p 563
iron deficiency anemia; anemia, pregnancy

28-12. c,e,f
p 563
iron deficiency anemia; erythropoiesis, pregnancy; Plummer-Vinson's syndrome

28-13. a,b,c,d,e,f
p 563
anemia, pregnancy; CBC, pregnancy; sickle cell preparation; ferritin

28-14. c
pp 564-565
iron deficiency anemia, treatment; iron replacement, pregnancy

28-15. a,e
pp 564-565
iron deficiency anemia, treatment; iron supplementation, pregnancy; ferrous sulfate

28-16. exchange transfusion
pp 565
anemia; exchange transfusion

28-17. a,b,c,d
p 565
acute blood loss anemia; obstetric hemorrhage; anemia, acute blood loss; blood loss, vaginal delivery

28-18. a,c,d
pp 565-566
anemia, chronic disease; anemia, pregnancy; iron supplementation, pregnancy

28-19. b,d,e,g
pp 566-567
megaloblastic anemia; folic acid, deficiency; vitamin B_{12}*, deficiency; anemia, pregnancy*

28-20. a,b,c
p 566
folic acid, deficiency; anemia, pregnancy

28-21. a,b
p 567
pernicious anemia

28-22. a
p 567
vitamin B_{12}*, deficiency; breast feeding; megaloblastic anemia, neonatal*

28-23. a,b,c,d,e
pp 567-568
hemolytic anemia, acquired; pregnancy-induced hypertension; hemolytic anemia, autoimmune; anemia, pregnancy; Coombs test; Clostridium perfringens *exotoxin*

28-24. b
p 568
paroxysmal nocturnal hemoglobinuria

28-25. a
p 568
hemolytic anemia, drug-induced; glucose-6-phosphate dehydrogenase

28-26. a,b,c,f,g
pp 568-569
aplastic anemia; leukopenia, pregnancy; anemia, pregnancy; thrombocytopenia, pregnancy

28-27. hemorrhage and infection
pp 569
aplastic anemia; infection, aplastic anemia; hemorrhage, aplastic anemia; anemia, pregnancy

28-28. sickle cell anemia; sickle cell-hemoglobin C disease; sickle cell-β-thalassemia
p 569
sickle cell anemia; sickle cell-hemoglobin C disease; sickle cell-β-thalassemia; hemoglobinopathies, pregnancy

28-29. a,b,c
pp 569-570
sickle cell anemia; neonatal mortality, sickle cell anemia; maternal mortality, sickle cell anemia; folic acid, supplementation; anemia, pregnancy

28-30. a,b
p 570
contraception, sickle cell anemia; sickle cell disease, contraception; oral contraception, sickle cell disease; intrauterine device, sickle cell disease

28-31. b,c,e,f
pp 570-571
sickle cell-hemoglobin C disease; iron supplementation; folic acid supplementation; exchange transfusion, maternal; pulmonary dysfunction, hemoglobinopathies

28-32. 1 = b; 2 = a
pp 570-571
sickle cell-β-thalassemia; perinatal mortality, sickle cell hemoglobinopathies; anemia, pregnancy; perinatal morbidity, sickle cell hemoglobinopathies

28-33. b
pp 571-572
sickle cell hemoglobinopathy, pregnancy; exchange transfusion, sickle cell hemoglobinopathy

28-34. b,c,d
p 572
sickle cell trait; bacteriuria, asymptomatic

28-35. a
p 573
hemoglobin C

28-36. a,b
p 573
hemoglobin C; hemoglobin E

28-37. a,b
p 573
hemoglobin C; hemoglobin E; iron supplementation; folic acid supplementation

28-38. a,b
p 573
hemoglobin C; hemoglobin E

28-39. b
p 573
hemolytic anemia, sickle cell anemia; hemolytic anemia, sickle cell-hemoglobin C disease

28-40. 1 = c; 2 = c
p 573
hemoglobinopathy, genetic inheritance

28-41. a,b,c
p 573
sickle cell anemia; fetoscopy; amniocentesis, genetic; chorionic villus biopsy

28-42. a,b,d
p 574
hereditary spherocytosis

28-43. genetic disorders that are characterized by impaired production of one or more globin peptide chains
p 574
thalassemias

28-44. a
p 574
α-thalassemia; hemoglobin Bart's disease

28-45. b
p 574
α-thalassemia; hemoglobin H disease

28-46. c
p 574
α-thalassemia; α-thalassemia minor

28-47. c
p 574
α-thalassemia; α-thalassemia minor

28-48. d
p 574
α-thalassemia; α-thalassemia, carrier state

28-49. a,b,d
pp 574-575
α-thalassemia; hemoglobin Bart's disease; α-thalassemia minor; sickle cell anemia, α-thalassemia; hydrops fetalis, nonimmune; anemia, pregnancy

28-50. c,d
p 575
β-thalassemia; β-thalassemia, minor; β-thalassemia, intermedia; infertility

28-51. a,b,c,d,e,f,g
pp 575
thrombocytopenia; aplastic anemia; hemolytic anemia, acquired; eclampsia; consumptive coagulopathy; lupus erythematosus; megaloblastic anemia

28-52. a,c,e
pp 575-576
immune idiopathic thrombocytopenia

28-53. c
pp 576-577
immune idiopathic thrombocytopenia

28-54. None of the listed treatments is an effective treatment for immune idiopathic thrombocytopenia.
p 577
immune idiopathic thrombocytopenia

28-55. fever; neurologic abnormalities; thrombocytopenia; renal impairment; hemolytic anemia
p 577
thrombotic thrombocytopenic purpura

28-56. eclampsia complicated by thrombocytopenia, overt intravascular hemolysis, and hemoglobinuria
p 578
thrombotic thrombocytopenic purpura; eclampsia, differential diagnosis

28-57. a,c,e
pp 577-578
thrombotic thrombocytopenic purpura; plasmapheresis; exchange transfusion, maternal

28-58. b
p 578
obstetric hemorrhage

28-59. a,b,c,e
p 578
hemophilia A; coagulation disorders, pregnancy

28-60. a
p 578
obstetric hemorrhage; Factor VIII, coagulation factors; coagulation disorders, pregnancy

28-61. b
p 578
hemophilia B; Factor IX, coagulation factors; coagulation disorders, pregnancy

28-62. c,d,e
p 579
von Willebrand's disease; Factor VIII, coagulation factors; coagulation disorders, pregnancy

28-63. d
p 579
coagulation disorders, pregnancy

28-64. c,d,e
pp 579-580
leukemia; Hodgkin's disease; polycythemia; erythropoietin

28–65. a
p 580
urinary tract diseases, pregnancy

28–66. d,e
p 580
urinary tract infection; cystitis; pyelonephritis, acute; bacteriuria

28–67. a,b,c,e
p 580
cystitis

28–68. d
p 580
urethritis; Chlamydia

28–69. e
pp 580-581
pyelonephritis, acute

28–70. a,b,c,d
p 581
pyelonephritis, acute; labor; placental abruption; appendicitis; myomata, infarction

28–71. Compression of the ureter by the enlarged uterus and ovarian veins results in a progressive dilation of the renal calyces, pelves, and ureters, accompanied by a decrease in tone and peristaltic action. These changes lead to urinary stasis, which increases the susceptibility to renal infection.
p 581
pyelonephritis, acute; bacteriuria; urinary tract, pregnancy changes

28–72. a,b,c,d,e
p 581
pyelonephritis, acute; anesthesia, effects; bladder overdistention; oxytocin, antidiuretic effect; catheterization, bladder

28–73. persistent, actively multiplying bacteria within the urinary tract without the symptoms of a urinary tract infection
p 581
bacteriuria, asymptomatic

28–74. a,d
p 581
bacteriuria, asymptomatic; sickle cell trait; urinary tract infection, pregnancy

28–75. a
pp 581-582
bacteriuria, asymptomatic; prematurity; low birth weight

28–76. c
p 582
bacteriuria, asymptomatic

28–77. a,b,e
pp 582
pyelonephritis, chronic; pyelonephritis, acute

28–78. c,d
pp 583-584
urinary tract infection, pregnancy; pyelonephritis, acute

28–79. e
p 583
gentamicin; ototoxicity; urinary tract infection, pregnancy

28–80. b
p 583
nitrofurantoin; hemolysis, maternal; urinary tract infection, pregnancy

28–81. c
p 583
tetracycline; jaundice, maternal; urinary tract infection, pregnancy

28–82. c
p 583
tetracycline; tooth discoloration, neonatal; urinary tract infection, pregnancy

28–83. a
p 583
sulfonamide; kernicterus; urinary tract infection, pregnancy

28–84. e
p 583
gentamicin; nephrotoxicity; urinary tract infection, pregnancy

28–85. d
p 583
chloramphenicol; aplastic anemia; urinary tract infection, pregnancy

28–86. e
pp 583-584
urinary tract infection, pregnancy; ampicillin; gentamicin

28–87. b
p 584
urinary tract infection, pregnancy; pyuria

28–88. b
p 589
renal tuberculosis

28–89. b,d
p 584
urinary calculi; hyperparathyroidism; urinary tract infection, pregnancy

28–90. a,b,c,d
pp 584-585
glomerulonephritis, acute; preeclampsia

28–91. a,c,d,e
p 585
glomerulonephritis, chronic; preeclampsia

28-92. a,b,c,d
p 585
nephrosis (nephrotic syndrome)

28-93. a,b,c,d,e,f,g
p 585
nephrosis; syphilis; glomerulonephritis, chronic; lupus erythematosus; diabetes; amyloidosis; renal vein thrombosis; heavy metal poisoning

28-94. b
p 585
nephrosis

28-95. c
p 586
acute renal failure

28-96. a,b
p 586
acute tubular necrosis; eclampsia; preeclampsia; septic shock

28-97. a,b,c
p 586
acute tubular necrosis; eclampsia; preeclampsia; blood replacement; septic shock

28-98. b,e
p 586
renal cortical necrosis; placental abruption; pregnancy-induced hypertension; preeclampsia; eclampsia; septic shock

28-99. b
p 587
renal failure, obstructive; oliguria; ureteral obstruction, pregnancy

28-100. a,b,d,e
p 587
hemolytic uremic syndrome, postpartum; thrombocytopenia

28-101. a,b,c,d,e
pp 587-589
renal transplantation; polycystic kidney; orthostatic proteinuria; nephrectomy; hemodialysis

28-102. a,c
p 589
rheumatic heart disease; congenital heart disease; cardiac disease, pregnancy

28-103. d
pp 589-590
cardiac disease, pregnancy

28-104. a,b,c,d
p 590
cardiac disease, pregnancy

28-105. a,b,c,d,e
p 590
cardiac disease, pregnancy

28-106. c
p 590
cardiac disease, class III; cardiac disease, N.Y. Heart Association classification

28-107. d
p 590
cardiac disease, class IV; cardiac disease, N.Y. Heart Association classification

28-108. a
p 590
cardiac disease, class I; cardiac disease, N.Y. Heart Association classification

28-109. b
p 590
cardiac disease, class II; cardiac disease, N.Y. Heart Association classification

28-110. a,b,c,d,e
pp 590-591
cardiac disease, pregnancy

28-111. a,b,c
p 591
cardiac disease, class I; cardiac disease, class II; infection, cardiac failure

28-112. b,c,d,e
p 591
cardiac disease, pregnancy; heart failure

28-113. maternal hypotension
p 591
cardiac disease, delivery, anesthesia, conduction; anesthesia, cardiac disease; hypotension, cardiac disease

28-114. a,d
p 591
cardiac disease; delivery, cardiac disease; anesthesia, cardiac disease

28-115. b
p 591
cardiac failure, labor

28-116. a,b,e
pp 591-592
cardiac failure, pregnancy

28-117. a,b,d
p 592
cardiac failure; cardiac decompensation; antepartum care, cardiac disease; furosemide

28-118. a,b,c
p 592
cardiac disease, class III; cardiac decompensation

28-119. cardiac decompensation must be corrected
p 593
cardiac failure; abortion, cardiac failure

28–120. correction of cardiac decompensation
p 593
cardiac disease, class IV: cardiac decompensation

28–121. a
p 593
prematurity; intrauterine death; hypoxia, maternal; abortion

28–122. b,c,d,e
p 593
cardiac disease, pregnancy; artificial heart valves, pregnancy; anticoagulation, pregnancy; heparin; abortion, spontaneous; low birth weight

28–123. just before delivery
p 593
heparin; artificial heart valves; anticoagulation, pregnancy; delivery, anticoagulation

28–124. a reverse of blood flow from the pulmonary artery to the aorta with the development of cyanosis
p 594
patent ductus arteriosus; congenital heart defects; pulmonary hypertension

28–125. a
pp 593-594
polycythemia, spontaneous abortion; abortion, spontaneous

28–126. b,d,e
p 594
cyanotic heart disease; polycythemia; tetralogy of Fallot; Eisenmenger's syndrome

28–127. a,b
pp 594-595
ischemic heart disease; coarctation of the aorta; cardiomyopathy; mitral valve prolapse

28–128. The deformed thoracic cage causes some areas of the lung to be emphysematous and others to be atelectatic. Both result in inadequate ventilatory capacity.
p 595
kyphosclerotic heart disease; cor pulmonale; kyphosis

28–129. a,b,c,d
p 596
kyphosclerotic heart disease; kyphosis; abortion, therapeutic

28–130. None of the cardiac arrhythmias is incompatible with a normal pregnancy outcome.
p 596
cardiac arrhythmias, pregnancy

28–131. a
p 596
pulmonary function, pregnancy; transverse thoracic diameter

28–132. b
p 596
pulmonary function, pregnancy; vertical chest diameter

28–133. b
p 596
pulmonary function, pregnancy; residual volume

28–134. a
p 596
pulmonary function, pregnancy; respiratory rate

28–135. a
p 596
pulmonary function, pregnancy; tidal volume

28–136. b
p 596
pulmonary function, pregnancy; plasma carbon dioxide, pregnancy

28–137. a
p 596
pulmonary function, pregnancy; oxygen consumption, pregnancy

28–138. a,b,c,d
p 596
pneumonia, pregnancy; infection, pregnancy; pulmonary function, pregnancy

28–139. a
p 596
thromboembolism; pulmonary infarction

28–140. a,d,e
p 597
asthma; goiter, fetal

28–141. a,b,c,d
p 597
asthma

28–142. b,d
pp 597-598
tuberculosis

28–143. Pyridoxine should be administered to avoid neurotoxicity in the fetus.
p 597
tuberculosis; isoniazid; pyridoxine

28–144. a
p 597
tuberculosis

28–145. b
p 598
sarcoidosis

28–146. a,c,d,e
p 598
cystic fibrosis; infertility

28–147. 1 = a; 2 = c
p 598
diabetes

28-148. a,b
pp 598-599
diabetes

28-149. a,b,c,d
p 599
diabetes; macrosomia; stillbirth

28-150. identification of fasting hyperglycemia on two or more occasions (plasma level of 105 mg/dl or higher)
p 599
diabetes

28-151. b
p 599
diabetes, class A; glucose tolerance test

28-152. g
p 599
diabetes, class A; glucose tolerance test

28-153. e
p 599
diabetes, class A; glucose tolerance test

28-154. d
p 599
diabetes, class A; glucose tolerance test

28-155. a,c,d
pp 599-600
diabetes; glucose tolerance test; diabetes, class A

28-156. a,b,c,d
p 600
diabetes; glucose tolerance test

28-157. a,b,c,d
p 600
diabetes; insulin, pregnancy; placental lactogen; estrogen; progesterone; placental insulinase

28-158. a,b,c
p 600
diabetes, pregnancy

28-159. a,b,c,d,e,f
p 600
diabetes, pregnancy; cesarean delivery; pregnancy-induced hypertension; infection; macrosomia; hydramnios; postpartum hemorrhage; preeclampsia

28-160. a,b,c,d,e,f,g
pp 600-601
diabetes, fetal effects; perinatal death rate; birth injury; respiratory distress; congenital anomalies

28-161. d
p 601
diabetes, fetal effects; macrosomia

28-162. a,b,c,d
p 601
diabetes

28-163. a,c,e
pp 601-602
diabetes, class A; diabetes, overt

28-164. b,c,d
p 602
diabetes; congenital anomalies

28-165. a,b,c,d,e
p 602
diabetes; gestational age

28-166. b
p 602
diabetes; glucosuria; insulin, diabetes management

28-167. Acetonuria usually indicates a need to increase the insulin dose.
p 602
diabetes; acetonuria; insulin, diabetes, management

28-168. None of these drugs is recommended for use in a pregnancy that is complicated by diabetes.
p 603
diabetes; tolbutamide; estradiol; stilbestrol

28-169. c
p 603
diabetes; fetal well-being; nonstress test

28-170. a,b,c,d,e,f
p 604
diabetes; induction of labor, diabetes

28-171. a,c,e
p 604
diabetes; delivery, diabetes; insulin, diabetes management

28-172. a,c,d,e
p 604
diabetes; perinatal morbidity, diabetes; respiratory distress; hypoglycemia, neonatal; hypocalcemia, neonatal; hyperbilirubinemia

28-173. b
p 604
diabetes; fetal development, diabetes

28-174. c
p 604
diabetes, contraception, diabetes, barrier methods

28-175. a,b,d
p 604
thyroid disease; endocrine system, changes in pregnancy

28-176. a,b,c,d,e
p 604
hyperthyroidism

28-177. a,b
p 605
hyperthyroidism

28–178. b
p 605
hyperthyroidism; propylthiouracil; propranolol; iodine; goiter, fetal

28–179. The dose is increased until the woman appears clinically to be only minimally thyrotoxic and the level of thyroxine in the blood is in the upper range of normal for pregnancy.
p 605
hyperthyroidism; propylthiouracil

28–180. a,b,c,d,e
p 605
propranolol; hyperthyroidism; fetal growth retardation; fetal distress; hypoglycemia, neonatal; hyperbilirubinemia, neonatal

28–181. a
p 605
hyperthyroidism; thyroidectomy

28–182. a
p 605
hyperthyroidism, breastfeeding

28–183. Maternal thyroid-stimulating immunoglobulins cross the placenta to cause hyperthyroidism in the fetus and newborn.
p 605
hyperthyroidism, neonatal; Grave's disease; thyroid-stimulating hormone; placental transfer

28–184. a
p 605
hyperthyroidism, neonatal; propylthiouracil

28–185. b
pp 605-606
thyroid storm

28–186. a,b,c
p 606
hypothyroidism, neonatal; cretinism; infertility; abortion, spontaneous

28–187. a,b
p 606
hyperparathyroidism; hypoparathyroidism; tetany, neonatal

28–188. a,c,e
pp 606-607
adrenal dysfunction; Addison's disease; Cushing's disease; aldosteronism; pheochromocytoma

28–189. a
p 607
pituitary disease; diabetes insipidus; pituitary microadenomas; bromocriptine

28–190. b,c
pp 607-608
epilepsy; phenytoin

28–191. a,b,c,d,e,f
p 608
phenytoin, fetal anomalies; mental retardation; craniofacial anomalies; distal limb dysmorphosis; cleft lip; cleft palate; congenital heart disease; hemorrhagic disease, newborn

28–192. b
p 608
valproic acid; craniofacial anomalies

28–193. a
p 608
carbamazepine (Tegretol); microcephalus

28–194. b
p 608
valproic acid; neural tube defects

28–195. b
p 608
valproic acid; skeletal anomalies

28–196. b
p 608
epilepsy; anticonvulsant medications, pregnancy

28–197. megaloblastic anemia, due to a deficiency of folic acid
p 608
megaloblastic anemia; epilepsy; folic acid

28–198. magnesium sulfate
p 609
magnesium sulfate; epilepsy, convulsions; eclampsia, convulsions

28–199. a,c
p 609
intracranial hemorrhage; therapeutic abortion, intracranial hemorrhage

28–200. h
pp 609-610
therapeutic abortion; Huntington's chorea

28–201. a,b,c,d,e
p 609
spinal cord lesion, pregnancy; labor, second stage; fetopelvic disproportion; urinary tract infection; autonomic hyperreflexia

28–202. a
p 609
multiple sclerosis

28–203. b,c,d,f
p 610
myasthenia gravis; labor, second stage; myasthenia gravis, newborn

28-204. a,b,c,d
p 610
myasthenia gravis, newborn

28-205. a,b,c,d
p 610
myasthenia gravis; quinine; magnesium sulfate; kanamycin; gentamicin

28-206. b
p 610
migraine

28-207. b,d
pp 610-611
psychosis; lithium; cardiac defects, neonatal; breast feeding

28-208. a,c,d,e,f
p 611
liver disease; palmar erythema; spider angiomata; albumin, serum

28-209. intrahepatic cholestasis; hepatocellular damage due to pregnancy-induced hypertension; acute fatty liver; hepatic dysfunction due to hyperemesis gravidarum
p 611
liver disease; intrahepatic cholestasis; pregnancy-induced hypertension; acute fatty liver; hyperemesis gravidarum

28-210. a,b,c,d
p 611
intrahepatic cholestasis

28-211. icterus, pruritis
p 611
intrahepatic cholestasis

28-212. b,c,d
p 611
intrahepatic cholestasis

28-213. a,b,c,d
p 611
acute fatty liver

28-214. a,d
pp 612-613
acute fatty liver; Reye's syndrome

28-215. epigastric or right upper quadrant pain
p 613
liver disease; preeclampsia

28-216. a,b,c,d
p 613
hyperemesis gravidarum; hepatitis; pyelonephritis; gasteroenteritis; cholestasis; peptic ulcer; jaundice, maternal

28-217. a,b,c,d,e
p 613
hyperemesis gravidarum

28-218. a,b,c,d,e
pp 613-614
hepatitis A

28-219. b
p 614
hepatitis A; gamma globulin

28-220. a,c,d,e,f
p 614
hepatitis B; immune globulin, hepatitis B

28-221. a,b
p 614
hepatitis A; hepatitis B

28-222. a,b
p 614
hepatitis A; hepatitis B

28-223. b
p 614
hepatitis B

28-224. It is an indication of the infectious state. It correlates with the number of circulating virus particles. It also relates to the vertical transmission (mother to fetus) of hepatitis.
p 614
hepatitis B

28-225. c
pp 614-615
non-A-non-B hepatitis; blood transfusion, hepatitis

28-226. a
p 615
non-A-non-B hepatitis; immune globulin

28-227. a,b
p 615
chronic active hepatitis

28-228. a
p 615
cirrhosis

28-229. a,b
p 615
gallbladder disease; cholelithiasis

28-230. the common occurrence of anorexia, nausea, and vomiting during pregnancy; the displacement of the appendix by the enlarging uterus; the occurrence of leukocytosis during pregnancy; presence of other diseases during pregnancy that may be confused with appendicitis (e.g., pyelonephritis, placental abruption)
p 616
appendicitis

28-231. c,d,f
p 616
appendicitis

28–232. a,b,c
p 616
peptic ulcer; preeclampsia; pancreatitis; abdominal pain, pregnancy

28–233. d
p 617
ulcerative colitis; regional enteritis

28–234. a,b,c,d,e
p 618
obesity; hypertension; diabetes; thromboembolism; aspiration; wound infection

28–235. b
p 618
obesity; weight reduction, pregnancy

28–236. a
p 618
obesity; gastric bypass; jejunoileal bypass

28–237. malar rash; discoid rash; photosensitivity; oral ulcers; arthritis; serositis; renal disorders; neurologic disorders; hematologic disorders; immunologic disorders; antinuclear antibody
p 618
systemic lupus erythematosus

28–238. b
p 618
systemic lupus erythematosus

28–239. a,b,c,d
p 619
systemic lupus erythematosus; azathioprine

28–240. c,d,e
p 619
systemic lupus erythematosus

28–241. neuropathy; convulsions; thrombocytopenia
p 620
systemic lupus erythematosus; preeclampsia; eclampsia

28–242. a,b,c,d,e,f,g
pp 619–620
systemic lupus erythematosus, fetal effects; fetal growth retardation; heart block; stillbirth

28–243. a
p 620
systemic lupus erythematosus; heart block, neonatal

28–244. b,c,d
p 620
systemic lupus erythematosus; contraception, systemic lupus erythematosus

28–245. It is a prothrombinase complex inhibitor, an IgG immunoglobin. It can be associated with lupus or exist in patients without lupus. It incites thrombosis, and may be associated with recurrent fetal loss.
pp 620–621
systemic lupus erythematosus; lupus anticoagulant

28–246. e
pp 621–622
rheumatoid arthritis; dermatomyositis; scleroderma; polyarteritis nodosa

28–247. b
p 622
Marfan's syndrome; aortic aneurysm

28–248. b
p 622
sexually transmitted diseases

28–249. a,d,e
p 623
syphilis

28–250. condyloma latum
p 623
syphilis; condyloma latum

28–251. a
p 623
syphilis, congenital; stillbirth; syphilis

28–252. a,c,d
p 623
syphilis; VDRL

28–253. a,d,e
p 623
syphilis, treatment; benzathine penicillin G; erythromycin; tetracycline

28–254. a,d,e
p 623
syphilis, treatment; gonorrhea, treatment; benzathine penicillin G; erythromycin; tetracycline

28–255. d
p 623
erythromycin; syphilis, treatment

28–256. a
p 623
benzathine penicillin G; syphilis, treatment

28–257. b
p 623
benzathine penicillin G; syphilis, treatment

28–258. b
p 623
benzathine penicillin G; syphilis, treatment

28–259. c
p 623
crystalline penicillin G; benzathine penicillin G; syphilis treatment

28–260. at least every 6 months for 3 years
p 624
syphilis

28–261. a,b,e
p 624
syphilis

28–262. a,d
p 624
syphilis, congenital

28–263. The chorion laeve has fused with the decidua parietalis; this obliterates the endometrial cavity and prevents disease transmission up into the oviducts.
p 624
gonorrhea; chorion laeve; decidua parietalis; salpingitis

28–264. a,b,c,d
pp 624
gonorrhea; cervix; urethra; Bartholin's glands; paraurethral glands

28–265. infection of the sexual partner; gonococcal arthritis; gonococcal endocarditis; gonococcal ophthalmia of the newborn; postpartum pelvic infection
p 624
gonorrhea; ophthalmia neonatorum

28–266. a
p 624
gonorrhea

28–267. a
p 625
gonorrhea; procaine penicillin, aqueous

28–268. b
p 625
gonorrhea, penicillin resistant; spectinomycin

28–269. a,f
p 625
gonorrhea; erythromycin; procaine penicillin, aqueous; Chlamydia

28–270. c,d
p 625
gonorrhea, disseminated infection; crystalline penicillin; ampicillin

28–271. c
p 625
crystalline penicillin; gonorrhea, neonatal

28–272. spectinomycin; cefoxitin; cefotaxime
p 625
gonorrhea, penicillin resistant; spectinomycin; cefoxitin; cefotaxime

28–273. The infant should be isolated and treated for 24 hours with IV penicillin. Eye care by an experienced practitioner is also important.
p 625
gonorrhea, neonatal; gonococcal ophthalmia

28–274. a
p 625
Chlamydia; lymphogranuloma venereum

28–275. type II
pp 625–626
herpes, genital

28–276. b,c,d,e
p 626
herpes, genital; cervix

28–277. b
p 676
herpes, genital; acyclovir

28–278. a,b,c
p 676
herpes, genital; cervical neoplasia

28–279. d,e
p 626
herpes, neonatal

28–280. the threat of fetal infection with transvaginal delivery and the attendant increase in perinatal morbidity and mortality
p 626
herpes, delivery; cesarean delivery, herpes; perinatal morbidity; perinatal mortality

28–281. c
p 627
herpes; cesarean delivery; neonatal care, herpes; breast feeding, herpes

28–282. a
p 627
chancroid

28–283. b
p 627
granuloma inguinale

28–284. a
p 627
chancroid

28–285. b
p 627
granuloma inguinale

28–286. a
p 627
chancroid

28–287. a
p 627
chancroid

28–288. b
p 627
granuloma inguinale; Donovan bodies

28-289. b,c,d,e,f
pp 627-628
varicella; varicella pneumonia; acyclovir; immune globulin

28-290. a,b
pp 628-630
mumps; abortion; prematurity

28-291. a,b,d
pp 628-630
rubeola; abortion; prematurity

28-292. c,e
pp 628-630
influenza; pneumonia

28-293. e,f
pp 628-630
common cold

28-294. c,f
pp 628-630
poliomyelitis

28-295. a
pp 628-630
scarlet fever; abortion

28-296. a,b,c
pp 628-630
typhoid fever; abortion; prematurity

28-297. a,b
pp 628-630
malaria; abortion; prematurity

28-298. None of these is an indication for therapeutic abortion.
pp 628-629
abortion, therapeutic

28-299. a,c,d,e
p 630
herpes gestationis

28-300. b,d
p 630
acne; papular dermatitis; alopecia; chloasma; melasma gravidarum

28-301. b,d,e
p 631
melanoma; placenta, metastatic tumor; fetus, metastatic tumor

28-302. a,b
pp 631-632
hiatal hernia; carpal tunnel syndrome; symphyseal separation

28-303. None of the statements about breast carcinoma in pregnancy is correct.
p 632
breast carcinoma

28-304. n
p 599
diabetes, White classification

28-305. k
p 599
diabetes, White classification

28-306. c
p 599
diabetes, White classification

28-307. f
p 599
diabetes, White classification

28-308. a
p 599
diabetes, White classification

28-309. h
p 599
diabetes, White classification

28-310. d
p 599
diabetes, White classification

28-311. i
p 599
diabetes, White classification

28-312. b
p 599
diabetes, White classification

28-313. e
p 599
diabetes, White classification

28-314. g
p 599
diabetes, White classification

28-315. j
p 599
diabetes, White classification

28-316. m
p 599
diabetes, White classification

28-317. o
p 599
diabetes, White classification

28-318. l
p 599
diabetes, White classification

29–1. insufficiently strong or coordinated uterine forces that cannot efface and dilate the cervix; voluntary muscle efforts in the second stage of labor that are inadequate to overcome the resistance of the birth canal; faulty fetal presentation or abnormal fetal shape; abnormalities of the birth canal
p 641
dystocia, causes

29–2. pelvic contraction accompanied by uterine dysfunction
p 641
dystocia; pelvic contraction; uterine dysfunction

29–3. a
p 641
uterine dysfunction; fetopelvic disproportion

29–4. a
p 641
cervical effacement; labor, latent phase

29–5. b
p 641
cervical dilation; labor, active phase

29–6. 1 = mild; 2 = strong; 3 = short; 4 = long; 5 = irregular; 6 = regular
p 641
labor, Friedman curve; labor, latent phase; labor, active phase; uterine contractions

29–7. c,d
p 641-642
uterine dysfunction; cervical dilation rates; protracted labor, active phase

29–8. b
pp 642-643
uterine dysfunction, hypertonic

29–9. a
pp 642-643
uterine dysfunction, hypotonic

29–10. a
pp 642-643
uterine dysfunction, hypotonic

29–11. b
pp 642-643
uterine dysfunction, hypertonic

29–12. a
pp 642-643
uterine dysfunction, hypotonic

29–13. b
pp 642-643
uterine dysfunction, hypertonic

29–14. a
pp 642-643
uterine dysfunction, hypotonic

29–15. 1 = >14 hr; 2 = <1.2 cm per hr; 3 = <2.0 cm per hr; 4 = >3 hr; 5 = >2 hr; 6 = >1 hr; 7 = no descent in the deceleration phase or in the second stage of labor
p 643 (Table 29–1)
abnormal labor; prolongation disorders, labor; protraction disorders, labor; arrest disorders, labor

29–16. 1 = therapeutic rest; 2 = oxytocin or cesarean delivery for urgent problems; 3 = expectant management and support; 4 = cesarean delivery for cephalopelvic disproportion
p 643 (Table 29–1)
prolongation disorder, labor; protraction disorder, labor

29–17. b
p 643
uterine dysfunction; dystocia

29–18. a,b,c,d
pp 643-644
uterine dysfunction

29–19. the patient must be in active labor; there must be no cephalopelvic disproportion
p 644
uterine dysfunction, hypotonic; cephalopelvic disproportion; oxytocin stimulation; augmentation of labor

29–20. Usually, spontaneous activity does not persist and the normal forces of labor are replaced by hypotonic uterine dysfunction.
p 644
uterine dysfunction, hypotonic; cephalopelvic disproportion; uterine rupture

29–21. a,b,c,d,e
pp 644-645
uterine dysfunction, hypotonic

29–22. normal diagonal conjugate; parallel pelvic sidewalls; ischial spines that are not prominent; sacrum not flat; angle of the subpubic arch not narrow; occiput presentation; fetal head descends through the pelvic inlet with fundal pressure
p 644
clinical pelvimetry; pelvis, noncontracted

29–23. b
p 644
uterine dysfunction, hypotonic; oxytocin, uterine dysfunction

29–24. Oxytocin has a potent antidiuretic action. Fluids may precipitate water intoxication that may lead to convulsions, coma, or death.
pp 644-645
oxytocin, actions; water intoxication

29–25. a,c,e
p 645
oxytocin, uterine dysfunction; uterine dysfunction

29–26. a,c,e
pp 644-645
uterine dysfunction, hypotonic; oxytocin, uterine dysfunction; labor, stimulation

29–27. a
p 645
oxytocin, uterine dysfunction; cesarean delivery

29–28. b
p 646
labor, latent phase; uterine dysfunction, hypotonic; labor, false

29–29. c
pp 646-647
prostaglandins; cervical ripening; induction of labor; augmentation of labor

29–30. a,c
p 647
uterine dysfunction, hypertonic

29–31. a,b,c,d
p 647
pushing; labor, second stage; voluntary expulsive forces

29–32. a,b,c,f
pp 647-648
precipitate labor; postpartum hemorrhage; amnionic fluid embolism

29–33. a,b,c,d
p 648
contraction ring; protracted labor; pathologic retraction ring, Bandl

29–34. Uterine contractions begin at or near term but then disappear without the birth of a fetus. The fetus then dies and is retained in utero.
p 648
missed labor

30–1. 1 = 33; 2 = 3 to 4 (6 to 7)
pp 651, 652 (Table 30–1)
breech presentation, incidence

30–2. a,b,c,e,g,h,i,j,k,l,m
p 651
breech presentation, incidence; grand multiparity; multifetal pregnancy; hydramnios; hydrocephalus; anencephaly; uterine anomaly; placenta previa; breech presentation, recurrent

30–3. increased perinatal morbidity and mortality; low birth weight; umbilical cord prolapse; placenta previa; fetal anomalies and perinatal developmental abnormalities; multiple fetuses; need for operative intervention, especially cesarean delivery
p 651
breech presentation, associated complications; perinatal mortality; umbilical cord prolapse; intrauterine growth retardation; multifetal pregnancy, cesarean delivery; fetal growth retardation

30–4. b
p 651
breech, complete

30–5. a
p 651
breech, frank

30–6. c
p 651
breech, incomplete

30–7. a
pp 651-652
breech, frank

30–8. b
p 652
abdominal examination, breech presentation; Leopold maneuvers

30–9. 1 = slightly above the umbilicus; 2 = below the umbilicus
p 652
fetal heart sounds, cephalic presentation; fetal heart sounds, breech presentation

30–10. a,b,d
p 652
vaginal examination, breech presentation

30–11. b
p 652
ultrasonography, breech presentation; x-ray, breech presentation

30–12. a
p 652
breech presentation, maternal mortality; maternal morbidity; maternal mortality

30–13. prematurity; congenital anomalies; birth trauma
p 652
breech presentation, perinatal mortality; breech presentation, perinatal morbidity; prematurity; birth trauma; congenital anomalies; perinatal mortality

30–14. e
p 653
brain injury, breech presentation

30–15. b
pp 654-656
breech presentation, perinatal mortality; cesarean delivery

30–16. b,c
p 655
breech presentation, perinatal mortality; umbilical cord prolapse

30–17. a
p 655
breech presentation, perinatal mortality

30-18. a
p 655
breech presentation, perinatal mortality; prematurity

30-19. a,c,d
pp 656-657
external version; antepartum hemorrhage; premature labor

30-20. a,c
p 657
breech presentation, vaginal delivery; asphyxia, fetal; accommodation, fetal head

30-21. large fetus (>3500 g); contracted or unfavorably shaped pelvis; hyperextended head; maternal or fetal indications for delivery when the mother is not in labor; uterine dysfunction; footling breech; premature fetus (>26 weeks) with the mother in labor or in need of delivery; severe fetal growth retardation; history of previous perinatal death or children with birth trauma; firm request for sterilization by the mother
p 657
breech presentation, cesarean delivery; cesarean delivery, breech presentation

30-22. b,d
pp 225-226; 658
pelvic shape, breech presentation

30-23. injury to the cervical spinal cord
p 658
hyperextended fetal head; spinal cord injury, fetal

30-24. b,c,d
pp 658-659
vaginal delivery, breech presentation; breech presentation, delivery

30-25. b
p 659
face presentation

30-26. a,c,d
p 659
face presentation; pelvic contraction; anencephaly; macrosomia

30-27. a,b,d
p 660
face presentation; cesarean delivery, face presentation

30-28. a,b,c,d
p 662
brow presentation; caput succedaneum

30-29. b
p 662
brow presentation; vaginal examination, brow presentation

30-30. a
p 659
face presentation; vaginal examination, face presentation

30-31. b
p 662
shoulder presentation; oblique lie

30-32. a
p 662
shoulder presentation; transverse lie

30-33. a,b,c,d
pp 663-664
shoulder presentation; transverse lie

30-34. b,d,f,h
p 663
shoulder presentation; prematurity; placenta previa; contracted pelvis; fetopelvic disproportion; transverse lie

30-35. spontaneous rupture of the uterus or traumatic rupture consequent upon late and ill-advised version and extraction
p 664
shoulder presentation; uterus, rupture; maternal mortality

30-36. a,b,c,d
p 664
shoulder presentation; maternal mortality; maternal morbidity

30-37. a,d
pp 664-666
shoulder presentation; postpartum infection; conduplicato corpore; cesarean delivery, shoulder presentation

30-38. b
p 666
cesarean delivery, shoulder presentation; destructive procedure; shoulder presentation

30-39. a,b,c
p 666
compound presentation; perinatal mortality

30-40. d
pp 666-667
occiput posterior position, persistent; forceps delivery; episiotomy; midforceps rotation; Scanzoni maneuver

30-41. a,d
p 667
occiput posterior position, persistent; episiotomy; perinatal mortality

30-42. a,b,c,d
pp 667-668
occiput transverse position, persistent; hypotonic uterine dysfunction; deep transverse arrest; cesarean delivery, deep transverse arrest

30-43. With platypelloid and android pelves, there may not be adequate room for rotation of the occiput to either the anterior or posterior positions.
p 668
deep transverse arrest; android pelvis; platypelloid pelvis

30-44. >4000 g
p 668
fetal macrosomia

30-45. a,c,e,f,g,h
p 668
fetal macrosomia; prolonged gestation; diabetes, maternal; multiparity

30–46. a,c,d
p 668–669
fetal weight measurement; perinatal mortality; fetal macrosomia

30–47. a
p 669
shoulder dystocia; fetal macrosomia

30–48. The head is delivered causing the umbilical cord to be drawn into the pelvis and then compressed when the shoulders cannot be delivered.
p 669
shoulder dystocia; umbilical cord compression

30–49. a,b
p 669
shoulder dystocia; ultrasonography

30–50. First, the Woods "screw method" is attempted. The operator applies pressure to the infant's posterior scapula to rotate it upward, the posterior shoulder then being delivered as an anterior shoulder as it passes beneath the symphysis. If that fails, attempt to sweep the posterior arm over the chest to deliver it, then rotate the shoulder to an oblique diameter to allow delivery of the anterior shoulder. If that fails, deliberate fracture of the fetal clavicle is recommended to allow delivery.
p 669
shoulder dystocia; fetal macrosomia

30–51. a,c,d,e
p 669
hydrocephalus, internal; cerebrospinal fluid, excessive; breech presentation; spina bifida

30–52. b,c,d
pp 671–673
hydrocephalus, internal; uterus, rupture

30–53. a,c
p 671
hydrocephalus, internal; x-ray

30–54. a,b,c,d
p 673
fetal abdomen, enlargement; ascites, fetal; kidney, fetal

30–55. b
p 674
fetal abdomen, enlargement; ascites, fetal

31–1. a,b,c
p 677
pelvic contraction; dystocia

31–2. a,b,c
p 677
pelvic inlet contraction; diagonal conjugate

31–3. c
p 677
pelvic inlet contraction

31–4. 1 = a; 2 = a
p 677
pelvic contraction

31–5. b,d
p 677
x-ray; fetal head size, measurement; dolichocephaly

31–6. a,b,c
p 678
dolichocephaly; multifetal pregnancy; breech presentation; oligohydramnios

31–7. a,c,d
p 678
face presentation; shoulder presentation; pelvic inlet contraction; umbilical cord prolapse

31–8. b,c,d,e,f
p 678
pelvic inlet contraction; cervix, dilation; intrapartum infection; rupture of the membranes, spontaneous; dystocia, complications; uterine rupture

31–9. a
p 678
pelvic inlet contraction; pathologic contraction ring; cesarean delivery, indications; uterine rupture

31–10. a,b
pp 679–680
pelvic contraction; intracranial hemorrhage, fetal; molding; caput succedaneum; station, clinical determination

31–11. a
p 680
vaginal delivery, pelvic inlet contraction; occiput presentation; pelvic inlet contraction

31–12. b
p 680
vaginal delivery, pelvic inlet contraction; breech presentation; pelvic inlet contraction

31–13. b
p 680
vaginal delivery, pelvic inlet contraction; fetal macrosomia; pelvic inlet contraction

31–14. b
p 680
vaginal delivery, pelvic inlet contraction; android pelvis; pelvic inlet contraction

31–15. a
p 680
vaginal delivery, pelvic inlet contraction; cervix, dilation; pelvic inlet contraction

31–16. b
p 680
vaginal delivery, pelvic inlet contraction; uterine dysfunction; pelvic inlet contraction

31-17. b
p 680
vaginal delivery, pelvic inlet contraction; pelvic inlet contraction

31-18. b
p 680
vaginal delivery, pelvic inlet contraction; asynclitism; pelvic inlet contraction

31-19. c
pp 680-681
pelvic inlet contraction; oxytocin; uterine rupture

31-20. The plane extends from the inferior margin of the symphysis pubis, through the ischial spines, and touches the sacrum near the junction of the 4th and 5th vertebrae.
p 681
midpelvis

31-21. ischial spines
p 681
midpelvis; interspinous diameter

31-22. 1 = 10.5; 2 = 11.5; 3 = 5.0
p 681
midpelvis, measurements

31-23. d
p 681
pelvic contraction, midpelvis; midpelvis, measurements

31-24. c
p 681
pelvic contraction, midpelvis; interspinous diameter; midpelvis, measurements

31-25. b
p 681
pelvic contraction, midpelvis; pelvimetry, x-ray; ultrasonography

31-26. a
p 681
pelvic contraction, midpelvis; pelvic inlet contraction

31-27. b,c,d,e
pp 681-682
pelvic contraction, midpelvis; forceps delivery; midforceps delivery; labor

31-28. an interischial tuberous diameter of 8 cm or less
p 682
pelvic outlet contraction; interischial tuberous diameter

31-29. 1 and 2 = interischial tuberous diameter; 3 = pubic rami; 4 = pelvic soft tissue, no bony margins; 5 = inferior posterior surface of the symphysis pubis; 6 = tip of the last sacral vertebra
pp 682-683
pelvic outlet; interischial tuberous diameter

31-30. b
pp 682-683
pelvic outlet contraction; pelvic contraction, midpelvis

31-31. perineal tears due to distention caused by the fetal head
p 682
pelvic contraction, outlet; perineum, tears; outlet dystocia

31-32. b
p 683
pelvic fracture; cesarean delivery, indications

31-33. 1 = cardiorespiratory compromise; 2 = midpelvic contraction; 3 = cardiorespiratory compromise and midpelvic contraction
pp 683-684
pelvic contraction, kyphosis; pelvic contraction, midpelvis; kyphosis

31-34. a
pp 684-686
abnormal pelvis; dwarfism, obstetric complications; lameness, obstetric complications

32-1. a,b,c
p 687
vulva, atresia; Condylomata acuminata; *dystocia, vulva*

32-2. d,e,f
pp 687-688
vaginal septa; vagina, atresia; Gartner duct, cyst; levator ani, tetanic contraction; vagina, annular stricture

32-3. a,b,c,d,e
p 688
cervix, stenosis; conization

32-4. a,b
p 688
cervix, stenosis; cervix, conglutination

32-5. a
p 688
cervical carcinoma, invasive

32-6. a
p 688
uterus, anteflexion; diastasis recti; uterine displacement

32-7. b
p 688
uterus, retroflexion; abortion, spontaneous; uterine displacement

32-8. b
p 688
uterus, retroflexion; sacculation; uterus, rupture; uterine displacement

32-9. a,b
p 688
uterus, anteflexion; uterus, retroflexion; cervical dilation, impeded

32-10. a,b,c,d
p 688
uterine displacement, management; uterine displacement, effects on pregnancy

32-11. c
p 689
uterus, myoma; myoma, intramural

32-12. b
p. 689
uterus, myoma; myoma, subserous

32-13. a
p 689
uterus, myoma; myoma, submucous

32-14. d
p 689
uterus, myoma; myoma, pedunculated

32-15. b,d
p 689
uterus, myoma; hemorrhagic infarction; myoma, submucous

32-16. a,b,d,e
p 689
hemorrhagic infarction; placental abruption; appendicitis; ureteral stone; pyelonephritis

32-17. d
p 689
myomectomy, pregnancy; uterus, myoma; dystocia, myomas, uterine

32-18. a,d
pp 690-691
ovarian tumors, pregnancy; torsion, ovarian tumors; teratoma, cystic; cystadenoma, mucinous

32-19. a,b
p 691
ovarian tumors, pregnancy; laparotomy, pregnancy

32-20. d,e
p 691
cystocele; enterocele; bladder distention, labor; rectum, tumors

33-1. a,b,c,d
p 697
obstetric lacerations, perineum; rectocele; cystocele; uterine prolapse; vaginal relaxation

33-2. b,d,e
p 697
obstetric lacerations, vagina; pelvic relaxation; urinary incontinence; periurethral laceration

33-3. a,b,c
pp 697, 703
genital tract, lacerations; retained placental fragments

33-4. a,d,e
pp 697-698
cervix, lacerations; obstetric hemorrhage; annular cervical detachment; leukorrhea

33-5. c,d,e
pp 697-698
obstetric laceration, cervical; leukorrhea; vaginal packing; cautery, cervical; cryotherapy

33-6. a
p 698
uterine rupture

33-7. 1 = cesarean section or hysterotomy; repaired previous uterine rupture; myomectomy incision to endometrium; deep cornual resection; excision of uterine septum; 2 = instrumented abortion; sharp or blunt trauma; silent rupture during previous pregnancy
p 698
uterine rupture, etiology; cesarean delivery; myomectomy; hysterotomy; abortion, induced; cornual resection

33-8. 1 = persistent, intense, spontaneous contractions; oxytocin/prostaglandin administration; intraamnionic injection of hypertonic solution; perforation by monitor catheter; external trauma, blunt or sharp; marked uterine overdistention; 2 = internal podalic version; difficult forceps delivery; breech extraction; fetal anomaly that overdistends the lower uterine segment; vigorous fundal pressure; difficult manual removal of placenta
pp 698-699
uterine rupture, etiology

33-9. d
p 699
uterine rupture, etiology; placenta accreta

33-10. b
p 699
uterine rupture, complete

33-11. a
p 699
uterine rupture, incomplete

33-12. b
p 699
uterine rupture, complete; uterine rupture, incomplete

33-13. d
p 699
uterine rupture; cesarean section scar, rupture; cesarean section scar, dehiscence

33-14. through the body of the pregnant uterus
p 699
cesarean section scar, classical; classical cesarean section

33-15. b,e
pp 700-701
cesarean section, classical; cesarean section, lower segment; uterine rupture, cesarean delivery

33-16. b
p 701
cesarean section scar, healing

33-17. b,c,e
pp 701-703
uterine rupture, complete; uterine rupture, incomplete; oxytocin; uteroabdominal pregnancy

33-18. a,b,c,d
p 703
uterine rupture, labor

33-19. a,b
p 703
uterine rupture, labor; hemoperitoneum

33-20. 50 and 75 percent
p 704
perinatal mortality, uterine rupture; uterine rupture, perinatal mortality

33-21. a,b
pp 704, 706
uterine rupture, management; hysterectomy; obstetric hemorrhage; oxytocin

33-22. vesicovaginal
p 706
vesicovaginal fistula

34-1. 500 ml
p 707
postpartum hemorrhage; obstetric hemorrhage; labor, third stage

34-2. hemorrhage after the first 24 hours following birth
p 707
postpartum hemorrhage, delayed; obstetric hemorrhage

34-3. b
p 707
postpartum hemorrhage; obstetric hemorrhage

34-4. a,b,c,d,e,f,g
p 707
postpartum hemorrhage; obstetric hemorrhage; hypotonic myometrium; uterine atony

34-5. c,d
p 707
postpartum hemorrhage, immediate; obstetric hemorrhage; uterine atony; hypotonic myometrium; cervix, lacerations; vagina, lacerations; retained placenta

34-6. a,b,
p 708
postpartum hemorrhage; postpartum hemorrhage, delayed; retained placenta; obstetric hemorrhage

34-7. c,d
p 708
postpartum hemorrhage

34-8. b
p 708
placental separation; labor, third stage

34-9. the condition (degree of contraction) of the uterus
pp 708-709
postpartum hemorrhage; uterine atony; genital tract, laceration

34-10. a,b,c
p 708
postpartum hemorrhage; labor, third stage; breech extraction

34-11. a,b
p 708
postpartum hemorrhage; labor, third stage; vaginal delivery

34-12. a,b,c
p 708
postpartum hemorrhage; labor, third stage; internal podalic version

34-13. a,b,c
p 708
postpartum hemorrhage; labor, third stage; previous cesarean section, vaginal delivery

34-14. failure in lactation, atrophy of the breasts, loss of pubic and axillary hair, superinvolution of the uterus, hypothyroidism, and adrenal cortical insufficiency
p 709
Sheehan's syndrome; pituitary, anterior; obstetric hemorrhage

34-15. b
p 709
Sheehan's syndrome; obstetric hemorrhage; postpartum hemorrhage, sequelae; pituitary, anterior

34-16. a
p 709
mechanism of Duncan; labor, third stage

34-17. b
p 709
mechanism of Schultze; labor, third stage

34-18. a,b,c,d,e
pp 709, 711
third stage, management; placenta, separation; manual removal, placenta; postpartum hemorrhage

34-19. b,c,e
pp 709, 711
postpartum hemorrhage; oxytocin; uterine massage; prostaglandins; uterine packing; bimanual compression, uterus

34-20. The posterior aspect of the uterus is massaged with the abdominal hand. The vaginal hand, which is formed into a fist with the knuckles in contact with the uterine wall, massages the anterior uterine surface.
p 711
bimanual compression, uterus; postpartum hemorrhage, management

34-21. perform bimanual uterine compression; obtain help; transfuse with whole blood; inspect the birth canal for lacerations; explore the uterine cavity for retained placental fragments and/or lacerations; add a second intravenous line so that oxytocin administration may be maintained along with blood transfusion; constantly monitor maternal cardiovascular status
p 711
postpartum hemorrhage, management

34-22. a
p 712
cervix, lacerations; vagina, lacerations; postpartum hemorrhage, management

34-23. Vigorous transfusion therapy should be begun prior to surgery to combat the often profound hypovolemia.
p 712
hysterectomy; postpartum hemorrhage, management; transfusion, indications

34-24. b
p 712
placenta percreta

34-25. a
p 712
placenta increta

34-26. d
p 712
placenta accreta, partial

34-27. partial or total absence of the decidua basalis; imperfect development of the fibrinoid layer (Nitabuch's layer)
p 712
placentation, abnormal; Nitabuch's layer; decidua basalis; fibrinoid layer; placenta accreta

34-28. b
p 713
abnormally adherent placenta; placenta accreta

34-29. a,b,c,d
p 713
placenta accreta; placenta previa; multiparity, grand

34-30. a,b,d
pp 713, 715
placenta accreta; placenta previa; postpartum hemorrhage; obstetric hemorrhage

34-31. a
p 715
placenta accreta; placenta increta; ultrasonography; hysterectomy

34-32. a,c,e
pp 715-716
uterine inversion; obstetric hemorrhage; postpartum hemorrhage

34-33. obtain anesthesia consultation; if the inversion is fresh, attempt to manually reposition the uterus; institute two intravenous systems (lactated Ringers and whole blood); remove the placenta only after the uterus is repositioned and transfusion has been initiated; manually compress the uterus; administer intravenous oxytocin (only after uterine reposition and placental removal)
pp 716-717
uterine inversion; obstetric hemorrhage; postpartum hemorrhage; transfusion

34-34. a
p 717
uterine inversion; laparotomy

35-1. the infection of the genital tract after delivery
p 719
puerperal infection

35-2. a,b
p 719
puerperal infection; puerperal morbidity

35-3. a,b,c,d
p 719
puerperal morbidity; puerperium, fever; breast engorgement

35-4. a,c,d,e
p 720
postpartum infection; puerperal infection; vaginal examination, intrapartum; obstetric lacerations; rupture of membranes

35-5. None of mentioned antepartum factors has been clearly shown to predispose to puerperal infection.
p 720
puerperal infection; transferrin; anemia; nutrition, pregnancy; coitus, pregnancy

35-6. a,b,c
p 720
puerperal infection; vaginal examination, intrapartum; obstetric trauma

35-7. The postpartum genital tract has several areas that are essentially open wounds, and are consequently susceptible to the entry of infectious organisms. These are the site of placental attachment and the cervix or the birth canal which may have lacerations and/or an episiotomy incision.
pp 720-721
puerperal infection; obstetric lacerations; implantation site, placenta; episiotomy

35–8. a,b
pp 721, 725, 727
puerperal infection; obstetric lacerations; vagina, lacerations; cervix, lacerations

35–9. a,f
pp 721, 725, 727
metritis; postpartum fever; puerperal infection; breast feeding

35–10. b
p 721
thrombophlebitis; ovarian veins

35–11. a
p 721
thrombophlebitis; ovarian veins

35–12. c
p 721
thrombophlebitis; uterine veins

35–13. a,c
p 721
thrombophlebitis; puerperal infection; pulmonary embolism

35–14. a
p 721
thromboembolism; sudden death, maternal; cor pulmonale; septic thromboembolism

35–15. a,b,c,d
p 721
metritis; pulmonary embolism; sepsis; puerperal infection; pneumonia; thrombus

35–16. a
p 728
pelvic thrombophlebitis; puerperal infection

35–17. b,c
p 728
puerperal infection; pulmonary embolization; thrombophlebitis; anticoagulation; venous ligation; heparin

35–18. a,b
p 728
puerperal infection; thrombophlebitis; septic pulmonary emboli; anticoagulation; heparin

35–19. 1 = b; 2 = a
p 721
peritonitis; pelvic cellulitis (parametritis)

35–20. a,b,c
p 721
peritonitis; pelvic abscess

35–21. lymphatic transmission of organisms from infected lacerations of the uterus or cervix; direct extension of infection from lacerations of the cervix into the connective tissue at the base of the broad ligament; secondary to thrombophlebitis (through necrosis and breakdown of vessel walls)
pp 721–723
puerperal infection; pelvic cellulitis; parametritis; cervix, lacerations; uterus, lacerations; pelvic thrombophlebitis

35–22. a,b
p 722
puerperal infection; pelvic cellulitis; parametritis; cervix, lacerations; uterus, lacerations

35–23. a,b,c,d
pp 722, 724
puerperal infection; pelvic cellulitis; parametritis; pelvic abscess; space of Retzius; cul-de-sac of Douglas, abscess

35–24. a,b
pp 724–725
puerperal infection; blood culture; bacteriology, puerperal infection

35–25. b
p 725
puerperal infection; bacteriology, puerperal infection

35–26. a,b,c,d,f
pp 724–725
pelvic cellulitis; parametritis; puerperal infection; puerperium, morbidity; puerperium, fever

35–27. c,d
pp 725–726
pelvic peritonitis; puerperal infection

35–28. b,c
p 726
toxic shock syndrome; Staphylococcus *sp.*

35–29. respiratory complications, especially atelectasis and pneumonia; pyelonephritis; intense breast engorgement; bacterial mastitis; thrombophlebitis; episiotomy infection; wound abscess after laparotomy
p 726
puerperium, fever; atelectasis; breast engorgement; mastitis; thrombophlebitis; episiotomy, infection; pyelonephritis

35–30. a,c,d,e,f
p 726
atelectasis; puerperium, fever; pyelonephritis; breast engorgement; mastitis

35–31. a
p 726
thrombophlebitis; puerperium, fever

35–32. a,b,c,d,e
p 727
cephalosporins; clindamycin; gentamicin; chloramphenicol; vibramycin; pseudomembranous colitis

35–33. a
p 727
pelvic cellulitis; parametritis

35–34. a,b,c,d
p 728
peritonitis; clindamycin; gentamicin; cephalosporins; paralytic ileus

36–1. b
p 731
thromboembolism; venous thrombosis

36–2. stasis
p 731
thromboembolic disease; stasis, vascular; venous thrombosis

36–3. b
p 731
thromboembolic disease

36–4. a
p 731
ambulation, puerperium; thromboembolic disease

36–5. a
p 731
thrombophlebitis; venous thrombosis

36–6. b
p 731
phlebothrombosis; venous thrombosis

36–7. b
p 731
venous thrombosis, superficial; venous thrombosis, deep; pulmonary embolism

36–8. b
p 731
venous thrombosis, superficial; anticoagulation

36–9. a,d,e
pp 731–732
venous thrombosis, deep; venous thrombosis, puerperium; venous thrombosis, antepartum; anticoagulation; milk leg

36–10. b
pp 732–733
warfarin (coumadin); coagulation factors

36–11. b
pp 732–733
warfarin (coumadin); congenital malformations

36–12. a
pp 732–733
heparin; thrombocytopenia

36–13. b
pp 732–733
warfarin (coumadin); placental transfer

36–14. a
pp 732–733
heparin; placental transfer

36–15. c
pp 731–732
warfarin (coumadin); venous thrombosis, deep

36–16. b,c
pp 732–733
pelvic vein thrombosis; ovarian vein thrombophlebitis; heparin

36–17. a,e,f
pp 733–734
heparin; warfarin (coumadin); protamine sulfate; coagulation factors; fetus, intrapartum hemorrhage

36–18. dose, route, and time of administration of heparin relative to delivery; magnitude of incisions and obstetric lacerations; intensity of myometrial contraction upon completion of delivery of fetus and placenta (presence or absence of uterine atony); presence of other coagulation defects
p 733
anticoagulation, intrapartum; heparin

36–19. a
pp 734–735
pulmonary embolism; inferior vena cava, ligation

36–20. 1 in 2700 and 1 in 7000 deliveries
p 735
pulmonary embolism, incidence

36–21. a,b,d,e
p 736
pulmonary embolism

36–22. b
p 736
pulmonary embolism

36–23. a,c,e
p 736
heparin; warfarin (coumadin); pulmonary embolism

36–24. Ligation of the inferior vena cava below the level of the renal veins but above the entry of the right ovarian vein plus ligation of the left ovarian vein below its entry into the left renal vein is usually indicated.
p 736
pulmonary embolism, recurrent; inferior vena cava, ligation

36–25. b,c,d
p 737
subinvolution; metritis; ergonovine; methylergonovine

36–26. b
p 737
cervical erosions, puerperium

36–27. abnormal involution of the placental site; a retained portion of the placenta forms a placental polyp, which detaches from the myometrium and results in bleeding
p 737
postpartum hemorrhage, delayed; placental polyp; involution of the placental site, abnormal

36–28. b
pp 737–738
oxytocin; postpartum hemorrhage, delayed

36–29. b,e
pp 738–739
hematomas, puerperium; vagina, hematoma; vulva, hematoma

36–30. a,b,c,d,e
p 739
bladder function, puerperium; urinary tract infection, puerperium

36–31. a,d
pp 739–740
breast engorgement; breast fever; breast binders

36–32. a,c,d
pp 739–740
lactation, suppression; bromocriptine

36–33. b,c,e
pp 740–741
mastitis; Staphylococcus aureus; *puerperal fever; breast engorgement*

36–34. a
p 740
mastitis

36–35. a,c,d
pp 740–741
mastitis, suppurative; bacterial interference; staphylococcal infection; epidemic, nursery

36–36. Bacterial interference is the deliberate inoculation with a nonvirulent bacterial strain in order to prevent subsequent colonization with a virulent strain.
p 741
bacterial interference

36–37. a,b,c,e
pp 740–741
mastitis; staphylococcal infection; penicillin G; mastitis, suppurative; breast abscess; nursing, mastitis

36–38. the clogging of a duct and the consequent accumulation of milk in one or more breast lobules
p 741
galactocele

36–39. b,c,d
pp 741–742
polymastia; nipples; nipples, depressed; nipples, fissures; supernumary breasts

36–40. a
p 742
Chiari-Frommel's syndrome; pituitary adenoma; amenorrhea; estrogen; galactorrhea

36–41. a,b,d
p 742
footdrop; obstetric paralysis

36–42. b
p 742
symphysis pubis, separation in labor; sacroiliac synchondroses, separation in labor

37–1. the accurate determination of gestational age
p 745
gestational age; fetal growth, appropriate

37–2. b,c
p 745
preterm fetus; premature fetus

37–3. a
p 745
term fetus

37–4. d
p 745
postterm fetus

37–5. c
p 745
preterm fetus

37–6. a
p 745
preterm fetus; fetal growth retardation; intrauterine growth retardation

37–7. b
p 745
fetal growth retardation; intrauterine growth retardation

37–8. 1 = 10th; 2 = 90th
p 746
fetal weight; gestational age; intrauterine growth retardation; fetal growth retardation

37–9. b
pp 746–747
fetal weight; gestational age

37–10. a
p 747
fetal growth retardation, prematurity; prematurity; intrauterine growth retardation

37–11. a,b,c
p 747
fetal weight, term pregnancy

37–12. 1 = 3335; 2 = 3280 to 3400 g
p 747
fetal weight, term pregnancy

37–13. c
p 747 (Fig. 37–2)
fetal growth rate

37–14. a
p 747
high-risk pregnancy

37–15. b
p 747
fetal distress, definition

37–16. a,e,f
pp 748–750
neonatal care; neonatal mortality rate; fetal weight

37–17. 1 = 100; 2 = not applicable; 3 = 97; 4 = 100; 5 = 76; 6 = 26; 7 = 62; 8 = 29; 9 = 40; 10 = 3
pp 749–750
neonatal mortality; birthweight, neonatal outcomes; handicaps, occurrence by birthweight

37–18. Is further intrauterine stay likely to be of benefit or harm to the fetus?
p 751
preterm birth; intrauterine environment

37–19. b
p 750
intrauterine environment; preterm birth; fetal growth retardation; intrauterine growth retardation

37–20. c,d,e,f
pp 750–751
preterm labor; incompetent cervix; rupture of the membranes; hydramnios; multifetal pregnancy

37–21. b
p 750
preterm labor

37–22. uterine contractions occurring at least every 10 minutes and lasting for 30 seconds or more; progressive dilation of the cervix
p 751
preterm labor; cervix, dilation; labor

37–23. b
p 751
preterm labor; labor, inhibition; tocolysis

37–24. None of these statements about the management of preterm labor is correct.
pp 751–752
preterm labor, management; bed rest, preterm labor; tocolysis; progesterone, preterm labor; ethanol, preterm labor

37–25. a,b,d
p 752
preterm labor, management; magnesium sulfate; patellar reflex, magnesium sulfate; tocolysis

37–26. a
p 752
β-adrenergic receptors

37–27. b
p 751
β-adrenergic receptors

37–28. b,c,d
pp 752–753
preterm labor, management; β-adrenergic receptors, stimulants; β-adrenergic receptors, agonists; epinephrine, myometrium; tocolysis

37–29. b
p 752
preterm labor, management; β-adrenergic receptors, agonists; ritodrine; tocolysis

37–30. b,c
pp 752–753
preterm labor, management; β-adrenergic receptors, agonists; ritodrine; terbutaline; tocolysis, complications

37–31. a,b
pp 752–753
preterm labor, management; β-adrenergic receptors, agonists; isoxsuprine; ritodrine; tocolysis, complications

37–32. b,e
pp 752–753
preterm labor, management; β-adrenergic receptors, agonists; ritodrine; fenoterol; tocolysis, complications

37–33. b,c
pp 753–754
preterm labor; antiprostaglandins; ductus arteriosus; diazoxide; tocolysis; tocolysis, complications

37–34. b
p 754
rupture of the membranes, premature

37–35. a
p 754
rupture of the membranes, preterm

37–36. a
p 754
labor; rupture of the membranes, premature

37–37. Perform one sterile speculum examination to document rupture of the membranes to determine effacement and dilation, presentation, and to rule out umbilical cord prolapse. If the gestational age is 33 weeks or less and if there are no maternal or fetal indications for delivery, use close observation without the administration of prophylactic antibiotics. If the gestational age is 33 weeks or greater, deliver either by induction, if possible, or by cesarean section. Labor and delivery should be managed to minimize maternal hypotension, fetal hypoxia, and infection.
p 754
rupture of the membranes, preterm; labor, induction; cesarean delivery; infection, intrapartum

37-38. membranes ruptured for more than 24 hours
pp 754-755
rupture of the membranes, prolonged

37-39. b
pp 754-755
neonatal mortality; rupture of the membranes, prolonged; rupture of the membranes, premature

37-40. a,b,c,d,e,f
p 755
surfactant; fetal lung maturation; chronic maternal disease; heroin addiction; sickle cell disease; hyperthyroidism; chorionamnionitis; placental infarction

37-41. b
pp 755-756
rupture of the membranes, preterm; fetal lung maturation

37-42. b,c,d,e
pp 755-756
glucocorticosteroids, fetal lung maturation; rupture of the membranes, preterm; surfactant; fetal lung maturation

37-43. a,c,e
pp 756-757
preterm labor; episiotomy; neonatal morbidity, prematurity

37-44. a
p 757
fetal growth retardation; neonatal mortality; intrauterine growth retardation

37-45. b
p 757
fetal growth retardation; maternal size, fetal growth retardation; intrauterine growth retardation

37-46. b
p 757
maternal size, fetal growth retardation; weight gain, fetal effects; intrauterine growth retardation

37-47. a,c,e,f,g,i,j
pp 757-758
fetal growth retardation; chronic maternal disease; cyanotic heart disease; smoking; alcoholism; cytomegalic inclusion disease; rubella; intrauterine growth retardation

37-48. a
p 758
fetal growth retardation; placental abruption, focal; intrauterine growth retardation

37-49. a
p 758
fetal growth retardation; placental infarction; intrauterine growth retardation

37-50. b
p 758
fetal growth retardation; placenta previa; intrauterine growth retardation

37-51. a
p 758
fetal growth retardation; chorangioma; intrauterine growth retardation

37-52. b
p 758
fetal growth retardation; circumvallate placenta; intrauterine growth retardation

37-53. a
p 758
fetal growth retardation; velamentous insertion, umbilical cord; intrauterine growth retardation

37-54. b
p 758
fetal growth retardation; intrauterine growth retardation

37-55. a,b,c,d
p 758
fetal growth retardation; multifetal pregnancy, fetal growth retardation; fetal infection, fetal growth retardation; prolonged pregnancy, fetal growth retardation; ectopic pregnancy, fetal growth retardation; intrauterine growth retardation

37-56. a
p 759
fundal height; fetal growth retardation; intrauterine growth retardation

37-57. a,b,d
p 759
ultrasonography; fetal growth retardation, symmetric; fetal growth retardation, asymmetric; intrauterine growth retardation

37-58. a
p 759
fetal growth retardation; oligohydramnios; intrauterine growth retardation

37-59. a
p 760
fetal growth retardation; delivery, fetal growth retardation; intrauterine growth retardation

37-60. d
pp 759-761
fetal lung maturity; preterm labor, management; bed rest, preterm labor

37-61. a
p 761
fetal growth retardation, fetal distress; fetal distress; intrauterine growth retardation

37-62. a,b,c,d
p 761
fetal growth retardation; cesarean delivery, fetal growth retardation; uteroplacental insufficiency, fetal growth retardation; hypothermia; hypoglycemia, neonatal; intrauterine growth retardation

37–63. b
p 761
fetal growth retardation, symmetrical; fetal growth retardation, sequelae; intrauterine growth retardation

37–64. a
p 761
fetal growth retardation, asymmetrical; fetal growth retardation, sequelae; intrauterine growth retardation

37–65. a
p 761
fetal length; fetal growth retardation, sequelae; intrauterine growth retardation

37–66. b
p 761
fetal growth retardation, sequelae; intrauterine growth retardation

37–67. b
p 761
postterm pregnancy

37–68. errors in the reported gestational age
p 761
postterm pregnancy; gestation age

37–69. a,b,d,e
p 761
postterm pregnancy; anencephaly, postterm pregnancy; ectopic pregnancy, postterm pregnancy; placental sulfatase activity, postterm pregnancy

37–70. a,b,c,d
pp 761–762
postterm pregnancy; fetal distress; meconium, aspiration

37–71. *Postterm and favorable for induction:* attempt induction of labor; if induction is unsuccessful and there is no sign of fetal distress, wait and repeat induction in 1 week. *Postterm and unfavorable for induction:* if at 42 or 43 weeks and there is no maternal indication for intervention, no history of decreased fetal movement, and no oligohydramnios, wait 1 week and reevaluate; if undelivered by 44 weeks, induce, if possible, or deliver by cesarean. *Possible postterm:* if there is no evidence of complications or oligohydramnios, evaluate the patient weekly.
p 762
postterm pregnancy, management

37–72. at the onset of labor; at delivery
p 762
postterm pregnancy

37–73. a
p 763
postterm pregnancy; meconium, aspiration; cesarean delivery

37–74. a
pp 763–764
postterm pregnancy; contraction stress test, postterm pregnancy; nonstress test, postterm pregnancy

37–75. a
pp 761–763
postterm pregnancy; oligohydramnios; fetal distress

38–1. Surfactant serves to stabilize the newly-expanded fetal lung alveoli by preventing their collapse during expiration.
p 769
surfactant; hyaline membrane disease; type II pneumocytes; respiratory distress syndrome

38–2. a,b,c
p 769
hyaline membrane disease; surfactant; respiratory distress syndrome

38–3. None of the statements about hyaline membrane disease is correct.
p 769
hyaline membrane disease; respiratory distress syndrome; neonatal death rate

38–4. a,b,c,d,e
p 769
hyaline membrane disease; grunting tachypnea; atelectasis, neonatal

38–5. a,b,c,d,e,f,g,h
p 769
hyaline membrane disease; pneumonia, neonatal; sepsis, neonatal; aspiration, neonatal; pneumothorax; diaphragmatic hernia, neonatal; patent ductus arteriosus; myocardiopathy, neonatal; respiratory distress syndrome

38–6. a,b,c,d
pp 769–770
hyaline membrane disease; oxygen therapy, neonatal; retrolental fibroplasia

38–7. a
p 770
hyaline membrane disease; neonatal mortality, hyaline membrane disease; respiratory distress syndrome

38–8. c
p 770
pulmonary hypertension, neonatal; oxygen therapy, neonatal; hyaline membrane disease

38–9. a
p 770
retrolental fibroplasia; hyaline membrane disease; hyperoxia, neonatal

38–10. b
p 770
tracheal abrasion, neonatal; hyaline membrane disease; endotracheal intubation

38–11. c
p 770
bronchopulmonary dysplasia; hyaline membrane disease; oxygen therapy, neonatal

38-12. a,b,c,d
p 770
bronchopulmonary dysplasia; hyaline membrane disease; hypoxia, neonatal

38-13. b,c,d
p 771
meconium, aspiration; pneumonitis, neonatal; fetal distress; atelectasis, neonatal; pneumothorax, neonatal

38-14. a
p 770
meconium, aspiration

38-15. The mouth and nares should be suctioned thoroughly just after delivery of the head and before delivery of the thorax (whether the delivery is vaginal or cesarean); as soon as possible after delivery, the vocal cords should be visualized and all meconium aspirated from the area; the stomach should be emptied to avoid the possibility of further meconium aspiration; ventilation of the lungs must not be unduly delayed while the above procedures are being accomplished.
p 771
meconium aspiration; resuscitation, neonatal

38-16. b
p 771
retrolental fibroplasia; blindness, neonatal

38-17. b
p 771
retrolental fibroplasia; hyperoxia, neonatal

38-18. a,b
p 771
anemia, neonatal; hematocrit, neonatal

38-19. a,b,d
pp 772, 778
hemorrhage, fetal-maternal; anemia, neonatal

38-20. varying rate of occurrence of antigens; variable antigenicity; insufficient placental transfer of antigen from fetus to mother; insufficient placental transfer of antibody from mother to fetus
p 772
hemolytic disease; Rh isoimmunization; placental transfer; antigenicity

38-21. a,c
p 772
Rh antigen; immunogenicity, Rh antigen

38-22. a
p 772
Rho(D) antigen; antepartum care, routine; Rho(D) isoimmunization

38-23. a,b,d
pp 772-773
Rho(D) isoimmunization; perinatal death, Rho(D) disease; Rho(D) immune globulin

38-24. a,b,c,d,e
p 773
Rho(D) isoimmunization; Rho(D) immune globulin

38-25. b
p 773
Rho(D) isoimmunization, prophylaxis; Rho(D) immune globulin; transfusion, maternal

38-26. a
p 773
Rho(D) isoimmunization; Rho(D) immune globulin

38-27. A single 300 μg dose should be given at between 28 and 32 weeks of gestation and again within 72 hours of the birth of a Rho(D)-positive infant; a single 300 μg dose should be given at the time of amniocentesis or whenever there is uterine bleeding (unless the routine dose at 28 to 32 weeks had just been given); if a massive fetal to maternal hemorrhage is recognized, immune globulin is administered according to the formula that a 300 μg dose will protect against a bleed of up to 15 ml of Rho(D)-positive fetal red cells.
p 773
Rho(D) isoimmunization; Rho(D) immune globulin, prophylaxis; fetal-maternal hemorrhage

38-28. b
p 773
Rho(D) isoimmunization; Rho(D) immune globulin, prophylaxis; Coombs test, direct

38-29. a,c
pp 773-774
Rho(D) isoimmunization; maternal-fetal bleed, isoimmunization; fetal-maternal bleed, isoimmunization; Rho(D) immune globulin

38-30. 1 = a; 2 = b
p 774 (Fig. 38-1)
acid-elution test; fetal-maternal bleed; fetal hemoglobin

38-31. a
p 774
fetal-maternal bleed; Rho(D) isoimmunization; Rho(D) immune globulin; Rho(D) antibody, maternal serum

38-32. b
p 774
Rho(D) isoimmunization; perinatal mortality, Rho(D) isoimmunization

38-33. past obstetric history; accurate determination of gestational age; determination of paternal Rho(D) zygosity; measurements of maternal antibody levels; spectrophotometric analysis of amnionic fluid samples; identification of other pregnancy complications
pp 774-775
Rho(D) isoimmunization

38-34. a
p 775
Rho(D) isoimmunization; antibody measurement, Rho(D) isoimmunization; hemolytic disease of the newborn

38–35. b
p 775
Rho(D) isoimmunization; amniocentesis, Rho(D) isoimmunization; Rho(D) antibody, maternal

38–36. a
p 775
amnionic fluid, bilirubin; bilirubin, absorption at 450 nm; Rho(D) isoimmunization

38–37. a
p 775
Liley zone; amniocentesis, Rho(D) isoimmunization; hemolytic disease; Rho(D) isoimmunization

38–38. c
p 775
Liley zone; amniocentesis, Rho(D) isoimmunization; hemolytic disease; Rho(D) isoimmunization

38–39. b
p 775
Liley zone; amniocentesis, Rho(D) isoimmunization; hemolytic disease; Rho(D) isoimmunization

38–40. a,b,e
p 776
Rho(D) isoimmunization; hemolytic disease, newborn; Coombs test, direct; Coombs test, indirect; Rho(D) antibodies

38–41. a,d,f
p 776
immune hydrops; Rho(D) isoimmunization; hematopoiesis, extramedullary; ultrasonography

38–42. lethargy; stiffness of the extremities; retraction of the head; squinting; high-pitched cry; poor feeding; convulsions
p 776
kernicterus; hyperbilirubinemia; Rho(D) isoimmunization; convulsions, neonatal

38–43. a
p 776
kernicterus; hyperbilirubinemia; anemia, neonatal

38–44. a
p 777
hyaline membrane disease; Rho(D) isoimmunization; respiratory distress syndrome

38–45. a,c
pp 776–777
intrauterine transfusion; respiratory distress syndrome; Rho(D) isoimmunization

38–46. None of these methods has proved to be both safe and effective.
p 777
Rho(D) isoimmunization

38–47. a
p 778
anemia, neonatal; Rho(D) isoimmunization; sinusoidal fetal heart rate

38–48. b
p 778
cesarean delivery; Rho(D) isoimmunization

38–49. a,b
p 778
Rho(D) isoimmunization; exchange transfusion

38–50. a,f
pp 778–779
ABO incompatibility; stillbirth

38–51. Mother is group O with anti-A and anti-B in her serum, and the fetus is group A, B or AB; there is the onset of neonatal jaundice within 24 hours of birth; there are varying degrees of anemia, reticulocytosis, and erythroblastosis; there has been the careful exclusion of all other causes of hemolysis.
p 778
ABO incompatibility; hemolysis, ABO incompatibility; isoimmune disease, newborn

38–52. a,d
p 778
ABO incompatibility; Coombs test; exchange transfusion

38–53. a
p 779
Rho(D) isoimmune disease; ABO incompatibility; hemolytic disease, newborn

38–54. a
pp 779, 782
nonimmune hydrops fetalis; hydrops fetalis

38–55. b
p 779
bilirubin, unconjugated; placental transfer

38–56. a,b,e
p 781
kernicterus; hyperbilirubinemia

38–57. a,b,c,d,e,f
pp 780–781
kernicterus; hyperbilirubinemia; sulfonamides; salicylate; furosemide; gentamicin; vitamin K, analogs; diazepam

38–58. a,b,c
p 781
breast feeding; breast milk jaundice; kernicterus

38–59. a,b,c
p 781
jaundice, physiologic; hyperbilirubinemia; phototherapy, newborn

38-60. a,b,c,d
p 781
jaundice, physiologic; kernicterus; hyperbilirubinemia; icterus

38-61. a,c,d
p 782
hyperbilirubinemia; phototherapy; exchange transfusion; phenobarbital

38-62. a,b,c,e
pp 782-783
hemorrhagic disease of the newborn; coagulation factors, vitamin K

38-63. consumptive coagulopathy (DIC); hemophilia; congenital syphilis; sepsis; thrombocytopenia purpura; erythroblastosis; traumatic intracranial injury
p 783
hemorrhagic disease of the newborn; consumptive coagulopathy; hemophilia; syphilis, congenital; thrombocytopenia purpura; birth trauma; erythroblastosis

38-64. a
p 783
hemorrhagic disease of the newborn; hypoprothrombinemia, neonatal; vitamin K_1

38-65. a,b
p 783
hemorrhagic disease of the newborn; vitamin K; breast feeding; placental transfer, vitamin K

38-66. a
p 783
autoimmune thrombocytopenia purpura

38-67. b
p 783
isoimmune thrombocytopenia purpura

38-68. b
p 783
isoimmune thrombocytopenia

38-69. a
p 783
autoimmune thrombocytopenia purpura

38-70. b
p 783
isoimmune thrombocytopenia

38-71. b
p 783
isoimmune thrombocytopenia

38-72. b,c,d,e
pp 783-784
polycythemia, neonatal; hyperviscosity, neonatal; hypoxia, neonatal

38-73. a,c,d,e
p 784
infection, neonatal; immunologic capacity, neonatal

38-74. a
p 784
infection, neonatal; group A β-hemolytic streptococci

38-75. c
p 784
infection, neonatal; staphylococci

38-76. b
p 784
infection, neonatal; group B β-hemolytic streptococci

38-77. b,e
p 784
staphylococci; infection, neonatal; umbilical cord, neonatal care

38-78. a
p 784
infection, neonatal; bacteriology, gram-negative infections

38-79. None of the statements about group B β-hemolytic streptococcal infection is correct.
pp 784-785
infection, neonatal; group B β-hemolytic streptococci

38-80. a
p 785
infection, neonatal; group B β-hemolytic streptococci

38-81. a
p 785
infection, neonatal; group B β-hemolytic streptococci

38-82. b
p 785
infection, neonatal; group B β-hemolytic streptococci

38-83. a
p 785
infection, neonatal; group B β-hemolytic streptococci

38-84. b
p 785
infection, neonatal; group B β-hemolytic streptococci

38-85. a
p 785
infection, neonatal; group B β-hemolytic streptococci

38-86. b
p 785
infection, neonatal; group B β-hemolytic streptococcal infection, neonatal; group B β-hemolytic streptococcal infection, maternal; penicillin, neonatal prophylaxis

38-87. a,b,c,e
p 785
diarrhea, newborn; Escherichia coli; *infection, neonatal*

38–88. a,b
pp 785–786
necrotizing enterocolitis; bowel perforation, neonatal; pneumotosis intestinalis

38–89. a
p 786
rubella; rubella vaccine

38–90. a,c,d,f
p 786
rubella; rubella antibody, IgM, rubella

38–91. 1 = 50; 2 = 25; 3 = 15
p 786
rubella; congenital abnormalities

38–92. eye lesions; heart defects; auditory defects; central nervous system defects; fetal growth retardation; hematologic abnormalities; hepatosplenomegaly and jaundice; chronic diffuse interstitial pneumonitis; osseus changes; chromosomal abnormalities
pp 786–787
congenital rubella syndrome; rubella, congenital; cataracts, neonatal; glaucoma; patent ductus arteriosus; thrombocytopenia, neonatal; anemia, neonatal; hepatosplenomegaly, neonatal

38–93. a
p 787
diabetes, juvenile; rubella, congenital

38–94. a
p 787
placental transfer; rubella; rubella vaccine

38–95. eating raw or undercooked meat; contact with infected cat feces; placental transfer from infected mother to fetus
p 787
Toxoplasma gonadii; *toxoplasmosis*

38–96. a,e
p 787
toxoplasmosis; chorioretinitis; Sabin-Feldman dye test; IgM, toxoplasmosis; infection, neonatal

38–97. a,c,e
p 787
cytomegalovirus; IgM, cytomegalovirus; infection, neonatal

38–98. a,b,c,d,e,f,g,h,i,j,k
p 787
infection, neonatal; cytomegalovirus; microcephaly; hydrocephalus; mental retardation; cerebral palsy; epilepsy; deafness; chorioretinitis; blindness; hemolytic disease; thrombocytopenia; hepatosplenomegaly

38–99. b
p 787
TORCH; antenatal testing

38–100. a,b
pp 787–788
Chlamydia trachomatis; *pneumonia, neonatal; conjunctivitis, neonatal; infection, neonatal; abortion; premature labor*

38–101. a,b,c
p 788
infection, neonatal; syphilis, congenital; osteochondritis, neonatal

38–102. a,b,c,e
pp 788–789
drug addiction, maternal; drug withdrawal, neonatal; fetal growth retardation; respiratory distress syndrome; low birth weight

38–103. b
p 789
drug addiction, maternal; drug withdrawal, neonatal; methadone

39–1. elimination of difficult forceps operations; correct management of breech presentations; virtual eradication of internal podalic version operations; liberalized use of cesarean delivery for the treatment of cephalopelvic disproportion
p 793
birth injury; forceps delivery; internal podalic version; cesarean delivery; cephalopelvic disproportion

39–2. b,d
p 793
birth injury; intracranial hemorrhage, neonatal; molding; fetal skull, compression

39–3. b
p 793
birth injury; intracranial hemorrhage, neonatal

39–4. a,b,c,d,e,f
p 793
intracranial hemorrhage, neonatal

39–5. atelectasis; birth asphyxia; meconium aspiration; diaphragmatic hernia; congenital heart disease; idiopathic respiratory distress syndrome; pneumonia
p 793
intracranial hemorrhage, neonatal; atelectasis; meconium aspiration; respiratory distress syndrome; diaphragmatic hernia; asphyxia, birth; congenital heart disease; pneumonia

39–6. periventricular; intraventricular
p 793
intracranial hemorrhage, neonatal; prematurity, neonatal complications

39–7. a,b,e
pp 793–794
intracranial hemorrhage, neonatal

39–8. b
p 794
cerebral palsy; birth injury; asphyxia, birth; fetal distress

39-9. b
p 795 (Fig. 39-3)
cephalohematoma

39-10. a
p 795 (Fig. 39-3)
caput succedaneum

39-11. b
p 795 (Fig. 39-3)
cephalohematoma

39-12. a
p 795
caput succedaneum

39-13. b
p 795
cephalohematoma

39-14. a
p 795
intracranial hemorrhage, neonatal; birth injury; cephalohematoma; coagulation defects, newborn; thrombocytopenia, newborn

39-15. a
pp 795-796
brachial plexus, injury; Duchenne's paralysis; Erb's paralysis; birth injury

39-16. b
pp 795-796
brachial plexus, injury; Klumpke's paralysis; birth injury

39-17. a
pp 795-796
brachial plexus, injury; Duchenne's paralysis; Erb's paralysis; birth injury

39-18. b
pp 795-796
brachial plexus, injury; Klumpke's paralysis; birth injury

39-19. a
pp 795-796
brachial plexus, injury; Duchenne's paralysis; Erb's paralysis; birth injury

39-20. b,c,d
pp 795-796
brachial plexus, injury; birth injury; breech presentation, brachial plexus injury; macrosomia, brachial plexus injury

39-21. b
pp 795-796
facial paralysis; birth injury; forceps delivery

39-22. a,c,d,e
p 796
birth injury; skeletal injury, newborn; shoulder dystocia

39-23. torticollis
p 796
torticollis; birth injury; sternocleidomastoid muscle, birth injury

39-24. b,c,d
p 796
congenital amputations; amnion, premature rupture; constriction bands

39-25. a,b,c,d,f
p. 797
oligohydramnios; talipes; hip dislocation, congenital; limb reduction, congenital; body wall deficiency, congenital

39-26. the shielding provided by the uterus and the amnionic fluid in which the fetus floats
pp 797-798
coincidental injury, fetus; trauma, in pregnancy

39-27. a
pp 797-798
coincidental injury, fetus; trauma, in pregnancy

39-28. b
p 798
congenital malformations; perinatal mortality

39-29. b
p 798
congenital malformations; developmental abnormalities; perinatal mortality

39-30. a
p 798
congenital malformations; stillbirth, developmental abnormalities

39-31. b
p 798
congenital malformations; developmental abnormalities

39-32. b
pp 799
embryonic development; developmental abnormalities; teratogenesis

39-33. b,e
pp 799-800
developmental abnormalities; congenital malformations; embryonic development; teratogenesis

39-34. a
p 799
congenital malformations; developmental abnormalities; supernumerary digits

39-35. e
p 800 (Table 39-1)
trisomy 13-15; chromosomal anomalies; congenital malformations

39-36. a
p 800 (Table 39-1)
Turner's syndrome; chromosomal anomalies; congenital malformations

39-37. d
p 800 (Table 39-1)
Down's syndrome (trisomy 21); chromosomal anomalies; congenital malformations

39-38. b,c
p 800 (Table 39-1)
Klinefelter's syndrome; Triple X syndrome; chromosomal anomalies; congenital malformations

39-39. 1 = 0.56; 2 = 6 to 7; 3 = about 60
p 800
chromosomal anomalies; abortion, spontaneous; stillbirth

39-40. 1 = b; 2 = a
pp 800-801
chromosomal anomalies; mosaic, genetic; trisomy

39-41. b
pp 800-801
chromosomal anomalies; mosaic, genetic

39-42. a,b,c,e,f
p 801
Down's syndrome; chromosomal anomalies; developmental abnormalities; amniocentesis, cell fraction

39-43. b,d
p 801
Down's syndrome; chromosomal anomalies; paternal age, genetic effects; karyotyping

39-44. 1 = 1/885; 2 = 1/365; 3 = 1/109; 4 = 1/32
p 801 (Fig. 39-3)
Down's syndrome; chromosomal anomalies; maternal age, effect on pregnancy outcome

39-45. a,b,c,e,f,g
pp 801-802
inborn errors of metabolism; phenylketonuria

39-46. a,c,d
p 802
birth defects; teratogenesis; phocomelia

39-47. a,b,c,d
pp 802-803
anencephaly; adrenal gland, fetal; pituitary gland, fetal; cerebrum, fetal; neural tube defects; developmental abnormalities

39-48. a,b,c,d
pp 802-803
anencephaly; ultrasonography; α-fetoprotein; birth defects; developmental abnormalities

39-49. b
p 803
anencephaly; postterm pregnancy

39-50. a,b,c
pp 802-803
anencephaly; hydramnios; placental abruption; laminaria; prostaglandins

39-51. a,b,c,d,e
pp 803-804
spina bifida; meningomyelocele; anencephaly; hydrocephaly; birth defects; developmental abnormalities; talipes

39-52. a,b,c,d
p 804
hydrocephaly; dystocia; spina bifida

39-53. a,b
p 804
renal agenesis; urinary tract obstruction; oligohydramnios; developmental abnormalities; congenital anomalies

39-54. a
p 804
renal agenesis; developmental abnormalities; congenital anomalies

39-55. a
p 804
renal agenesis; pulmonary hypoplasia; developmental abnormalities congenital anomalies

39-56. a
p 804
renal agenesis; developmental abnormalities; congenital anomalies

39-57. congenital heart disease
p 804
congenital heart disease; developmental abnormalities

39-58. 1/1000 live births
p 804
developmental abnormalities; talipes; congenital anomalies

39-59. b,c,d,e
p 805
developmental abnormalities; congenital dislocation of the hip; congenital anomalies

39-60. Simple ligation of the stalk with a silk thread is usually sufficient; if the base of the supernumerary digit is broad or the digit well developed, surgical removal may be necessary
p 805
developmental abnormalities; polydactyly; congenital anomalies

39-61. a,c,e,f
p 805
developmental abnormalities; cleft lip; cleft palate; congenital anomalies

39–62. An omphalocele is a peritoneal sac covered with amnion and filled with intestine.
p 805
developmental abnormalities; omphalocele; congenital anomalies

39–63. a,b,c,e
p 805
developmental abnormalities; omphalocele; α-fetoprotein; congenital anomalies

39–64. b
p 805
inguinal hernia, neonatal

39–65. a
p 805
umbilical hernia, neonatal

39–66. a,b
p 805
inguinal hernia, neonatal; umbilical hernia, neonatal; congenital anomalies

39–67. imperforate anus
p 805
developmental abnormalities; anal atresia

39–68. b
p 805
sacrococcygeal teratoma

39–69. b
p 806
genetic counseling

39–70. detailed history from before conception to delivery (especially potential exposure to teratogens); photographs of infant; radiographic skeletal survey of infant; chromosomal analysis of blood from heart or a great vessel; complete autopsy of the infant
p 807
perinatal mortality, developmental abnormalities

39–71. a
pp 807–808
genetic inheritance, dominant genes; congenital anomalies, evaluation

39–72. b
p 808
genetic inheritance, dominant genes

39–73. the ratio of carriers who phenotypically express the genetic trait to the total number of individuals who carry the gene (expressed as a percentage)
p 808
penetrance; genetic inheritance

39–74. expressivity
p 808
expressivity; genetic inheritance

39–75. a,b,c,d,f
p 808
multifactorial inheritance; polygenic inheritance; cleft lip; spina bifida; anencephaly; congenital heart defects

39–76. a
p 808
developmental abnormalities; genetic inheritance; congenital anomalies

40–1. d
p 811
contraception; fertility

40–2. b
p 811
contraception; fertility; ovulation, onset

40–3. a,b,c
p 811
contraception; ovulation; amenorrhea; menopause

40–4. 1 = 2.4; 2 = 4.6; 3 = 9.6; 4 = 17.9; 5 = 18.6; 6 = 23.7
p 812 (Table 40–1)
contraception; failure rates, contraceptives; oral contraceptives, failure rate; intrauterine device, failure rate; condom, failure rate; diaphragm, failure rate; rhythm method, failure rate

40–5. a
p 811
contraceptives, failure rate

40–6. a,c,d
pp 812–813
oral contraceptives; estrogen-progestin contraceptives; ethinyl estradiol; progestin, oral contraceptives

40–7. a,b,c
p 813
oral contraceptives; estrogen-progestin contraceptives; withdrawal bleeding

40–8. b
pp 813–814
oral contraceptives; estrogen-progestin contraceptives

40–9. b
pp 813–814
estrogen-progestin contraceptives; oral contraceptives; ethinyl estradiol; mestranol

40–10. b
pp 813–814
estrogen-progestin contraceptives; oral contraceptives; progestin

40–11. a,c,d,e,f
p 814
estrogen-progestin contraceptives; oral contraceptives; endometrial carcinoma; ovarian carcinoma; rheumatoid arthritis; menstruation; blood loss, menstruation

40–12. a
p 814
estrogen-progestin contraceptives; oral contraceptives; oral contraceptives, side effects

40–13. a
pp 814–815
estrogen-progestin contraceptives; oral contraceptives

40–14. b
p 815
estrogen-progestin contraceptives; oral contraceptives; hepatitis

40–15. a,c
p 815
estrogen-progestin contraceptives; oral contraceptives; oral contraceptives, side effects; hepatic focal nodular hyperplasia

40–16. 1 = b; 2 = b
p 816
estrogen-progestin contraceptives; oral contraceptives; blood loss, menstrual; dysmenorrhea

40–17. a,d,e,f
pp 816–817
estrogen-progestin contraceptives; oral contraceptives; stroke, oral contraceptives; hypertension, oral contraceptives; myocardial infarction, oral contraceptives; thromboembolic disease, oral contraceptives

40–18. thromboembolism, current or past; cerebrovascular accident, current or past; coronary artery disease; impaired liver function; liver adenoma, current or past; breast cancer; hypertension; diabetes; gallbladder disease; cholestatic jaundice during pregnancy; sickle cell hemoglobinopathy; surgery completed within 4 weeks; major surgery on or immobilization of a lower extremity; patient over 40 years of age; smoking
p 818
estrogen-progestin contraceptives; oral contraceptives, contraindications; thromboembolism; cerebrovascular accident; coronary artery disease; liver function, impaired; liver adenoma; breast cancer; hypertension; diabetes; gallbladder disease; cholestatic jaundice; sickle cell hemoglobinopathy; smoking

40–19. a
p 817
estrogen-progestin contraceptives; oral contraceptives; ovulation

40–20. a,b,c,d
p 818
estrogen-progestin contraceptives; oral contraceptives; cervical mucorrhea; myomas, uterine; vulvovaginitis

40–21. b
p 818
breast feeding; estrogen-progestin oral contraceptives; oral contraceptives

40–22. higher incidence of irregular bleeding; higher pregnancy rate
p 818
oral contraceptives; progestin contraceptives

40–23. a,b,c,d,e
pp 818–819
progestins, injectable; lactation; amenorrhea; anovulation

40–24. stilbestrol
p 819
oral contraceptives; stilbestrol

40–25. inserted only once; complete protection against pregnancy; not spontaneously expelled; no adverse effects that necessitate removal; after removal, it would have induced no changes detrimental to pregnancy
p 820
intrauterine device

40–26. chemically inert device made of nonabsorbable (radioopaque) material; device from which there is a continuous elution of a chemically active substance
p 820
intrauterine device

40–27. None of the devices have achieved all the "ideal" criteria.
p 820
intrauterine device; contraception

40–28. c
p 820
Progestasert; intrauterine device; contraception

40–29. a
p 820
Lippes Loop; intrauterine device; contraception

40–30. b
p 820
Cu7; intrauterine device; contraception

40–31. a
p 820
Copper T; intrauterine device; contraception

40–32. d
p 821
Progestasert; intrauterine device; contraception

40–33. The precise mechanism of action is not known. The primary action seems to be interference with successful implantation. Effectiveness increases with size and extent of contact with the endometrium.
p 820
intrauterine device, action; contraception

40–34. b
p 820
intrauterine device, action; contraception; copper; Cu7

40-35. a
p 820
intrauterine device, complications; contraception

40-36. b,c,d
p 821
intrauterine device, complications; contraception; pelvic inflammatory disease

40-37. a,c
p 821
intrauterine device, complications; contraception

40-38. b
p 821
intrauterine device; actinomyces, intrauterine device; contraception

40-39. b,c
pp 821-822
intrauterine device, lost device; ultrasonography; intrauterine device, extrauterine; contraception

40-40. a
p 823
intrauterine device; pregnancy, intrauterine device

40-41. a,b,c,e
p 823
intrauterine device; pregnancy, intrauterine device

40-42. 1 = b; 2 = c
p 823
intrauterine device; abortion, intrauterine device; pregnancy, intrauterine device

40-43. b
p 823
intrauterine device; ectopic pregnancy; contraception

40-44. a,c,e
pp 823-824
intrauterine device, insertion; abortion, intrauterine device; puerperium, intrauterine device

40-45. a,b,c,d,e,f,g
p 824
intrauterine device, contraindications; gonorrhea; cervical stenosis; dysmenorrhea; contraception

40-46. b,a,d,c,e,g,f
p 824
intrauterine device, insertion; contraception

40-47. a,c
p 824
intrauterine device, expulsion; contraception

40-48. d
p 824
Lippes Loop; intrauterine device; contraception

40-49. b
p 824
Cu7; intrauterine device; contraception

40-50. b
p 824
Copper T; intrauterine device; contraception

40-51. a
p 824
Progestasert; intrauterine device; contraception

40-52. b,c
pp 824-825
condoms; contraception, barrier

40-53. b,c,e,f
p 825
contraceptives, intravaginal

40-54. b
p 825
contraceptives, intravaginal; congenital malformations, contraceptive use

40-55. to the superior surface along the rim and centrally
p 825
contraceptives, barrier; diaphragm; spermicide

40-56. a,b
p 825
contraceptives, barrier; diaphragm

40-57. b
p 826
contraceptives, sponge

40-58. a,c
p 826
contraceptives, breast feeding; breast feeding

40-59. calendar; temperature; cervical mucus (Billings)
p 826
contraception; rhythm method, contraception; cervical mucus

40-60. c,d
p 827
contraception, surgical; tubal sterilization

40-61. a
pp 827-828
Irving procedure, tubal sterilization; tubal sterilization

40-62. b
pp 827-828
Pomeroy procedure, tubal sterilization; tubal sterilization

40-63. c
pp 827-828
Parkland procedure, tubal sterilization; tubal sterilization

40-64. d
pp 827-828
Madlener procedure, tubal sterilization; tubal sterilization

40-65. e
pp 827-828
fimbriectomy; tubal sterilization

40–66. a
pp 827-828
Irving procedure, tubal sterilization; tubal sterilization

40–67. b
pp 827-828
Pomeroy procedure, tubal sterilization; tubal sterilization

40–68. c
pp 828-829
sterilization, surgical; postoperative care, surgical sterilization

40–69. The three principal surgical techniques are ligation and resection; application of rings/clips; and electrocoagulation.
p 829
sterilization, surgical; sterilization, nonpuerperal

40–70. a,b,c,d
p 829
tubal sterilization, complications

40–71. general anesthesia without endotracheal intubation
p 829
tubal sterilization, complications; mortality, tubal sterilization; anesthesia

40–72. a,b,c,d,e
p 829
tubal sterilization; morbidity, tubal sterilization

40–73. b
p 829
tubal sterilization; posttubal ligation syndrome

40–74. b
p 830
tubal sterilization, reversal

40–75. a,b,c,d
pp 830-831
hysterectomy, sterilization

40–76. b
pp 830-831
sterilization, surgical; tubal sterilization; hysterectomy, sterilization

40–77. a,b
pp 831-832
vasectomy; sterilization

40–78. microsurgical technique; length of time after vasectomy; presence of sperm granulomas
p 832
vasectomy, reversal

40–79. d
p 832
contraception, male

41–1. extraction of the fetus
p 837
forceps delivery

41–2. blade; shank; lock; handle
p 837
forceps

41–3. 1 = b; 2 = a
p 837
forceps, cephalic curve; forceps, pelvic curve

41–4. a
p 837
forceps, fenestrated

41–5. b
p 837
Kielland forceps

41–6. a
pp 837, 838 (Fig. 41-1)
Simpson forceps

41–7. b
p 837
Barton forceps

41–8. a
pp 837, 838 (Fig. 41-2)
Tucker-McLane forceps

41–9. c
p 837
Tarnier forceps

41–10. 1 = perineal floor; 2 = anteroposterior; 3 = vaginal introitus
p 837
forceps delivery; low forceps delivery

41–11. a,b,d
pp 837-838
forceps delivery; midforceps delivery; low midforceps delivery; engagement, fetal head

41–12. a
p 838
forceps delivery; low midforceps delivery

41–13. None, high forceps delivery has no place in modern obstetrics.
p 838
forceps delivery; high forceps delivery

41–14. a
p 838
midforceps delivery; perinatal morbidity, midforceps delivery; perinatal mortality, midforceps delivery; maternal morbidity, midforceps delivery

41–15. a,b,c,d
p 838
forceps delivery; low forceps delivery

41-16. traction; rotation
p 838
forceps delivery

41-17. a,b,c
p 838
deep transverse arrest; midforceps delivery, deep transverse arrest; cesarean delivery; oxytocin stimulation; augmentation

41-18. a,b,c,d,e,f,g
p 839
forceps delivery, indications

41-19. a,b,c,d
p 839
forceps delivery; low forceps delivery, elective

41-20. Prophylactic forceps may be beneficial to minimize maternal strain and to prevent cerebral injury to the fetus.
pp 839-840
forceps delivery; forceps delivery, prophylactic; low forceps delivery, elective

41-21. b
p 840
forceps delivery; forceps delivery, prophylactic; low forceps delivery, elective; low birth weight infant, forceps delivery

41-22. head engaged (preferably deeply engaged); vertex or chin anterior presentation; position of the head precisely known; cervix completely dilated; membranes ruptured; no disproportion between the size of the head and the pelvic inlet, midpelvis, or outlet
pp 840-841
forceps delivery

41-23. b,c
p 841
forceps delivery; low forceps delivery

41-24. a,b,c,d,e,f
pp 841-842
forceps delivery; fetus, position

41-25. 1 = a; 2 = b
p 842
forceps delivery; pelvic application, forceps delivery

41-26. a
p 842
forceps delivery; pelvic application, forceps delivery

41-27. insufficient expulsive forces; resistance of the perineum
p 842
forceps delivery; low forceps delivery

41-28. a,b,e
p 843
forceps delivery; low forceps delivery

41-29. occiput anterior—blades should be equidistant from the sagittal suture; occiput posterior—blades should be equidistant from the midline of the face and brow
p 843
forceps delivery; low forceps delivery

41-30. b
p 843
forceps delivery; low forceps delivery

41-31. a,b,d
pp 843-845
forceps delivery; low forceps delivery; Ritgen maneuver; episiotomy

41-32. a,b,c
p 846
forceps delivery; midforceps delivery

41-33. a
p 846
forceps delivery; midforceps delivery; occiput posterior position

41-34. b
p 847
fetal head, manual rotation; occiput posterior position, manual rotation

41-35. b
p 847
fetal head, manual rotation; occiput posterior position, manual rotation; forceps delivery

41-36. a
p 847
forceps delivery; midforceps delivery, occiput posterior position; Kielland forceps

41-37. a,b,d
pp 847-848
forceps delivery; midforceps rotation; Scanzoni maneuver

41-38. b,c,e
pp 848-849
forceps delivery; midforceps rotation; Kielland forceps

41-39. Barton forceps
p 849
forceps delivery; midforceps rotation; Barton forceps

41-40. a,b,c,d
p 849
forceps delivery; midforceps delivery, indications; fetal distress, forceps delivery; umbilical cord prolapse, forceps delivery

41-41. 1 = a; 2 = b
p 849
forceps delivery; maternal morbidity, midforceps delivery; perinatal morbidity, midforceps delivery

41-42. b
pp 849-850
forceps delivery; perinatal morbidity, midforceps delivery; cerebral palsy, midforceps delivery

41-43. hollow of the sacrum (also called the mentum posterior)
p 850
forceps delivery; face presentation

41-44. a
p 850
forceps delivery; trial forceps

41-45. b
p 850
forceps delivery; failed forceps

41-46. a
p 850
forceps delivery; trial forceps

41-47. malposition of the fetal head; incomplete dilation of the cervix; disproportion; inexperience of the operator
p 850
forceps delivery; failed forceps

41-48. a,b,c
p 850
vacuum extraction

41-49. scalp abrasion; scalp laceration; cephalohematoma; intracranial hemorrhage; death
p 851
vacuum extraction; cephalohematoma; intracranial hemorrhage, neonatal

41-50. None of these procedures is commonly used in the United States.
p 851
Dührssen incision

42-1. a,b,d
p 855
breech presentation, labor; breech presentation, vaginal delivery

42-2. b
p 855
breech presentation, labor; breech presentation, vaginal delivery

42-3. b
p 855
breech extraction, partial; breech presentation, vaginal delivery

42-4. a
p 855
breech delivery, spontaneous; breech presentation, vaginal delivery

42-5. c
p 855
breech extraction, total; breech presentation, vaginal delivery

42-6. an obstetrician skilled in breech deliveries; a gowned associate to aid in the delivery; an anesthesiologist; an individual able to perform infant resuscitation; someone available to render general assistance
p 856
vaginal delivery, breech presentation; breech presentation, vaginal delivery

42-7. a
p 856
perinatal mortality; perinatal morbidity; breech presentation, vaginal delivery

42-8. cesarean delivery; total breech extraction
p 856
cesarean delivery, breech presentation; breech extraction, total; fetal distress; breech presentation, cesarean delivery

42-9. a,d,e,f
p 856
breech extraction; breech presentation, complete; breech presentation, incomplete; episiotomy, breech presentation

42-10. a
p 856
breech presentation, vaginal delivery; breech extraction; breech presentation, complete; breech presentation, incomplete

42-11. (1) Rotate the trunk until the anterior arm and shoulder appear at the vulva; deliver the anterior shoulder and arm; rotate the body in the reverse direction to deliver the other shoulder and arm; (2) deliver the posterior shoulder first by drawing the fetus over the maternal groin; then depress the fetal body to deliver the anterior shoulder and arm
pp 856-857
breech extraction, delivery of shoulders; breech presentation, vaginal delivery

42-12. a
p 857
breech extraction; breech presentation, vaginal delivery

42-13. a,c
p 857
breech extraction, delivery of arm; breech presentation, vaginal delivery

42-14. a,c,e
p 858
breech extraction; nuchal arm; breech presentation, vaginal delivery

42-15. a
p 858
Mauriceau maneuver; breech extraction; breech presentation, vaginal delivery

42-16. a,b,c,d,e,f
p 858
Mauriceau maneuver; breech extraction, delivery of the head; breech presentation, vaginal delivery

42-17. a,b,c
p 858
breech extraction, frank breech; Pinard maneuver; breech decomposition

42-18. a
p 859
breech extraction, forceps; Piper forceps; breech presentation, forceps delivery; breech presentation, vaginal delivery

42-19. Suspending the fetus keeps the arms out of the way and prevents excessive abduction of the trunk.
p 859
breech extraction, forceps; Piper forceps; breech presentation, forceps delivery; breech presentation, vaginal delivery

42-20. Dührssen's incisions should be made if the aftercoming head is trapped by an incompletely dilated cervix and the fetus cannot be delivered by traction and manually forcing the cervix over the occiput.
p 859
aftercoming head, entrapment; Dührrsen incisions; breech presentation, vaginal delivery

42-21. a,c
p 862
breech presentation, vaginal delivery; anesthesia, breech delivery

42-22. risks due to manipulation: infection, rupture of the uterus, laceration of the cervix, perineal tears, extension of the episiotomy; risks due to anesthesia: uterine atony, postpartum hemorrhage
p 862
breech extraction, maternal risks

42-23. 1 – a; 2 – b
p 862
breech extraction, maternal risks; breech extraction, fetal risks

42-24. a,b,c,d,e,f
p 864
breech extraction, fetal risks

42-25. In a version operation, the presentation of the fetus is altered artificially.
p 864
breech presentation; version operation

42-26. b
p 864
podalic version

42-27. a
p 864
cephalic version

42-28. c
p 864
external version

42-29. d
p 864
internal version

42-30. c,d
p 864
breech presentation; external cephalic version

42-31. b,d
pp 864-865
breech presentation; external cephalic version

42-32. a,b,c
p 865
breech presentation; external cephalic version

42-33. b,c,d
p 866
breech presentation; internal podalic version

43-1. incisions in the abdominal and uterine walls
p 867
cesarean delivery

43-2. b
p 867
cesarean delivery

43-3. Cesarean delivery is used when it is believed that further delay would compromise the fetus and/or the mother, yet vaginal delivery is unlikely to be accomplished rapidly and safely.
p 867
cesarean delivery, indications

43-4. a,b,c,d
p 867
cesarean delivery, indications; breech presentation; fetal distress; dystocia; cesarean delivery, repeat

43-5. b
p 867
cesarean delivery; perinatal mortality

43-6. b
p 868
cesarean delivery; neonatal mortality; neonatal morbidity

43-7. b
p 868
breech presentation, vaginal delivery

43–8. e
pp 868–869
cesarean delivery, maternal mortality; cesarean delivery, maternal morbidity; cesarean delivery, neonatal morbidity; breech presentation; transverse lie

43–9. a,b
pp 869–870
cesarean delivery, repeat; repeat cesarean delivery, timing

43–10. the date of onset of the last menstrual period (LMP); results of serial fundal heights initiated in the first half of pregnancy; the time that the fetal heart was first heard with a fetoscope; the estimated size of the fetus
p 870
repeat cesarean delivery, timing; gestational age, determination

43–11. None of these is an *absolute* contraindication to cesarean delivery.
p 870
cesarean delivery, contraindications

43–12. b,d
pp 870–871
vaginal delivery subsequent to cesarean delivery

43–13. The classical cesarean section incision is a vertical incision into the body of the uterus above the lower uterine segment and reaching the uterine fundus.
p 871
cesarean delivery; classical cesarean section, incision

43–14. b
p 871
cesarean delivery, lower segment vertical incision

43–15. a
p 871
cesarean delivery, lower segment transverse incision

43–16. b
p 871
cesarean delivery, lower segment vertical incision

43–17. a
p 871
cesarean delivery, lower segment transverse incision

43–18. b
p 871
cesarean delivery, lower segment vertical incision

43–19. a
p 871
cesarean delivery, lower segment transverse incision

43–20. a
p 871
cesarean delivery, lower segment transverse incision

43–21. a
p 871
cesarean delivery, lower segment transverse incision

43–22. a
p 871
cesarean delivery, lower segment transverse incision

43–23. a,b,c,d
p 871
cesarean delivery, preparation

43–24. a,c
p 871
cesarean delivery, anesthesia; cesarean delivery, preparation; anesthesia, obstetric

43–25. a
pp 871–872
cesarean delivery, vertical abdominal incision

43–26. a
p 872
cesarean delivery, abdominal incision; Pfannenstiel incision

43–27. a,b,c,f
p 872
cesarean delivery, abdominal incision; Pfannenstiel incision

43–28. size and presenting part of the fetus; the degree and direction of uterine rotation
p 872
cesarean delivery

43–29. b
p 872
cesarean delivery, bowel laceration

43–30. The loose reflection of peritoneum above the bladder margin is grasped with forceps in the midline and sharply incised; scissors then develop the incision laterally, aiming cephalad at the lateral ends; the lower peritoneal flap is then bluntly dissected away from the myometrium; the separation of the bladder should not exceed 5 cm in depth.
p 872
cesarean delivery

43–31. a,b
p 874
cesarean delivery, uterine incision

43–32. The placenta must be either incised or detached. Especially if the placenta is incised, the cord should be clamped as soon as possible to minimize fetal hemorrhage.
p 874
cesarean delivery, management of placenta; cesarean delivery, fetal hemorrhage

43-33. After the retractors are removed, a hand is slipped into the uterine cavity between the symphysis and the fetal head; the head is gently lifted while gentle transabdominal fundal pressure is exerted; the shoulders are then delivered using gentle traction and fundal pressure; the body follows readily.
p 874
cesarean delivery, delivery of infant

43-34. An assistant can apply upward pressure through the vagina with a sterile gloved hand.
p 874
cesarean delivery, cephalopelvic disproportion

43-35. c,d,e,f
pp 874-875
cesarean delivery

43-36. b
p 875
cesarean delivery, delivery of the placenta

43-37. a,c
p 875
cesarean delivery, uterine incision; multifetal pregnancy, cesarean delivery

43-38. advantages: ease of fundal massage; ease of visualization; exposure of adnexa; disadvantages: discomfort; possibility of vomiting with epidural or spinal anesthesia; displacement of a tubal ligation ligature
p 875
cesarean delivery, uterine repair

43-39. b
p 875
cesarean delivery, uterine repair

43-40. a,b,c
p 875
cesarean delivery, uterine repair

43-41. A running-lock suture is begun just beyond one angle of the incision; each stitch penetrates the entire thickness of the myometrium without withdrawing the needle after it has entered; one or two layers of suture can be utilized; the running-lock suture is continued just beyond the opposite angle of the incision.
p 875
cesarean delivery, uterine repair

43-42. b
p 878
cesarean delivery, uterine repair

43-43. a
p 878
cesarean delivery, tubal sterilization

43-44. The entire fallopian tube is visualized; the mesosalpinx is perforated with a hemostat; the tube is ligated proximally and distally with 0 chromic suture to remove a segment at least 2 cm in length; tissue is sent for histologic examination; the site of the section is observed for bleeding.
p 878
cesarean delivery, tubal sterilization; tubal ligation

43-45. b,c,d
p 878
cesarean delivery, abdominal closure

43-46. b
p 878
cesarean delivery, abdominal closure

43-47. a
p 878
cesarean delivery, abdominal closure

43-48. d
p 878
cesarean delivery, abdominal closure

43-49. c
p 878
cesarean delivery, abdominal closure

43-50. a,b,c,d,e
p 878
cesarean delivery; transverse lie; placenta previa; cervical carcinoma, invasive; uterine myoma; cesarean delivery, classical

43-51. e
pp 878-879
cesarean delivery; cesarean delivery, classical

43-52. b
p 879
cesarean delivery, extraperitoneal

43-53. a,b,c,d,e,f
p 879
cesarean delivery, postmortem

43-54. a,b,c,d,g
p 879
cesarean hysterectomy, indications; uterine atony; placenta increta; intrauterine infection

43-55. damage to the urinary tract; increased blood loss
p 879
cesarean hysterectomy

43-56. b
p 880
cesarean delivery, blood loss

43-57. c
p 880
cesarean hysterectomy, blood loss

43-58. b,e
pp 879-880
cesarean hysterectomy

43-59. b
pp 20; 880
cesarean hysterectomy; uterine artery, anatomic relationships; ureteral injury, cesarean hysterectomy

43-60. the uterine arteries and veins
p 880
cesarean hysterectomy, supracervical

43-61. a,b,c,d
p 880
cesarean hysterectomy, total

43-62. An "open" vagina may promote drainage and thereby, possibly, avoid hematoma or abscess formation.
p 880
cesarean hysterectomy; vaginal cuff

43-63. c
p 881
cesarean hysterectomy, reperitonealization

43-64. a,c,d
p 881
cesarean delivery, preoperative care

43-65. c,d
p 881
cesarean delivery, fluid management

43-66. blood loss through the vagina or bleeding concealed in the uterus
p 881
cesarean delivery, blood loss; concealed hemorrhage, cesarean delivery; external hemorrhage, cesarean delivery

43-67. d
p 881
cesarean delivery, recovery room care

43-68. a,b,c,d
p 881
cesarean delivery, postoperative care

43-69. meperidine 50 to 100 mg (depending on the size of the patient) every 3 hours as needed; morphine 10 mg every 3 hours as needed
p 882
cesarean delivery, postoperative care; analgesia, cesarean delivery

43-70. hourly for 4 hours, then every 4 hours
p 882
cesarean delivery, postoperative care

43-71. a,b,c,e,f,g
p 882
cesarean delivery, postoperative care

43-72. b
p 882
cesarean delivery, postoperative care; cesarean delivery, management of fluids

43-73. b
p 882
cesarean delivery, postoperative care; oliguria, cesarean delivery

43-74. a
p 882
cesarean delivery, postoperative care

43-75. b
p 882
cesarean delivery, postoperative care

43-76. a
p 882
cesarean delivery, postoperative care

43-77. c
p 882
cesarean delivery, postoperative care

43-78. b,c
p 882
cesarean delivery, postoperative care

43-79. a
p 882
cesarean delivery, postoperative care

43-80. c
p 882
cesarean delivery, postoperative care

43-81. d
p 882
cesarean delivery, postoperative care

43-82. d
p 883
cesarean delivery, postoperative care; anemia; transfusion, cesarean delivery; transfusion, postoperative

43-83. b,c,d
pp 739; 882
cesarean delivery, postoperative care; breast feeding; bromocriptine

43-84. fourth or fifth
p 882
cesarean delivery, postoperative care

43-85. For the first week, activities should be limited to self-care and care of the infant with assistance; the return visit for postpartum evaluation should be during the third postpartum week.
pp 882-883
cesarean delivery, postpartum care

43-86. b,c
p 883
cesarean delivery, prophylactic antibiotics; infection, cesarean delivery; febrile morbidity, cesarean delivery

TOPICS INDEX